W9-CMH-216

EFFECTIVE PROGRAM PRACTICES FOR AT-RISK YOUTH

A CONTINUUM OF COMMUNITY-BASED PROGRAMS

James Klopovic, M.A., M.P.A.
Michael L. Vasu, Ph.D.
Douglas L. Yearwood, M.S.

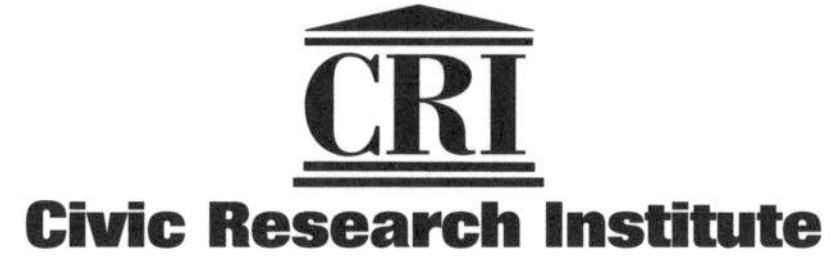

Civic Research Institute
4478 U.S. Route 27 • P.O. Box 585 • Kingston, NJ 08528

By Civic Research Institute, Inc.
Kingston, New Jersey 08528

Printed in the United States of America

Library of Congress Cataloging in Publication Data
Effective program practices for at-risk youth: A continuum of community-based programs/
James Klopovic, M.A., M.P.A., Michael L. Vasu, Ph.D., Douglas L. Yearwood, M.S.

ISBN 1-887554-35-1

Library of Congress Catalog Card Number 2003103321

Dedication

To my dearest daughters, Cindy and Nicole; you always inspire me no matter the circumstance. You are always loved. And heartfelt thanks, thanks which can never be repaid, to the Schues, Carolyn and Tom. And to my "Mum" who makes so many things possible. To the many more who contributed time, expertise, advice, and commentary, thanks again and again.

— J.K.

I would like to dedicate this book to my wonderful daughter Colleen.

— M.L.V.

This book is dedicated to my loving wife, Natalia, and to my parents, Clarence and Deanna, for their enduring support, devotion, and encouragement throughout my career. A special note of thanks to Vladamir for his persistent and meticuolous attention to the early drafts of this manuscript.

— D.L.Y.

About the Authors and Contributors

James Klopovic, M.A., M.P.A.

James Klopovic is an author and policy analyst concerned with strategic planning, community development and grants writing and administration. Mr. Klopovic has over thirty-five years of experience in the public sector at the federal, state, and local levels. He has authored and coauthored numerous publications concerning community development and the effective, efficient delivery of public services. He is currently Policy Analyst, The Criminal Justice Analysis Center, The Governor's Crime Commission, North Carolina. He is involved in various research and development projects that focus on prevention, performance, and public service delivery systems for the future. He resides and writes in Durham, North Carolina.

Michael L. Vasu, Ph.D.

Michael L. Vasu is the Director of the Social Science Research and Computing Lab and a professor in the graduate program in Public Administration, in the Department of Political Science and Public Administration at North Carolina State University (NCSU). He is the author of *Politics and Planning* (Chapel Hill: University of North Carolina Press) and the coauthor of *Organizational Behavior and Public Management* (New York: Marcel Dekker). He has published extensively in the areas of public policy, social science computing, and public opinion research methodology. Dr. Vasu is one of the authors of the award winning software package SocStatSim. He has been qualified, and has served, as an expert witness in the U.S. Federal Courts (electoral simulation) and North Carolina State Courts (Public Policy Research Methodology). He is the former President of the Southern Association for Public Opinion Research.

Dr. Vasu has conducted a numerous national polls, directed research, and done management and political consulting for public and private sector clients. His clients include the North Carolina Governor's Crime Commission, North Carolina Administrative Office of the Courts, the U.S. Department of Justice, and numerous local governments.

Douglas L. Yearwood, M.S.

Douglas L. Yearwood is the Director of the North Carolina Criminal Justice Analysis Center. He received is master's degree in criminal justice from North Carolina Central University. He is a Certified Public Manager and also holds an Advanced Law Enforcement Planner Certification. In addition to governmental reports he has published book reviews and articles in *Justice Research and Policy*, the *American Journal of Police*, the *Journal of Gang Research*, the *Journal of Family Violence*, the *FBI Law Enforcement Bulletin*, *The Criminologist*, *Federal Probation*, *Domestic Violence Report*, and *American Jails*. He currently serves as Secretary/Treasurer for the national Justice Research and Statistics Association.

James R. Brunet, Ph.D.

James R. Brunet teaches in the political science and public administration department at North Carolina State University. He expects to receive his doctoral degree in May 2003. His research interests cover the foundations of public administration and the administration of justice in the United States. He is currently investigating the determinants of employee drug testing policies in law enforcement agencies. His work appears in a variety of scholarly outlets including *State and Local Government Review*, *Review of Public Personnel Administration*, *Justice System Journal*, and *Western Criminology Review*.

Irvin B. Vann. Ph.D. (Cand.)

Irvin B. Vann is a Doctoral Candidate in Public Administration at North Carolina State University, concentrating in Geographic Information Systems (GIS). His academic and professional interests include GIS policy, research methods, organizational behavior and ethics in the public sector.

Meredith B. Weinstein, Ph.D.

Meredith B. Weinstein is a Visiting Assistant Professor of Political Science and Public Administration at North Carolina State University. Her expertise includes research methodology, juvenile delinquency, and perceptions of crime. She has written and consulted on the development of juvenile delinquency prevention programs.

Preface: Thoughts on "Effective Practices for At-Risk Children"

Difficulties in society usually can be traced back to the neighborhood, the home, the individual, even the nursery, and society's ineffectiveness in addressing obvious shortcomings in the social fabric before they become expensive, intractable problems. When we do not address problems (upstream), our prisons fill, social service calendars are booked well in advance, and an unending train of people need public assistance. Why is this when we are at our best when coming to the aid of our fellow Americans, especially in a crisis? One of the problems is that we need to "see" that crisis before we act. It is tough to see a fellow citizen going sour when he or she is just entering kindergarten; often it is easier when he or she drops out of school, or heads to court; however, at this point it is much too late. So it is that the idea for this book arose and that a decade of working with local governments and seeing, firsthand, how difficult it is to muster an appropriate response at an appropriate time for appropriate people and wondering about a better way, a practical and feasible way, to help people reach their potentiality followed.

Why have a book like this at all—one that attempts to make sense of the real confusion of bringing the community together to heal and strengthen itself. Goodness knows libraries are filled with thoughts and directives on how to go about the process. Entire governmental agencies are constructed with a mission to do the same. Also, the work is some of the most difficult, some of the most frustrating, some of the least productive ever undertaken. Of those who attempt it, few really succeed. The simple answer is that there is a sensible, productive way to go about making communities stronger. There is a way to enable communities to address their own problems their own way in their own time with a large measure of their own sweat. It is neither simple nor easy, but it is possible for the collective strong of heart. And because it is possible, the process of making strong communities has to be undertaken; the payback is inevitably worth the cost.

This book reflects the experiences of many communities—what practitioners have found to be effective practices. It is a way, proven by the people actually making it happen, to build stronger communities that are more capable of helping their neighbors become content and productive. It is a way to build infrastructure ahead of and as persistent as the difficulties any community wants and needs to address. It is a way to build permanent answers to problems that seem to defy solution.

This book is an idea, not *the* idea for gathering and focusing the knowledge base from good works, able talent, and real concern for promoting the common good. It allows all levels of government, all sectors, to participate while being guided by a large dose of local determination. The actual path taken to stronger communities is as unique as the community that accepts the challenge. It is an answer to the problems of bringing the community together in a logical way, with a logical process, and a series of field-proven actions. It allows the targeting of limited resources to the people who need it most while it is defined to reach the entire neighborhood, especially our younger neighbors. It focuses on programs that make a difference. It orders and organizes the complex and confusing task of problem solving at the grassroots level. It makes making a difference possible.

What we hope happens as a result of reading this volume is that community by community people see the advantages of building a strong collaborative organization. This permanent operation, this partnership, then guides the best performance-based ideas to make the greatest difference. This difference is made by answering specific needs of our neighbors, usually our youngest, as they progress along the path of success as an individual and as a contributing member of society. This path of development that we all must follow offers the most opportune times for guidance, sometimes as little as the right word at the right time, that makes all the difference between success and failure. Yet many times the opportunity is not taken because we are not prepared to take advantage of it. The developmental continuum outlined in this volume is a way to be prepared when opportunity presents itself.

The process of being prepared, of collaborating, partnering, and building, is done slowly with permanency in mind. It is achieved by tactfully offering assistance when and where needed instead of waiting until the community and the individual suffer the disappointment and disgrace of downfall and failure. We will never eradicate social blight such as juvenile delinquency, teen pregnancy, drug abuse, domestic violence, and the ultimate expression of failure, crime. But we can make a profound difference in the way things are. All that is needed is to begin.

— J.K.

Table of Contents

Part I

The Developmental Continuum—Enabling the Community to Help At-Risk Youth

by James Klopovic, M.A., M.P.A. and Douglas L. Yearwood, M.S.

We have a genuine opportunity to leave a lasting legacy, a bricks- and-mortar heritage that strengthens community and people. It is not just the beginning of a new millennium; we have a confluence of individuals and events that make improvement possible. We have a historically resilient economy that has given us historic prosperity and will continue to do so. Science is giving us new hope not only for the productive capacity to continue this prosperousness but for a better and better quality of life, which is also getting longer. We have a new consciousness. People at all levels, in all sectors of the country, realize that only through working together can we really progress.

Our politicians see the wisdom of facilitating the things and processes necessary to build or repair our communities. State and local leaders agree. More important, there is growing strength at the community level to construct strong neighborhoods that benefit everyone. And there is more and more awareness of how to help those most in need. The process of building strong communities is where we need to focus our creativity, our energy, our resources, and our talents. When we build strong communities we build a true legacy of a better tomorrow. And building a better tomorrow starts with our youth.

But to get there we need to understand the way certain things are. We need to confront our critical failings. We need to ask probing questions. We need to consider realistic answers. And, most important, we have to resolve to move in a productive direction. So let us think analytically and critically about how we currently try to address social ills, especially social dysfunction, with a view to understanding how to do things more productively. Thus, if building a better tomorrow starts with building strong communities for our youth, addressing services for youth at risk is crucial.

There is real reason to have a continuum of developmentally appropriate, performance-based services for youth. Chapter 1 makes the case for working with children as early as possible, considerably before there is any indication of trouble such as difficulty in school or involvement with the juvenile justice system. There are increasing societal difficulties which compound the problem of doing preventive work with children. The economy will ebb and flow, creating funding uncertainties. Local governments have a tough time providing basic services and really struggle to support services for youth especially since it is difficult to determine the outcome of such programming. Furthermore, there are common misconceptions that confound the work of helping children. Chapter 1 redefines collaboration, value, prevention, problem solving, the continuum of services, and program success. This redefinition allows for new thinking that anticipates and answers the difficulties of working with at-risk youth.

The developmental continuum is the focus of Chapter 2. Communities need to be enabled to construct a series of services that answer the developmentally appropriate needs of all youth and especially at-risk youth. When building such targeted services, program staff and leadership need to consider why and how to go about this community building. Action progresses productively when it follows a prescribed, performance-oriented path of effective practices that have been proven by past and continuing use in the field, doing the job of helping children stay on the path to productive citizenry.

Chapter 1

The Need for a Continuum of Performance-Based Services for Youth

PARAMETERS: THE NEED FOR PREVENTIVE SERVICES

Children and Juveniles Need Appropriate Help on the Path to Independent Adulthood

Most needy and at-risk children succeed at life. In fact, teens finish high school in greater numbers than their parents. Colleges have ever more diverse graduates. Record numbers of young adults volunteer. Pot smoking is down from the 1970s. And more teens list sports and exercise as favorite pastimes today (Whitman, 1997, pp. 24–27). Furthermore, the Census Bureau's National Crime Victimization Survey reports some of the lowest victimization rates in the history of the survey. But these promising circumstances beg the obvious: Why do so many children and families still struggle often with unhappy results? Furthermore, it is an established fact that if one does not commit serious violent behavior by the age of 20, it is unlikely one will ever become a serious violent offender (Elliot, 1993, p. 4). So what is being done to stop violent behavior before we ever hear about the unfortunate adult outcome? Why do we still spend so much on social services, social aid, crime, and victimization if crime rates have improved and children are doing better? The fact is, even when most children do well, significant numbers need certain and well-timed services to keep them on track.

Communities Need Organization and Focus

The community is first to suffer the result of a citizen surviving on the fringes of society, living hand-to-mouth and, worse yet, resorting to public assistance or crime. The community is closest to the problem yet most times is least equipped to confront it. Failure of collaborative efforts is legendary. Furthermore, a hallmark of the public sector is austerity.

Why isn't there a way to make collaborative efforts and partnerships work permanently and on a wide enough scale to cause material change? More and more people suffer the reality that there is just not enough money to go around even in good economic times, especially when considering assessed needs and the service-to-needs gaps. So we have to "cooperate" to get things done. But cooperation today means that people come to the table to see what they can get to make sure their own project or job gets started or survives. Productive cooperation is difficult to achieve; just ask those attempting it. It is not bad; it is just the way things are. People focus on what organizations have that can be plundered, which is clearly a frustrating occupation as an agency, especially one in the public sector, is not structured to efficiently address need, nor does it have enough money, resources, people, and time in the first place. That is the nature of bureaucracy, especially public organizations, and the bureaucracy will never have enough of anything for reasonable demands.

In this environment the community suffers first and last. It is more cost-effective to deal with the problem upstream, ahead of social dysfunction, yet most effort and funding go downstream, after a problem manifests. This then suggests that communities at the grassroots level must be as organized as possible to conduct the business of making the community whole and well by refocusing effort ahead of problems, when the causes of those problems are relatively easy to address—the upstream approach.

Need to Change Public Institutional Focus

The institutions we construct compel us to continue to strengthen them at the expense of other worthy social infrastructures. It is part of the nature of the criminal justice system, for example. We build strong courts, corrections, and law enforcement systems to be able to confront crime, which is a graphic example of expense to society and failure of the individual; clearly, though, we must continue that. The system *is* good, but our system shines only *after* the crime is on the books, only *after* the criminal acts. More important, society suffers *before* the "system" can operate because the crime is the long-delayed visible result of a lengthy process of failure on the part of the criminal.

Addressing crime and victimization, for example, is an endless occupation because there will never be a lack of crime, and criminals, or people living marginal lives. So we build stronger, bigger, better, more of the same institutions as the problem either defies solution or grows. There seems to be no end because there is no end. True, we must have these institutions and help them work as well as possible. But how much is enough? It is not wrong to continue to strengthen these systems, but some resources must be devoted to lessening the need for them. Our institutions are designed to react, not to prevent; true prevention happens in the community.

Public institutions are forever in the cycle of sanctioning youth after the crime-criminal cycle begins, for example, in an act of lawlessness or disruption to the well-being of the community. So it is that boot camps were supposed to "prevent" crime. What do they prevent when the ticket to camp is the commission of a crime? Our current thinking on prevention is to cure a sickness, which is never-ending work. No matter if we are in medicine, commerce, education, or criminal justice—we are constantly repairing. And we are good at it, or at least we convince ourselves we are good at it. In other words, in order for us to "show our stuff," we have to wait for society to be wronged, for an individual to be in the care of the system or at least under the jurisdiction of the system. Society has suffered, neighborhoods have suffered, people have suffered, and all continue to suffer. This can be termed the pathological model of prevention, the repair of a sickness. Using our example of the criminal justice system, would it not be better not to have the crime and criminal in the first place? The difficulty is that there is little systemwide problem resolution at the community level with this focus, that is, focusing on strengthening the individual to avoid the problem altogether.

Institutions, public and private, need a continuum of performance-based services to target and keep risk-based populations on track to the ultimate societal goal (i.e., productive citizenship). This is also a change of thinking. Much literature, research, and programming, if forward-thinking at all, call for productive adulthood as the goal of the public service effort. But the goal should be productive citizenship. The former suggests that productivity alone is success. There are too many working poor who are employed and struggling, as will their children in many cases. The latter concept, productive citizenship, implies that the individual is capable of returning effort to the common good of the community. The individual is qualified for and gainfully employed to the best of his or her ability in a career that provides for basic needs and wants and a better tomorrow. The individual has a foundation of morals and a sense of how to help the community succeed. His or her children, in turn, can aspire to the same because they have the means and the example. This is not a dream, there are growing numbers of communities that are developing new capabilities to prepare their own for the demands of citizenship.

SOCIETAL FACTORS IMPACTING SOCIAL SERVICE INFRASTRUCTURE

We need to step to the horizon and take a peek beyond. There is a confluence of factors, a social sea change, that only complicate our ability to provide basic services.

Economy

While historically our economy is prosperous, it is also cyclical. As the economy expands and contracts, unemployment will rise and fall with all the attendant difficulties of boom and bust, not the least of which will be a bust-related rise in crime and need for public assistance while there is diminished capacity to provide it.

Ecology

This is a unique dynamic. The complications of our degraded or fragile ecology complicate the ability to provide basic services. An issue of *Time* magazine was devoted to the state of our ecology and how we can save planet earth (Linden, 2000, p. 24). Our ecosystems, the web of life, are fraying, according to Linden. Our coastal/marine systems are casualty to pollution, overfishing, and climate change. Freshwater is victim to conversion and diversion, overuse, pollution, and invasions by harmful species. The picture here is grim. Agricultural lands are spoiled by chemicals and soil degradation. Grasslands are being degraded and converted to alternative uses. And forests are over harvested, fire-cleared, and shrinking according to Linden. So what does this have to do with the struggle at the local level of government? Everything. Local governments are left to struggle with basic problems and basic services delivery, such as clean water, waste disposal, safety and security, and education, exacerbated by the expense of having to deal with the degradation of our natural resources. And local governments are concerned with providing the basics in ever more difficult circumstances. The point needs to be made that these problems only worsen with time. The next few years will be witness to that.

Release of Ex-Offenders to the Community

One issue of *U.S. News and World Report* featured an article on the "record flow of ex-offenders with nowhere to go" (Glasser, 2000) except to be "dumped" back into the communities and the lifestyles that produced them in the first place. The prison system grew by 60+ percent in the 1990s to about 1.9 million inmates. While they are serving longer sentences, 95 percent of them will reenter society; three-quarters of them will still have a drug and/or alcohol problem. A Baltimore suburb of 5,000 had to absorb 900 ex-convicts in one year according to the article, and this scene will repeat again and again. There are no clear answers here except that this movement will continue to drain limited resources.

Growth of Minority Populations

Minority communities continue to explode. California is now a white minority state. Another example is Siler City, North Carolina. According to the local chamber of commerce, Siler City had no Latinos in 1990; ten years later, Latinos are a majority of those working the poultry industry. This trend tracks the growth of the haves and have-nots. Minorities of today repeat the process of immigrant assimilation with success over time, but only after a pattern of initial difficulties. The Latino community is having a particularly difficult time. Latinos suffer a surprising number of crime victimizations, especially unreported incidents, because they are not familiar or comfortable with U.S. criminal justice, especially law enforcement. Other minorities, for example, eastern Europeans, have their own struggles. One fact is certain, their numbers increase. The problems with more and more families surviving on the fringes of society will only darken in the next few years.

Returning to the Community

Troubled youth still have no vehicle to reenter the mainstream. What community does not struggle helping its teens with difficulties return to the path toward good citizenship? We seek community-based alternatives and are inevitably frustrated at a lack of success, a lack of ability to reach target populations, and certainly a lack of funding. Would it not be better to decrease the need for reentry in the first place?

Put all this together and there are real difficulties providing basic services. Things may indeed be improving with the general state of our children, but it is not nearly enough. Furthermore, these improvements in our social condition, especially as we observe our children, can arguably be attributed to the economy and factors other than the concerted effort of public service providers. This in turn begs the question, "What should we be doing to effect a better outcome for more of our citizens?" The at-risk juvenile who is ignored penalizes society by regressing, incident by incident, to being a marginal citizen or, in the worst case, a ward of the state on assistance or incarcerated. Targeted, research-based, performance-oriented action is an answer, but how do we go about it?

REDEFINING THE TERMS OF ENABLING THE COMMUNITY

Every generation faces the dire realities of the difficulties of correcting social, familial, and individual problems. Elaborating on some of them only sets the stage for obvious answers defined by the times. What we are talking about here is a new way of thinking about the same business of making communities as strong as they can be by directing resources and energy to the people who need it most, when they need it, and how they need it. Simply, we must challenge—indeed, redefine—the terms of this business.

Collaboration to Create Value

Collaboration needs to be revisited. It is plain to see that individual agencies, organizations, even sectors cannot realize needed success in the community unless resources and talent are pooled. But this coming together needs to change fundamentally from being a resources grab to a process of value building. It is best described by an analogy. Imagine a community coming together to assemble the wherewithal for an agreed endeavor. The means to realizing this project are symbolized by a pie. The current mentality has collective leadership gather at the table to divide that pie according to need so each person can do a little more of what he or she currently is doing. Some get a bigger slice than others; many get none; often the pie is divided arbitrarily. This is not wrong; it is just the way it is.

The new way of thinking about building community projects means coming to the table to actually make the pie; something which is a composite of multiple talents guided by a common, beneficial goal. All the collective body has at the outset of building the project is an empty pie tin. Each participant needs to contribute flour, sugar, butter, spices, fruit, utensils, heat, sweat, expertise, supervision, and especially inspiration, accordingly and willingly. When they leave the table a beautiful and delectable pie remains, ready for the county fair. Not only is value created, but a new process of collaboration evolves. It is one in which an agency has to give rather than get to have a play in doing good for the neighborhood. Value is created when the sharing of assets leads directly to effect, result, and benefit. With that example more people see possibilities and want to get involved. Tangibles are created not consumed.

Focus on Wellness, Not Curing an Illness

We need to move from seizing upon a sickness to "cure" to instead advancing healthy communities via individual betterment. In other words, we need to change from the current mind-set of curing a problem or sickness after it happens to keeping systems and people healthy before the individual and society suffer the ailment or, in this case, the crime or dysfunction. This is moving from pathology—sickness—to health—the promotion of knowledge, skills, behaviors, and attitudes for social competency and adult independency. It changes the focus on the immediacy of crisis to the long-term view of building problem solving infrastructure ahead of a problem. We need not respond with a repair; we strengthen by assisting natural ability. Although this is a much more difficult way of doing business, it is not a dramatic tactic. Certainly it is much harder to think this way, but this view helps focus limited resources where they are needed most, to really attack root causes of dysfunction which ensures the health and social, behavioral, and physical well-being of the individual. Then, individual well-being as a productive citizen is how neighborhoods in turn become healthy.

The focus on wellness instead of illness also gives those involved a realistic view of the herculean amount of work true prevention requires. But this insight is healthy, as real progress justifies and overshadows the drudgery and frustration. Furthermore, building ahead of problems leaves a legacy of bricks and mortar, of organization and process, of strategy and realistic ideas for subsequent teams of professionals and public careerists who assume the responsibility of keeping the neighborhood wholesome and productive. Social problems are a moving target; if anything, they change as society evolves. Thus the answer to each problem not only has to be as permanent as the dysfunction, but it must evolve with it. Furthermore, when constructed properly, that answer confronts the problem and, in fact, evolves ahead of the problem rather than constantly trying to catch up to the galloping dynamic of the issue attacked.

Enable the Community by Building Ideas, Not Filling Lists of Services

We should redirect the focus from institutional response to one that also concentrates on enabling the community. We need to adjust, as necessary, from an emphasis on institution strengthening with more services in response to increasing demand to shared emphasis of keeping institutions strong and supporting productive ideas that are ahead of the problem and, most important, at the township level. This implies a circular flow of ideas, resources, and expertise with the emphasis on bottom-up generation of information and ideas. The change of thinking here is to recognize the primacy of locally generated ideas, information, and action. Currently, the public sector is largely top down, after-the-fact problem solving; there is a tendency to grab for the latest service, especially if it is one with a little renown. The process, loosely defined, is similar to filling a shopping cart. Institutional leadership takes inventory of what services are offered, notes where certain projects fit, then plugs them in. A complicating factor is that these services are, likewise, designed to resolve a problem already in existence, not to keep the problem from manifesting in the first place.

This top-down way of doing business ignores the fact that communities do have successful ideas that work at systemic problem resolution. We need our social services institutions—that goes without saying. But we do not need people saying, "Well, it works in Boston; so it will work in Lumberton, North Carolina." Perhaps it is better to change the thinking to, "We have a great idea in Boston; let's see what the folks of Lumberton have to say about it." The change is subtle but significant, from top-down to bottom-up with the intention of nurturing ideas that work, not imposing a service because it is convenient. This also implies that all parties need to be prepared to work together for a long-term collaborative effort to create the value of a network of services that really make measurable, real differences. There is a certain campaign mentality to this new way of enabling the community.

What we also need is a significant effort, not total, but a noticeable push toward building bricks-and-mortar projects, infrastructure, in our neighborhoods based on ideas generated from the heart of the community that complement our institutional responses. Our neighborhoods are where our problems and our answers lie.

Strengthen, Don't Problem-Solve

Too much has been said about solving problems after the fact. It is much easier to hammer the crime and the criminal because action is predictable and dramatic. Although we will always need good social troubleshooters, much more effort needs to be turned from going after a problem to productively strengthening what already exists before there is the difficulty that calls for a reactive, expensive social response. There is much more to work with and the result is much more productive, especially over time, when we look for the resiliency everyone and every community has. When we mention resiliency we are talking about innate competencies, assets, and strengths. What is more rewarding is that the most productive strength-based work is done with children. It is productive in that so little effort is needed to keep a child on track in school, in the neighborhood, and at home with the obvious attendant success as an adult after a successful childhood and primary education.

Redefine the Comprehensive Strategy to Be a Developmental Continuum of Services

Currently the Federal Office of Juvenile Justice and Delinquency Prevention defines a comprehensive strategy as follows:

> An effective continuum of services in a community offers a range of programs and services that provide the "right resources for the right kid at the right time." The services meet the dual objective of promoting the healthy development of children and youth and ensuring the safety of the community. (Coolbaugh & Hansel, 2000, p. 2)

This is a good definition of the strategy for promoting youth development, but then we must consider the suggested programming. Most recommended projects are for troubled, older youth, such as intervening in delinquent behavior or some sort of sanctioning even if it is community based. In other words, action taken is after problems arise. What has been prevented? The cycle of offense and institutional intervention is well on its way when current socially therapeutic strategies are invoked.

Conversely, the more productive, forward-thinking organizations and sponsored services recognize that there are specific needs for each developmental age group of children in their particular communal environment. The developmental continuum recognizes these needs as seamless. Most strategies do not propose answering the very different needs each of us has on the way to productive citizenship. Even if they address the needs of a specific age group of people, that is where it stops. Any benefit is lost if the individual reverts to difficulty in the next stage of development.

A service or even a range of services cannot simply address a specific need one time. The service has to address needs as they evolve, over time. It is obvious that the preschooler needs different assistance than does the middle-schooler. Furthermore, the developmental continuum needs to have a network of services ready before the child passes through the predictable stage of growth through which we all must pass. And these services must be built for the long haul; they must be an institutionalized part of the network of social services at the local level of government.

These local "institutions" would not be just any casual operation to be taken lightly. They would be designed with the purpose of standing in the face of root causes of community dysfunction. They would not only be effective, efficient, and permanent, they would be in sufficient number to address the requirements of the total population in need. Furthermore, they would be diverse enough to address the continuum of problems faced by our youth, especially youth with barriers to success. This is an enlightened change of thinking from institutional reaction to nourishing local innovation that builds on individual strengths with a seamless progression of guidance.

REDEFINE PROGRAM SUCCESS

We need to rethink the definition of success. Outcome is not success; success is citizenship. There has been a refreshing "revolution" in the public sector, which has been looking to the private sector for how to determine whether effort is effective. Now we are increasingly aware that numbers are not enough. People are beginning to see the difference between an input and an output and that there are degrees of output. Now we need to take the next logical step. We need to redefine and push toward success when considering the collective public's efforts to rectify social dysfunction. We want the collective public to embrace citizenship. Yes, "results" are good, especially when those results are defined in terms of promoting beneficial character and talent. But even that is still not good enough. A person can be productive in a menial job and not be involved in the public institutional network yet still remain a marginal person. The goal of projects, programs, and ideas should be to help the individual attain productive citizenship. This does not imply that all people can avoid public assistance. It does mean that, given the opportunity and appropriate assistance, successful maturation results in a person who is equipped to succeed in the family, in the community, and in the workplace.

This is even a change of thinking from the arguably reasonable request that the investment of public resources, talent, and time produce a benefit to the individual and community. It asks that services and effort assist the individual in developing the talent, skills, and character to be able to return resources to the community. This then is the measure of success needed for the development of ideas that lead to public services designed to cure what we see as blights on the neighborhood.

References

Coolbaugh, K., & Hansel, C. J. (2000, March). The comprehensive strategy: Lessons learned from the pilot sites. *Juvenile Justice Bulletin*.

Elliott, D. (1993). *Youth violence: An overview.* Denver: Center for the Study and Prevention of Violence, Institute of Behavioral Science, University of Colorado.

Glasser, J. (2000, May). Ex-cons on the street. *U.S. News and World Report*, pp. 18–20.

Linden, E. (2000, May). Condition critical. *Time Magazine*, pp. 18–24.

U.S. Department of Justice. (2001). Criminal victimization 2000: Changes 1999–2000 with trends 1993–2000 [On-line]. Washington, DC: Office of Justice Programs, Bureau of Justice Statistics. Available: *http://www.ojp.usdoj.gov/bjs/pub/pdf/cv00.pdf.*

Whitman, D. (1997, May). The youth "crisis." *U.S. News and World Report*, pp. 24–27.

Chapter 2

General Guidelines for Estabishing a Continuum of Services for Youth

What we want is a vision for our public effort. Citizenship is our goal. Simply, we want productive citizens, citizens who are reaching their potential and free to make choices of how to successfully pursue career, family, and community. That is, they have been given the tools to pursue a promotable career as their potential dictates; they are contributing members of a capable nuclear family if they so choose; and they are engaged in promoting wellness for the community if they also so choose. This is not merely helping people to be problem free. It is attaining competence and character. Yes, it is a tall order, but it is not an excuse to avoid the pursuit of citizenship as the goal of a public service or project. If projects begin with this purpose in mind—that of developing citizens—more likely than not they will succeed—not all the time, but certainly the results will be better, and often unexpectedly rewarding for having tried. Stating a lofty goal is actually simple. The difficulty is in how we go after it.

What is needed is a plan, a suggestion for the many ways to realize a communal, worthy goal—a suggestion for how we can realize the vision with respect to the changing socioeconomic reality of neighborhood dysfunction and the evolution of society. But first more of the strategy of that plan:

- *Mission.* Develop a continuum of research-based community alternatives targeted and sequenced to the developmental stage and individual need of children in general with the emphasis on the at-risk family and child.
- *Goal.* Stabilize performance-based projects built and sustained by local performance-based operational organizations.
- *Strategy.* Grow this permanent capacity to the assessed locale and target population of greatest need.
- *Tactic.* Develop small, targeted, sustainable, productive projects with return on investment as resources and expertise from all sources and local resolution determine.

This vision and strategy suggest certain criteria which, in turn, recognize a new way of defining, of thinking about, delivering public services:

- *Local determination.* It is essential that the people next to the problem have the largest say in how to attack the problem. This does not mean complete control goes to local efforts; it does mean there is collaboration and partnership as defined previously.
- *Performance-based.* Any project undertaken must have a monetary return to the community. That is, on the way to helping the individual and community reach potential, there has to be at least a cost savings and preferably a dollars-and- cents profit. This does mean some projects that have an intrinsic value and seem to do good will not measure up, but resources are too limited to do otherwise.
- *Permanency.* Projects undertaken must stabilize in the community based on stable funding and efficient, effective operations. This means the emphasis is first on enabling capacity, then on service provision, in that order.
- *Long-range focus.* Immediacy must be superseded by a view to tomorrow. The project must begin and be institutionalized with the express purpose of growing to close the service-to-needs gap. Just doing a project one time, hoping to make a difference, will not do. There needs to be a determined march to systemic improvement with a network of expanding projects over time.

- *Targeted.* Services must be targeted to those who need and can benefit most from those services. Project purpose can address general needs; in fact, that it does address a general client base is preferred. But after the general definition, it must have a concomitant needs-based focus as a primary interest.

The plan then is to help the local communities sustain an effort but with the aforementioned aims and criteria in mind. If such an effort is sustained over the first five years it should be stable and thus continue. Then this kind of endeavor holds the greatest potential in addressing immediate problems such as juvenile delinquency, violence, drug abuse, teen pregnancy, academic failure, and more. Furthermore, it should see the successful passage of our youth through childhood, adolescence, and young adulthood to the vision of productive citizenship. The next question becomes one of process. Just how do all these grand plans come about?

THE CONTINUUM OF SERVICES

The community of this new millennium should gradually build a permanent network of developmentally appropriate services ahead of dysfunction and social blight if it is to succeed in being a place where people want to live and thrive. Each service will be performance-based and emanate from a platform of operations, a partnership, at the local level of government. While services are built with permanency in mind, they are also subject to constant assessment that determines and adjusts the fit with the dynamic nature of public service delivery and society.

Much of what is suggested here is common sense. Thus, why rehash the obvious? Simple: Because the obvious is not being done. People have a smattering of understanding about how things progress, but many projects—if not most—just survive from one financial crisis to the next with minimal effect and at great expenditure of public funds and trust. The trick then becomes to combine the *what*—a justified, effective idea—with the *how*—a detailed, logical sequence of field-proven activities to build effectual service delivery. The best test of this practical guide, this suggested path to success, is evidenced by the practitioner's reaction to the concept, "Oh yes, I know that; but I haven't thought of it that way, let me get busy on it." The evident is made obvious and, more important, possible.

The continuum provides a "safety net," a pyramid of programming as the child develops and as the need for focused attention arises. The construct of the pyramid is apropos as the large foundation graphically demonstrates the proportionate dedication of resources to the earlier stages of development and programming. The continuum does not wait for things to go wrong; it anticipates pitfalls and is there to guide the way to success. The idea is to design activities for general populations but target limited services at appropriate stages of child development to avoid the escalation of difficulties youth may experience. This is to augment institutional response, which should be used only after the failure of community involvement. In truth, the community-based continuum reduces the need for expensive institutional involvement. Actually, it does not matter *what* actions are taken provided that each is performance-based and addresses a developmental need. The wider the array of working ideas the better.

Whereas psychiatry and psychology may differ on the stages of development, we defer here to practicality to define stages of growth. We simply follow the child through school. Consequently, in this volume we address the needs of children in preschool, elementary, middle, and high school; these classifications work as well as any if only that the characteristics of each stage are nearly universally understood. Certainly it makes it easier to talk in those terms and there is much less confusion. This introduction to the continuum suggests new ways of thinking about community development.

RETHINKING HOW TO ENABLE THE COMMUNITY

Providing this new continuum of action is actually simple in concept but not easy in execution. Certain notions about community must be carefully considered if not reconsidered.

Policy

Programming must consider sanctioned youth and emphasize nonsanctioned youth to correct the imbalance of resource flow from after-the-fact reaction to true prevention ahead of the problematic event. Policy should balance the flow of resources first to prevention as we have defined it and then to sanctioning. Both are needed but with a little more harmony.

Critical Partnerships by Sector

The delivery of public services now and in the future must be a true collaboration that creates value which not only initiates an idea but works to ensure its long-term survival. Local leadership should seek to build a certain number and blend of agencies, a critical mass of collaboration of interested and vital parties, to ensure project stability and productivity.

- Facilitate *public sector* inter- and intra-agency partnerships to share expertise and resources.
- The *private sector* has interest in and must materially fund and support (with hard dollars and volunteers) community wellness efforts.
- The *private nonprofit* sector, as exemplified by the faith community and foundations, must continue their interest in neighborhood health (citizenship) and must assert their prominence in the community with collaborative efforts based on continuum projects.

Funding the Trade-off

Starting a project is not a matter of choosing one or another; it is a matter of choosing one at the expense of not doing the other. That is the trade-off. Measure performance to justify and allow continuum projects to compete with other basic services in an environment of limited resources. This does not mean that a continuum service will win every time at the budget hearing. It means that budgeting officials will make the best decision about what to fund based on logical, factual justification and what is best for their constituents.

Leadership

Consider continuum leadership on two levels: The policy or oversight body and the project director must be committed, involved, and skilled. This may seem obvious until it is investigated. Leadership is many times transitory, over-committed, and not trained. This will not do if meaningful change is to occur. The same applies to senior staff of service delivery operations.

Measurements

"Measure what you want, get what you measure" is a common expression. We need to move to true results-based delivery of public services. It is difficult, but more can and needs to be done. The fact is, as evidenced by field investigation, most evaluation efforts are basic and ineffective. Most projects still count the number of people served, for example, and have little material understanding of how to measure necessary changes in behavior which are mentioned as the basic objectives of the project in question. At a minimum, the well-working project must consider results, a statement of monetary effectiveness, and process.

- *Impact.* Is the project changing lives for the better? Counting numbers will no longer do. Material improvements in the individual and community must be documented.
- *Cost-effectiveness vs. cost-benefit.* Cost-benefit calculations should be reserved for only a select few public projects, those with sectorwide, or larger, implications. Most projects, especially those in the community, should have as a basic element of evaluation, the development of a cost-effectiveness statement. All that is needed is a simple statement that a project pays more than it costs to make a compelling case for being part of the services network, to maintain funding, and to ensure adequate resources. The funding battle may still be lost, but it will be extremely painful for decision makers to say no when the numbers say yes.
- *Process.* "Control your operations, control your destiny." The emphasis of project daily operations must be on process because it is by under-

standing process that the service evolves from idea to stable service delivery system. Presently, most local project staff are occupied by numerous distractions such as winning the next grant or pursuit of "quality" or simply delivering the service regardless of necessary operational infrastructure and support. A project must be strong before it reaches out. Furthermore, a daily study of process promotes basic and necessary learning to improve the operational base and respond to a dynamic public and social system.

Public service delivery systems must rigorously measure and report results and monitor processes with the purpose of continuously learning about and improving operations. Either the project produces, or it changes operations to produce, or it is abandoned. When such a philosophy is adopted by sponsoring agencies, there is a demonstrable shift in operation energy, efficiency and effectiveness, and a requisite refocusing from output to results.

RETHINKING THE WELL-WORKING PROJECT

We need to end the cycle of continuously struggling to keep a project alive because of a misunderstanding of what a healthy project is. For example, many local projects move from one funding crisis to another rather than concentrating on impact and process data to ensure more reliable streams of resources. Others begin immediately with a statement of quality, then they get distracted by a single-minded pursuit of it while the basics of project building go wanting. We need to plan, begin, and grow permanent projects with specific target populations in mind. Thus, every project, the community infrastructure against community problems, should be conceived, built, and cultivated with the following hierarchy in mind. Though there is purpose to this order, each factor is defined by the others, and all work together for a common end—the permanent, well-working project.

- *Stability*. This needs to be put as simply as possible: A firm plan for permanence must based on a steady funding stream; if there is not, one should not begin. It matters not how many lives one could change, or how efficient one is, or how good one looks if the project does not exist.
- *Accessibility*. Each idea brought to fruition must target specific clientele and locale. First, the project must target the neediest group. It targets by conducting a hard-hitting assessment that will yield a full profile of the population in question. This is vital as that understanding will determine program effect, effect demonstrates impact, and from impact comes justification for limited resources. Also, it is necessary to understand the service area of the target group. The purpose here is to define the physical limits of the service so as not to dissipate the effort by trying to do too much for too many, which usually foreshadows failure. The project

must be large enough to generate support and small enough to measure. A specific group and realistic service area determine how one gets services out the door. A project is no good if it skims a few lucky winners off the top of the pool. The truly productive project penetrates horizontally throughout the area of need and vertically to all of the defined target group. Infrastructure must be accessible by bringing the service to the individual or the individual to the service.

- *Quality*. The pursuit of "quality" actually detracts from the health and permanence of the local project if only because everyone has a unique idea of what quality is and how to attain it. Therefore, we settle the argument by suggesting that public service delivery quality is experience and a history of providing services that change lives for the better. Quality is last in the hierarchy for a specific reason. First, quality is not forgotten; it is integral to the other essential elements of project health, stability, and accessibility. It is just that quality needs to be defined in terms of permanency and reaching a target group. Ordering quality first has a tendency to command all attention, all resources. When quality is number one, it becomes the commanding mantra at the expense and exclusion of other vital priorities. Practitioners tend to focus on delivering a good service because that is what they have been trained to do, whereas, the task is much larger than that. Quality is surely not disregarded; it is just defined in terms that promote stability and accessibility.

Ideas, collaboration, infrastructure, project health, individual improvement, and bricks and mortar in the community are what define the new thinking, the new work of the community for this new century. The going will be tough and slow but worth it. To get going we have to have a way, a construct, a process to think about and guide project building. For that we suggest thinking about project development in terms of how local municipalities and projects work.

BUILDING THE MODEL PROGRAM

The model program balances the dichotomy of direction and order with freedom of local decision making. While this is an ideal, more and more communities have demonstrated that it is most achievable. This way of building public-sector service delivery systems has its roots in an analysis of the decision-making process. At the risk of oversimplification, the decision to act comes when there is justification of an idea and a logical way to proceed. As elemental as this may sound, good answers to both the why and the how of a decision are rarely present, and for good reason, when action is taken. When it comes to decision time, limited funding, politics, and experience are large determining factors; the logic of pointed analysis is often a luxury.

Our model suggests processes for how to make better decisions to commit to an idea and how to enhance chances of success once committed. The difference between this construct and others is "choice." It recognizes that although an idea may come from out of town, the realization of it is as unique as the town and group that try it. That is the way it has to be; prescribing an idea is a prescription for failure. This "why" and "how" of decision making need a little explanation.

Goal of the Performance-Based Model

Simply, the model seeks to move local municipalities to action via informed decision making. Further, via logical, factual argument, the model fosters political will that moves to action and commitment. This is where commitment leads to the betterment of the target population, and that measured betterment is demonstrated as youth move to productive citizenship. Commitment is seen in the dedication of the following:

- *Money*. Funding must be permanent to avoid the self-defeating cycle of always beginning by having to search for funding every year, thus never realizing potential and the ability to make material differences in the community.
- *Resources*. Ample logistics and project support is in place for the planned services.
- *People*. Human resources are ready, skilled, knowledgeable, and dedicated.
- *Time*. This is the most precious commodity. When people are willing to invest their time just about anything is possible.

Basics of the Decision—The "Why"

The "why" is the justification that allows the action to compete in the tradeoff game with basic services. Here we are talking about proof that a course of action will pay off. More and more the public sector has to be concerned with performance. We are expected to provide more than simple process evaluation. Public servants, elected, appointed, and professional careerists, have to understand how to achieve positive and lasting results from all that is undertaken. This is assuming a performance orientation. For this understanding we need to differentiate several levels of performance:

- *Efficiency*. Doing things well. This is just putting things into work.
- *Effectiveness*. Doing the right things well. This is done by having realistic objectives and measures that help direct initial effort to provide meaningful change in communities or agencies. Lives are bettered.

- *Impact.* Impact or results are material and make systemic improvements; thus, individuals and communities are bettered.

Performance Measurement. We also need to consider the fairness of our yardsticks. It may be all right to assess an agency or entity on its general climate with standard measures, but a local municipality should be judged on political, economic, and social characteristics or dimensions of performance that government officials can influence. Therefore, measures have to be outcome oriented and locally devised to determine whether, in fact, social improvement has been accomplished. Moreover, they must be realistic in that stakeholders, those working on the problem, have certain influence with those measures.

Performance measurement is a result of rigorous evaluation, not merely an observation or a feeling that good is being done. The preferred way to accomplish this is to help project stakeholders build performance measurement into all phases of the endeavor rather than focusing only on the terminal process of just getting started. The broader purpose is to develop an outcome orientation in general rather than to leave project participants with short-term expectations of compliance issues only. If we expect results, outcome, and impact, that is what will happen. The chain of outputs is a simple tool, a logic model, to help communicate and understand the concepts of performance assessment.

The Chain of Outputs. The chain of outputs (Swiss, 1991) has many pluses. The best is its simplicity. People, no matter who or where they may be working, understand what can be confusing terms. The importance of the chain lies in the fact that people can graphically see how to measure performance for their particular project. Figure 2.1 illustrates this chain. There are many advantages, which are elaborated later. When considering the chain of outputs, look at it as a tool to describe how work translates to the goal of the project at hand. There is a great difference between input and output. Many times in project development the two are confused. The distinction must be made to avoid the trap of working very hard on inputs that lead in the wrong direction—or lead nowhere—and at the expense of moving toward real results, the intended output. The chain of outputs is a simple graphic to illustrate that there is a real difference between daily activities and making a difference by effecting positive change, preferably some measurable improvement in the community. For now, we need a common understanding of what performance is along the chain of outputs.

- *Measuring how hard we work—Efficiency for the short term*:
  - *Input.* Inputs are what we consume. They are the things are quite easy to measure. Thus, they can easily distract from measuring meaningful effect. These may be dollars for salaries, time spent, reams of paper used, gasoline, and the like. *Just because inputs are expended does not mean important change will happen.*

Figure 2.1
Chain of Outputs

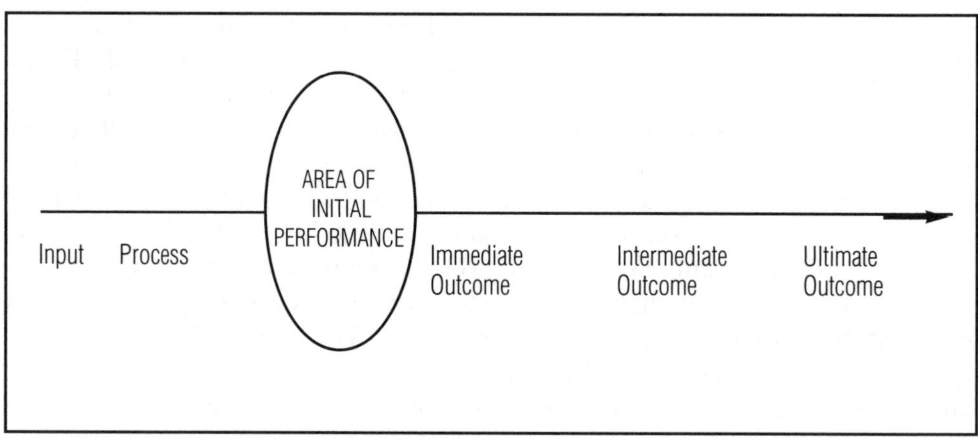

— *Process*. These are the things that go on *inside* the organization. They are essentially procedures or some initial numbers affecting our professional infrastructure. As with inputs, *just because there are procedures doesn't mean anything significant will happen.*

- *Measuring what matters—Effectiveness for the long term:*

— *Immediate outcomes.* Here we begin to show the initial effect on our target populations. This may be the number of clients seen by a crisis center, for example. Again, numbers do not mean much, but here is where we start demonstrating some results on people *outside* our professional systems. The connection is important to make.

— *Intermediate outcomes.* These are actually early results that demonstrate our client group will probably improve as a direct result of the project. They may be improvements in percentages or rates of change that predict the eventual success of a project. (Note the circled area on the chain in Figure 2.1. We can expect initial measures somewhere in the range depicted. Again, the importance is that measures from the initial year or two of the project's life have to be connected to more meaningful results. This avoids, as much as possible, an effort starting off with a great burst of activity and even greater expense while headed in no particular direction with no particular result. Projects without this sense of purpose usually fade away. The chain then attempts to ensure that initial performance is indeed an indicator of long-term, ultimate, benefit.)

— *Ultimate outcomes.* Here the community is made better. For example, in criminal justice terms, neighborhoods are safer and more secure.

Improvement may be measured, either quantitatively through reducing crimes or arrests, for example, or qualitatively through citizen satisfaction surveys. It is not enough that professionals working in the system *feel* accomplished; the recipients of the effort have to *confirm* by word and behavior that improvements have been made.

The importance of the chain is twofold. First, it graphically demonstrates the real difference between input and output. This distinction is vital to determining results, as there is less tendency to become satisfied with easy-to-achieve numbers when leadership and clients demand to see real improvement. Second, and probably more important, is the focusing effect of the chain. People can easily be distracted from their real purpose just by the crush of the work at hand. When work is defined along the chain, inputs have to connect to outputs. People can see the progress to project goals.

Outcomes are important to understand for another reason: to win initial and continuing commitment. The measures along the chain are important, but a better, if not more compelling, case for the project is made by the drama of a cost-effectiveness statement which demonstrates return on investment—a bona fide outcome. We have seen the effect of a brief, organized presentation to a town council that put the argument in terms of what the municipality would get from the project, not what it would cost. The presentation simply and elegantly outlined the project, presented charts of positive trends, discussed the positives and negatives of proceeding, showed the dollars and cents of it, and quoted a few beneficiaries. The project was handily written into the budget. This tactic works more often than not. Another advantage of justification based on performance is that a baseline of measures and expectations is established. Subsequent requests for support simply update progress and savings.

Still, it is difficult to show ultimate outcomes, especially in the public sector. But, with the chain, we can reasonably ask for indicators of initial performance and know that the project is well on its way to doing what it set out to do. If the chain of outputs is used to understand project performance for as many public projects as possible, it will improve project survival rates and the project development process over time. The chain is the mechanism for understanding, even ensuring, that initial effort connects to long-term goals. Without *it*, it is easy (actually commonplace) for rigorous activity to be headed nowhere.

Basics of the Decision—The "How"

Justifying one's idea for service is not nearly enough. Justification for local project development must be part of a package that includes a detailed plan of action—the "how" of making the idea a reality. There must be a sense of direction or all work is largely a waste. The problem is where to begin. Furthermore, if a project begins well, participants wonder, "Where do we go from here?" More important, people also wonder whether they are making a difference.

Public service delivery is difficult. We do not have the simple measure of profit to tell us we are on track, as does the private sector. Sometimes the client and his or her wishes are elusive. And many times there is no precedent for what we are attempting. Even after we begin a project, there are myriad details and many masters to add to the confusion. What is needed is a way to order the chaos of community advocacy and development. A way is the order and process suggested by Exhibit 2.1, The Project Life Cycle: A Guide to the Process of Community Development for Public Services, at the end of the chapter).

Building a project is not simply a start-up; a project is a sequence of phases and never-ending process improvement if it is done correctly and has notable effect. If one contemplates the development and maturation of just about any project it does indeed have a beginning, a middle, and an end or, in this case, when the project works well, a continuation. We have found that some of the most effective project development occurs when stakeholders think in terms of planning, operating, and then expanding their service. There is definite purpose in each phase and in the entire construct.

Unfortunately, most projects in the public sector, especially those that seek to work on social dysfunction, never get past the initial stages of operation. The way they begin is the way they continue, processes never really improve, funding is always a life-and-death battle just to keep going, let alone expand, and, worst of all, they never really reach their intended clientele in ways and numbers necessary to make a real difference in the community. The project is stuck at continuously beginning because there is no plan to grow. The fact is, the real goals of a project are realized in the expansion phase, which few such local public service projects ever reach.

The project life cycle is not completely mechanical, it has an organic character; that is, it is flexible and completely up to interpretation by its users. It actually evolves with the project to which it is applied. While the project life cycle is laid out linearly, in outline form, the application of it is not lockstep through each action item, one after the other. The outline merely orders necessary work that in actuality is synergistic; most suggested actions are happening simultaneously yet in concert with one another. Some steps need to be revisited depending on the phase of development, especially concerning funding, for example. The process is meant to keep project staff and leadership focused on necessary detail and keep the project on track as a stable, well-working part of the community.

The stable, productive project as a vital, permanent part of local services is the goal of developing a project or service using the project life cycle. Part 2 of this volume, on building local partnerships, describes an actual life cycle sketched out with effective practices used in real community development. This also serves as the best way to illustrate the project life cycle, by implementing it in action, in a real situation. Following is an introduction to each phase of the project life cycle:

- *Planning the service delivery system.* Planning means thinking about the project. This phase of development is necessarily long and detailed. It is meant to stimulate critical thinking, collaboration, and action that anticipates operational difficulties and enhances the chance of successful start-up. The process is vital as there are an enormous number of tasks that must have attention, so many so that it is common for project staff to be distracted by their numbers or by unproductive busy work. The important thing to remember about planning is that it is necessary, as elementary as it may sound. Many projects in the public sector breeze past planning or ignore it all together and begin work by delivering the service, only to find they are discontinued down the line for many reasons that can be traced back to a lack of planning. The attention to correct detail of the planning phase determines the strength of the operational phase and lays the groundwork for the all-important expansion phase.
- *Operating the service delivery system.* Operating the service delivery system means doing the project. It is in this phase that the plan comes alive and evolves. The operation focuses on building project stability *while* delivering the service. The service is important, but not until the infrastructure that supports it is in place and running well. Consequently, we talk about a strategy for human capital development, not merely describing an organizational chart, for example; there is a big difference in this way of thinking. The focus is on the long term, on systems and processes that are built to perform and expand when the time is right. "Permanence," "effect," and "client satisfaction" are buzzwords of the operational day in the performance-oriented service delivery system.
- *Expanding the service delivery system.* This phase closes the service-to-needs gap. This is where all such projects need to be. The purpose of a lengthy and at times brutal planning process, and a long experience of working the project just to get it right, pays off by being able to answer to the true needs of clients. At start-up, the project only begins to answer a need, to resolve a problem; by definition it cannot answer the assessed need communitywide. In fact, it is impossible to measure the impact of initial efforts because so little of the systemic need is met. That is the reason to be able to expand to the areas of need and to the clientele of need—to have a crack at making noticeable, communitywide improvement. Clearly, there can be no expansion unless there is the real work of planning and working out the daily flow of work for the project.

Another aspect of the life cycle is its cyclicality, it never ends. If applied correctly, it becomes completely tailored to the people, environment, and project at hand, especially when it is reapplied to coincide with project maturation. Progress through each phase only provides a vantage point from which to begin the process again, but this time from a loftier peak. In other words, the project life cycle has an evolutionary characteristic. For, example, leadership in planning is quite different from leadership during operation and expansion of the effort as it progresses and inevitably matures. Thus leadership progresses from the work of designing the vision, to promoting it, to redesigning it as the maturational phase demands. The life cycle makes that distinction so project stakeholders are aware of it and can anticipate the need to change and have some experientially based suggestions for how to change.

Furthermore, the life cycle concept promotes learning about and the ability to grow with a dynamic environment—even to grow ahead of it. It is not based on any one person or any one group of people; it is based on the promotion of an idea via a process which lives beyond the terminal involvement of stakeholders. People come and go, but the idea and the operational systems remain. This is actually a hallmark of the progressive community of the future: local capacity to achieve community wellness. There is another aspect of the life cycle that makes it a real development tool, that of effective practices.

EFFECTIVE PRACTICES—FIELD-TESTED ACTION

It is not enough to have a logical process to guide project building; two additional important elements are required: choice and proven action. Choice comes in electing how to go about executing the process of development based on the uniqueness of the community. Proven action is in the form of effective practices. We often hear the argument, "How do you know these actions are effective? Where is the proof?" The actions suggested are known to be effective because they have been and are working for the people who are doing the job of project development. They are effective because they work in an environment similar to one in which project replication is being considered. Again, the idea is proposed, and the precise interpretation of how to realize it is completely up to the new team of stakeholders interpreting the process for their sets of boundaries and opportunities. The life cycle then becomes most practical as there is not only order but specific, proven ways to put each action item into motion.

Thinking about project development in terms of process is an effective way to pull order from chaos. Most people know what to do; what matters is when to do it and how to go about it without being distracted by unnecessary details. The life cycle of effective practices does not fit the usual descriptors of suggestions on how to strengthen the community and deliver services. It is not the way to attack a problem; it is simply a suggestion of practical ideas to enhance the successful resolution of the problem one chooses to tackle.

The truth is that only the people strapping on the harness of community activism are in a position to determine what is best for them. The best outsiders can do is suggest the most promising activities of what others have learned. Thus, effective practices relate only that which has worked for those undertaking a similar challenge. A useful guide is only as useful as it is practical and used. We hope that this volume becomes dog-eared with use and the change of hands, and that there is more to the thinking behind this construct of working to build local services.

People, no matter what sector, no matter what the task, want to know and need to know why they should invest their time. Once they have that answer, they need to know how to go about making their project happen. Effective practices are laid out that way. The first part of the model concerns itself with the "why" by looking essentially at the justification in the literature, with the depth of relevant benefits and possible proof of effectiveness via a review of specific evidence. The second half of the model is the "how": the detailed process of how to get the job done that follows the maturation of the project. Together they energize, ideally compel, action. In the least, by an organized elaboration of the experiences of real people doing similar work, mistakes previously made are usually avoided. And workable suggestions for the really thorny, tough issues are detailed as related from the crucible of the field. When mistakes are made, they are novel and not the catastrophic, project-ending type. In other words, the chances of success are greatly enhanced. Success here means the project remains standing tall, secure in the community, doing good work, ready to serve for as long as the problem lasts and the service is vital.

THE DEVELOPMENTAL CONTINUUM: PROVIDING GUIDANCE WHEN AND HOW IT IS NEEDED

There is another vital element to the building and delivering of effective public services especially for at-risk youth aimed at relieving social dysfunction: the developmental continuum. It is not enough to have a justified plan to start a project. It is not enough even to have a proven idea, built on proven action. And it is not enough to have the community infrastructure to support performance-based service projects that have permanency. The community needs all that and services that address the developmental needs of youth as they progress to the goal of the community, productive citizenship.

Growth, learning, and progress to maturity, or lack of it, are gradual and continuous; thus programming must be the same. Even if a community is fortunate enough to see a project through all phases of development and it successfully expands to meet assessed need, that well-working service must link to the next developmentally appropriate service as determined by the client. Maturation does not stop even though the service might. The benefit of answering an age-appropriate need is realized only if we address the next stage of developmental need. The logic of this construct of public policy is made much more sensible by the fact that little effort is needed to keep young people on the path to success.

While the professions may argue about the various stages of human development, it is practical to define specific support in terms commonly used in public education. Thus we speak of the various stages of development as that of preschool children, elementary, middle, and high school youth. It is convenient and it works because people largely understand or can understand the dynamics and needs of each stage. The community has to recognize these needs and design services for each group, which answers a critical failing of most social services—that of being terminal, of dealing only with a specific clientele which is overwhelmingly older youth and most often after they are in some sort of difficulty. This, then, is the final element to building social services infrastructure, building a sequence of services that guides youth development.

The continuum of services for at-risk youth is built one step at a time. Individual projects are begun as resources for project stability become available. The local community begins by understanding how to build a continuum, then begins their progression of services one program at a time. The remainder of this volume details an example of a such a progression of services. It is certainly not meant to be the series of choices. What matters is that the community undertakes to build the organizational capacity to support a network, a sequence of their projects. When there is a continuum of services that is built to last, that penetrates to targeted clients and proliferates to communities of greatest need, the choice of the idea is less important. What matters is that there is action and that the progression of needs are being met.

A SUGGESTED DEVELOPMENTAL CONTINUUM

A true developmental continuum evolves over time. It would be ideal but unrealistic to put into place an entire network of developmentally focused services all at once. Some communities talk of experimenting with an incubator site where pilot projects are started for each developmental stage. The goal would then be to assess and facilitate project evolution until the network for each stage is robust and closes the service-to-needs gap. Still, the community needs time to figure itself out. It needs time to really change the way the business of community empowerment and development is done. The work of creating function from dysfunction is long term and unique. That is why the continuum presented in this volume is just one series of ideas that serves as an example, based on projects that in fact are in the community doing the work of guiding our children to productive citizenship.

- *The local partnership.* The local partnership has a dual purpose. Not only is it the support organization for continuum services, but it focuses on the first level of developmental need, that of preschoolers, up to the age of 5. The developmental need met is school readiness.
- *Engaging elementary school students and parents.* This covers the needs of the elementary years, from about ages 5 to 11. Action seeks to engage parents in the work of helping children acquire social, academic, and behavioral skills to continue success patterns in the home, neighborhood,

and school. Parents are a focus at this stage as it has been observed that parents are particularly influential during the elementary school years, arguably because it is the last opportunity for an at-risk parent to reach an at-risk child and help halt the downward spiral of failure. Here the goal is strengthening social, behavioral, and academic skills capability.

- *Alternative schools.* This model offers community programming for the middle school years, from about ages 12 to 14. Again, the focus is on academic and social success but with an array of alternative school and extended day opportunities depending on the variety of needs for the preteen and young adult.
- *Juvenile day treatment.* Finally, we offer a project description for high school–age youth who may have more serious barriers to success. These are typically young adults from ages 15 to 18. This is a way for the community to return juveniles to the mainstream.

Your continuum may be different.

The importance of community capacity built on research-based, performing projects is no less than the shaping of public service delivery systems. No more can individual institutions, individual sectors answer the public need. Only by true collaboration on seamless, sequential action targeted to the neediest children can we address difficulties that ruin chances at becoming independent, productive citizens. It is through citizens capable of success in career and family that we have communities that continue to thrive and nurture the next generation.

USE EFFECTIVE PRACTICES

The best way to go about using an effective practices model is to learn from the detailed practical lessons. Understand the long-term sequential nature of the business of building a viable public delivery system. Plan your own plan. Then ultimately act on that plan and resolve to make it work. We hope also to motivate simply by relating the message of possibility, that "it" can be done; to embolden the timid and to direct the assertive. Mainly, we hope to show a way through an avalanche of detail and necessary drudgery to accomplishment and reward via doing work worth doing.

We suggest that it will be helpful, when looking at the following chapters that document how various communities are working on real-world problems, to keep in mind the concepts of a developmental continuum of services and of project development according to the program life cycle. While doing so, ask yourself how these concepts can be applied to your particular community. Although there is no promise that making a particular program a reality will be easy or simple, there is a promise that good things will come from the effort.

Furthermore, we need a new way of doing the business of local activism to enable and strengthen community, a bottom-up commitment to act. And this enthusiasm to build community should be based on a new construct of collaboration and partnership:

- *Local infrastructure.* That the local municipality establishes the performance-based organizational platform on which to build a partnership of agencies and resources from which to offer services. This means that there is local determination and generation of ideas and, in mustering the necessary action, resources, expertise, and will of the public, private, and private nonprofit sectors.
- *Performance-based.* That all operations and services have a measurable contribution to the overall goal of nurturing citizenship. Performance recognizes the trade-off of doing one activity at the expense of another; thus, every endeavor has to return a measure of well-being to the community.
- *Developmentally appropriate continuum of services.* That the services answer the range of developmental needs from birth to the goal of productive citizenship at young adulthood with a seamless network of developmentally appropriate services. And that those services penetrate to the assessed needs of the community in general and specifically to defined client groups.

The developmental continuum then is the new construct by which we can redefine community advocacy and activism. It is forward thinking in that it is constantly evolving and constructed with permanency in mind. It is a model by which people can come together and know their effort is fruitful. It acknowledges that although we need to collaborate to survive and prosper, each neighborhood is unique and has a right to tackle its own issues. It also recognizes our interdependence—the real necessity to work together to make ideas work permanently. The continuum also recognizes that success with this way of proceeding requires patience and understanding; but it is . . . a beginning.

References

Swiss, J. E. (1991). *Public management systems; monitoring and managing government performance.* Englewood Cliffs, NJ: Prentice-Hall.

Exhibit 2.1
The Project Life Cycle: A Guide to the Process of Community Development for Public Services

Every successful project, one that becomes permanent and establishes an experience of service that makes life better, goes through a determined process of development: the life cycle. By conceiving a public service as a delivery system, project leadership can see and execute the sequence of essential actions that must be taken to build sustaining structure around the service. The idea is to conceive, conduct, and expand with permanence in mind. Going through the process is neither easy nor simple because it is time-consuming and often frustrating. Not going trough the process courts failure and certainly misses the promise of a good idea, that of being able to expand the service beyond the beginning to eventually close the service-to-needs gap and make a real difference with people and in our communities.

Note: In the outline that follows, asterisks denote critical items. Although every step is important to the process of project building, critical items are highlighted to ensure focus in essential milestones and tasks. These items must be considered and answered to ensure, as much as possible, program success.

I. Phase I: Planning Your Service Delivery System—Thinking About Your Project

A. *Assemble Key Leadership
   1. Establish a working relationship with key collaborators
   2. Establish consensus of purpose

B. Develop a Governance Structure
   1. Define roles, duties, and responsibilities of leadership
   2. Set up administrative support
   3. Establish an operational plan for governance
   4. Orient working groups

C. *Conduct a Needs Assessment
   1. Analyze relevant data
   2. Define the problem
   3. Define the target population
   4. Define the target area
   5. Research resources
   6. Determine project needs

D. *State Vision, Mission, Goals, and Objectives (consider project hierarchy of characteristics)
   1. Stability: established permanent funding
   2. Accessibility: services reaching those who need it
   3. Quality: an experience of service that changes lives for the better

E. *Outline Impact Analysis and Process Evaluation Plan
   1. Define measure(s) of success
   2. Define methodologies

3. Establish benchmarks

F. *Create Resource Development and Financial Management Plans
   1. Develop a plan for permanent funding
   2. Establish fiscal policies and procedures and a budget
   3. Establish lines and modes of communication for project fiscal matters

G. *Develop a Collaborative Marketing Plan for Essential Support and Partnerships
   1. Describe your collaboration
   2. Outline your partnering process
   3. Involve key stakeholders— corporate and noncorporate, internal and external clients

H. Develop a Long-Range Plan for Essential Services
   1. Define basic terms
   2. Detail the planning process—short, mid-range and long term objectives
   3. Plan for performance
   4. Structure continuous planning
   5. Conceptualize essential services
   6. Plan the character of service—stability, accessibility, and quality

I. Establish an Implementation Plan According to Your Vision and Mission
   1. Write the performance-based implementation plan
   2. Develop a practical board skilled in implementation

J. *Profile Key Staff
   1. Describe your project director
   2. Describe your staff and your service providers

K. Outline Key Project Staff Roles, Duties, Responsibilities, and Professional Human Capital Development Process
   1. Consider your key positions
   2. Outline your human capital development process

L. Prepare the Project Site
   1. Decide location
   2. Describe the facility
   3. Plan for automation and well-equipped office space

II. Phase II: Operating Your Service Delivery System—Doing Your Project

A. *Develop Organizational Structure and Your Human Capital
   1. Design a functional organizational structure
   2. Develop human capital

B. Hire Staff Collaboratively

C. Orient and Train Key Staff—Concentrate on Career Professional Development

1. Orient staff thoroughly
2. Specify a plan for career/professional development

D. *Justify Resources: Emphasize Permanent Funding Via a Development Campaign

1. Conduct organized, comprehensive fund raising
2. Develop a research-based project performance presentation

E. Develop Key Services According to Need, Stability, Accessibility, and Quality

1. Define characteristics of key services
2. Generate performance-based services
3. Ensure that each service contributes to stability, accessibility, and quality

F. Incorporate Analysis and Evaluation

1. Promote performance and improvement
2. Implement performance analysis
3. Implement process improvement

G. Integrate Into Existing Environment

1. Develop and execute the plan to integrate into your existing environment
2. Orient key stakeholder groups

H. Establish Mechanics of Communication

1. Design and use internal communication mechanisms
2. Design and use external communication mechanisms

I. Write Operational Guidelines

III. Phase III: Expanding Your Service Delivery System—Closing the Gap

A. Stabilize Your Initial Effort

1. Ensure performance orientation and narrow your scope
2. Ensure client focus
3. Ensure efficient/effective operational procedures, especially human capital development

B. Secure Permanent Funding

1. Strengthen your funds development campaign

C. Establish a Long-Range Planning/Guidance Body

1. Orient, train, and develop the board for expansion

D. *Determine Your Service to Needs Gap

1. Establish the reassessment process
2. Conduct the needs assessment

E. *Detail Your Expansion Strategy
   1. Revisit/restate vision, mission, and goals
   2. Identify essential people and resources
   3. Establish a time line
F. Involve Key Support Via Consensus
   1. Prepare for essential public relations and awareness
   2. Remake essential collaborations and partnerships
G. Expand Sequentially According to Will and Resources

Part II

Effective Local Partnerships—Building a School Readiness Program via the Life Cycle Community Services Development Model

by James Klopovic, M.A., M.P.A. and Douglas L. Yearwood, M.S.

The local partnership is an excellent organizational infrastructure for the delivery of public, needs-based, targeted services. The advantage of the partnership is that it is the focal point for local leadership to guide local control of limited resources where they are needed most. The disadvantage is that a partnership is difficult to begin, let alone stabilize, in the community due to real complexity and the need to be widely inclusive. There needs to be a way to begin and guide local community services development. That way is via a document that organizes essential activities along a proven and understandable process that moves people from idea to measurable improvements in individual lives and thus in the community as a whole. We call this an *Effective Practices* manual. This process of practices is referred to as effective practices because each suggested activity is based on everyday work of people in the field, people successfully doing the job of delivering the chosen service. It is a simple tool to help people focus limited money and, especially, time. It also allows for choice. Effective practices are only suggestions; project staff have to define what is best for them for every decision at hand as long as they have a proven path to follow. This effective practices document presents a way to organize, or even simplify, this complex and difficult, yet vital, task of developing, stabilizing, and expanding community services.

There are now many superior examples of flourishing local partnerships to prepare children for school, which are aided by helpful oversight and funding from like-minded state leadership; we have looked to examples of successful local partnerships in North Carolina to derive the general strategies and principals set out here, which can work in any jurisdiction. As with all large, collaborative, long-term projects, when broken down into essential elements they become understandable and no longer seen as insurmountable.

The partnership focus needs to be on school readiness as the first part of the continuum of developmentally appropriate services on the communal path to developing capable citizens. Such an effort has to begin and end with children. While the community builds the partnership infrastructure, it is also delivering basic services that ensure that a child is ready, emotionally and physically, and has enthusiasm for school. The view must be long term as a break in the attention paid to child/youth development can derail any progress the child has made. For clarity we review basic school readiness services as employed by N.C. Smart Start, a program to prepare children, ages birth to 5, for formal schooling. The local partnership, then, is the means by which essential services are delivered. While services offered are as unique as the governmental entity employing them, early on, school readiness is determined by similar, basic physical, emotional, and social early childhood needs. The life cycle model of community development is then applied to services that respond to the developmental needs of the child on the path to capable adulthood and citizenship as defined by individuals and their uniqueness as persons and the community that defines them.

The conceptual mechanism for understanding how to go about building the local partnership is the Project Life Cycle (see Exhibit 2.1, in Part I, Chapter 2). Every long-term public service delivery system has a beginning, a middle, and a continuation. Thus, the life cycle is defined in three phases: (1) planning; (2) operating; and (3) expanding the partnership. Each phase has a series of unique and necessarily recurring actions that offer a process to follow. What is unique about this process of building is that it offers a path of choices proven effective by practitioners who have and are doing the work. The reason to proceed is there, the proven way is suggested; all that remains is for a local champion to say it is time to begin.

Before any service is offered at the local level of government, it has to have an infrastructure of support services that provides the business platform from which services, especially services for children can be offered. Chapter 3 discusses the interrelationship and mutual support of state and local collaborations to offer services for children that get them ready for school. The benefits of targeted services for our youngest neighbors are numerous and supported by meaningful results from many effective partnerships in North Carolina. Making sure children are ready for school, for example, pays incalculable returns by having children stay in school and out of public social services or the criminal justice system. Chapter 3 further discusses the concept of the life cycle model for the development of partnerships and the subsequent services offered through them. Project staff learn the business of community infrastructure building by considering the task in terms of planning, operating, and expanding an idea with a long-term view of building permanent answers to community problems.

Before the first service is offered a rigorous and focused planning process must be accomplished. Chapter 4 begins the explanation of the Life Cycle of a project by elaborating the steps involved in planning your local partnership. The example of preparing children for school is used as it is the goal of the first series of services in the continuum of services for at-risk children and emphasizes the need to have very solid business practices in place before those services are offered. Planning is daunting and complex enough even when adequately done. It is too easy to be busy about the wrong things and therefore head nowhere. The purpose of this particular elaboration of planning is to offer a proven way to progress.

Chapter 5 discusses the daily operations of a partnership. Many action items suggested in planning now take on the characteristics of an up and running business. Plans give way to action to provide support and services. All of this is to assist the community in maturing their community development efforts beyond the planning stage to the stage of advancement where they can think about expanding. This is the stage of project maturation to which public services should arrive but few do. Progress through the Life Cycle is a way to reach the necessary goal of being a permanent part of the local service infrastructure and expanding to meet the assessed need.

Project expansion is elaborated in Chapter 6. Extending services to the assessed need in a community is a stage rarely achieved by a project because the work of stabilizing a project is rarely considered in the planning and operating phases of project maturation. Consequently, real effect in the community, effect that addresses community dysfunction in material ways, just does not happen. Yet, this is the goal of every project, to make a real, measurable differences in the lives of the folks in their neighborhoods.

For clarity, Chapter 7 outlines the services that need to be in a school readiness initiative: child care and education, health care and education, and family services. Note that each developmental stage for a child—preschool, elementary school middle school, and high school—has an overall goal, for example school readiness as the first comprehensive goal. How a local community chooses to construct the services that accomplish that goal is as individual as the community. What is constant is the process by which that community achieves those goals. Chapter 7, which suggests school-readiness services completes the first service project model in the continuum of developmentally appropriate services for children that of being prepared, mentally and physically for school.

Chapter 3

Justifying Local Partnerships—They Don't Cost; They Pay

Do you ever wonder why so many people spend so much energy on righting the wrongs of society, or of a neighborhood, with little in the way of results we can see or feel? We work, we spend, and we struggle in the face of a prison population that has risen year after year for almost three decades and crime remains higher than when we locked up one-sixth of this number (Sentencing Project, 2001). Schools become fortresses and we still suffer, in disbelief, when we have to witness disasters such as those at Columbine and Osaka and know we have not seen the last. We follow on the nightly news the case of a young person gone terribly wrong, yet his or her kindergarten teacher remarked many years before that something needed to be done for the youngster and it wasn't. It is not a matter of what we do; we know what to do. It is a matter of when and especially how we go about doing these things that make the difference.

In fact, the life cycle model for local Smart Start partnerships detailed in Part II began by looking at what was being done at the local level of government to work with children in general, as well as special efforts being made for the neediest children. The local partnership was designed to be the operational platform from which the community could launch performance-based services to target locally defined needs. After a few visits to some localized efforts, it became clear that what people did to address problems and needs depended on how the community built its capacity to support good ideas. In other words, success depends on relationships, especially when partnerships form to address the developmental needs of children. A good term to use is "collective efficacy" (National Institute of Justice, 2001). According to Sampson and Raudenbush (2001), collective efficacy is cohesion among neighborhood residents combined with shared expectations for informal social control of public space. This cohesion is a major social process that, to the authors, is manifest in the local Smart Start partnership. Our analysis of local partnerships looks at the process of how communities organize and build infrastructure to support ideas that make a difference. It serves as a suggestion for how to make a difference. The path to building a partnership will be unique to our environment; what is important, though, is that we do follow a logical and sequential process.

This initial part of the continuum aims not to duplicate the wealth of good information that anyone can get from a probe of the world wide web, the bookstore, and the people working successful projects. Many resources already exist—for example, the North Carolina Partnership for Children's Website link: Smart Start Tool Kit (*www.smartstart-nc.org*). While the life cycle of project/program development is not a laundry list of merely neat things to do, we do order and detail the most effective, field-proven strategic and daily operational practices that enhance the chances of ultimate success. References such as the Smart Start Tool Kit are great founts of ideas from which a well-done effort can draw. Together they outline a proven process, good resources, and good ideas that, when combined with determination, form the basic elements of success.

A strong, permanent local collaboration is a necessary underpinning that begins the network of preventive services that really saves children from going wrong. Soon we will have more children under the supervision of the criminal justice system than we have enrolled in college. Robin Karr-Morse points out that Goldman Sachs, the investment firm, predicts a spending increase of $2–$3 billion more for prisons per year! Right now the correction industry has 523,000 employees, which puts it just behind General Motors. One in twenty of today's babies will spend time behind bars (Karr-Morse & Wiley, 1997). We all know the numbers or variations of them. These facts, and volumes more, beg the question, "What have we really done, to prevent these numbers in the first place?" We need an answer, if only to stop the hemorrhaging of the huge sums of tax dollars these numbers represent, not to mention the grief, both individual and collective, represented by an occupied jail cell.

The pity of a life gone wrong is that in many, even most cases, something could have been done to keep that young life on track. We know who they are. Every teacher, every child-care provider, every neighbor sees them. They see the child who is inadequately fed and clothed. They see parents who are having trouble coping with raising their children, parents who are too overwhelmed to show love and care for them. They see youngsters who, even early on, give in to boredom and escape to juvenile pressures, the media, and drugs. Study after study, as well as common sense, attests to the simplicity of these economical and effective early measures that can keep a child feeling good in school and at home. Well-timed and consistent efforts such as prenatal care, extra classes, tutoring, and mentoring have proven successful. The fact is, the later we wait to "treat" a problem, the more it will cost and the less effective that treatment is. Put another way, "Is it better to deal with a child struggling a little with reading and long division or with the young adult struggling with gang involvement and a criminal record?" If we know what to do, why are so many communities fighting to make a material difference in the neighborhood, in the classroom, in the labor pool?

The answer is that too few communities are doing the laborious, long-term, exasperating, yet rewarding, work of laying foundations (e.g., parenting education that has, as a component, parents reading to their children). Although it sounds simple enough, it is not that easy. It is complex and nettlesome work. That is why we see so few successful attempts at building partnerships. But we do have many successes to provide examples. Therein lies hope. This model is not a "blueprint" or a "road map" or "best" practices. These trendy workshop titles have difficulties, the largest being that they promise solutions and fall far short of stated expectations. Also, our model is not meant to take the place of existing research, observations, and testimony from people making partnerships work. Although it provides some detail of the volumes of long-range work for a significant number of citizens, another message should also be clear: The work is productive. It is productive because it deals with children at arguably the most critical moments in their lives. More often than that, a successful collaboration provides examples for how to build the community no matter the goal undertaken.

The Editor-in-Chief of *U.S. News and World Report* observed: "Achievement springs not simply from the quality (of schooling) but also from a child's family and community. For example, children from low-income households enter school with as little as one-fourth the vocabulary of middle-class students. Teachers matter. Incentive and sanctions matter—and providing resources matters" (Zuckerman, 2001, p. 64).

In this volume we attempt to capture the process of providing meaningful resources, and to give communities an idea of the nature and extent of this type of large community undertaking. Why? Because it can be done; it has to be done. Without an understanding of an organized way to proceed, communities are left to flounder and opportunities are lost, never to be regained. Far greater than the cost of losing dollars is the cost of losing young lives. It is an expense that we do not have to suffer.

INTERRELATIONSHIP OF LOCAL PARTNERSHIPS AND STATE AGENCIES

The Chicken or the Egg?

We cannot begin a discussion of local partnerships without understanding their interrelatedness to state structure, hierarchy, or oversight agency. It is a matter of the chicken or the egg—which comes first, the state oversight agency or the local partnership? Basically, each is more potent because of the other.

Still, local partnerships must be solid and a permanent part of local public service infrastructure. State support does not reach its potential unless there is local level capacity to translate resources to real benefit. Certainly, a well-working local collaboration is that much stronger with state support, but local organization must first be well led, well staffed, performance oriented, and dynamic. Thus we need to understand, briefly, how the state positions itself to be a part of something that is greater than the sum of the parts.

Smart Start, which promotes school readiness and is organized and administered by the North Carolina Partnership for Children, is a proven example of how state government works closely with local communities to make a permanent, material, measured difference. In its winning application for the Innovations in American Government Award, Smart Start is defined as a "comprehensive, public-private initiative where communities pool resources and bring their best ideas to the table." Where it "creates a decentralized framework of result-driven accountability and decision-making." Easier said than done but well worth the effort. Smart Start is a careful blend of state guidance and local control that has a handsome return on investment.

The overall goal is school readiness, but much more happens. Partnerships seek to build capacity in child care and other services for young children, and to improve the condition of young children in general. The logic is that success early on means intermediate success at home, in school, and in the community, which eventually leads to success as a productive citizen. A second powerful goal is the driving force of performance-based programming. No proposal for service, no idea, is undertaken unless it makes a direct and material contribution to the local vision and mission. Each project must maintain its contribution, day by day. If not, project staff are given a chance to mend productivity. If effectiveness cannot be proven, the effort is abandoned. So what is this approach that enables our children to succeed, especially those with barriers to success?

The state provides tactful oversight and guidance, much akin to parental care, by defining and supporting a comprehensive approach. About 70 percent of effort and resources are devoted to child care that is accessible, affordable, available, and of higher quality. The remaining 30 percent flows to child health and family support services, including parenting education. This network of local partnerships, and the state agency collaborative oversight, binds vision and service that contribute to community well-being, which is the reason for government in the first place. Local communities are free to determine their direction and partner as they see fit. The state, via an organization of task-specific commissions, boards, and subcommittees, provides healthy guidance that minimizes interference and bureaucracy. Over time, a well-working partnership provides a model for the living, breathing process of community infrastructure building. One success leads to others. In this volume, we attempt to define the factors of a productive working relationship, so others can replicate the process.

The Character of Partnering

It is helpful to understand the character of partnering from the state perspective. Smart Start is characterized by dynamic tension, balancing the seemingly incompatible tasks of:

- Providing structure and guidance and promoting local control and decision making;
- Building on best practices and encouraging creativity;
- Providing strong leadership and promoting collaboration;
- Offering support and helping a community become more self-sufficient;
- Addressing the needs of the neediest and conveying the message that Smart Start is for all young children and families in the state; and
- Creating a strong local presence and informing citizens about how Smart Start at the state level touches their everyday lives. (Dombro, 2001, p. 22)

There is as much art as there is science in building a partnership. It evolves over time by thinking deeply on how to work together, then, ultimately, jumping in and making mistakes. People working with ideals, vision, mission, beliefs, and common purpose inevitably make mistakes while they create opportunities for necessary improvement and positive evolution.

Child care improves as teacher education, staff capacity, and subsidies increase. Children are demonstrably healthier as preventive health care and education reaches them in increasing numbers, and families strengthen as medical services and education reaches them. But we must remember that Smart Start, or any similar program, is just that, a start. The critical flaw in this foundation building is that true success comes from what follows—that is, how the community continues to develop its children, especially those at risk. But with a good start, it is much simpler, efficient, and effective to keep children in school, out of court, and on track to reaching their potential. One of the first things asked about such an endeavor is, "Why do it at all? What is the justification for our taking on a really Herculean responsibility?"

WHY EARLY INTERVENTION IS IMPORTANT AND HOW TO PROMOTE IT

The need for a local collaborative effort is not as much for what it overtly does—that is, channel limited resources to priority needs—but rather for how it builds infrastructure that prevents difficulties for the community and actually promotes community wellness. The focus is on positive measures that stop the causes of a problem rather than the negative, more common tactic of reacting when something goes wrong. When people and agencies come together in a well-oiled, machine-like fashion guided by passion and common purpose, they fulfill the promise of government and the citizen activist; the community improves. When working for and with children, the promise provides for the betterment of its children, especially the youngest of children, with well-timed, necessarily persistent assistance. The earlier this assistance is provided, the better.

It is now well documented that the first five years in a child's life are critical to brain development, physical development, growth of social integration skills, and increase in the feelings of personal worth (Zalkind, 2001). Research indicates that from birth to age 5, 85 percent of a child's intellect, personality, and social skills is formed. Basic emotional and social responses are learned, including that all-important characteristic, the ability to trust. By the age of 3, most of the child's working vocabulary is in place (Zalkind, 2001). Why shouldn't human, monetary, and capital resources be enthusiastically channeled in great measure to this proven and timely need? The problem is not the desire to do so; the difficulty is the channel itself. The community must be prepared to manage, with effect, these resources.

A strong partnership is defense against the built-in political nature of government funding, which is short term and nearly whimsical depending on who views the problem and the fact that those people, the ones who disburse funds, change regularly. Dealing with growing children and the inevitable difficulties that come with childhood requires a long-term proposition. Consequently, answers must have long-term focus. This is the antithesis of the lengthy, complicated, and political nature of resource acquisition for the public sector. A project must contend with competing demands for money during the budgetary process and be on the oppressive, inevitable, budgetary cycle. If grant funds are sought, usually federal and state requirements are imposed for spending purposes. And all sources of public funding are controlled by stringent oversight.

Demographics continue to morph nearly year to year. In North Carolina, for example, 67 percent of mothers work and quality child care costs more than the state's public colleges. Nationally, as of 1999, fifty-eight teenage girls got pregnant every day (Loeber & Farrington, 2000). State and federal support of proven programs to combat these ills falls dramatically short of the need which we are only beginning to understand. Each year police make more than 250,000 arrests of children age 12 and younger, a surprising number are for more and more serious offenses according to researchers from the Washington, DC, Office of Juvenile Justice and Delinquency Prevention (Loeber & Farrington, 2000). OJJDP analysts further state that these child delinquents (between the ages of 7 and 12) have a two- to threefold risk of becoming tomorrow's serious, violent, and chronic juvenile offenders who then are at a much greater risk of becoming adult serious offenders.

The same report goes on to describe the intervention that best addresses persistently disruptive children and child delinquents. That (ideal) intervention should:

- Be integrated across services;
- Focus on children before age 13;
- Apply multimodal interventions, addressing more than one risk factor domain (e.g., individual, child, or family); and
- Screen for and address the multiple problems of the child, as necessary.

By incorporating these factors, a local partnership can address local issues based on its understanding of the risks children face and work on the strengths every child has. These strengths are commonly called protective factors. The elevation of these assets with the minimization of risks means positive development. The problem is that most children have only about eighteen of forty available assets (Search Institute, May 1999).[1] We are only beginning to understand the true nature and extent of what it is to really nurture the development of our children. Much more about the problems, needs, and numbers of our at-risk children will become evident as more infrastructure is built at the local level and, by being close to the problem, more realistic facts surface.

A well-working partnership is a primary stand against the reality that there is never enough money, people, and time to address the true needs of our youngest citizens when they need it most. Most communities struggle just to provide basic services and only dream about answering basic needs of their youngsters. Many times, however, the political will is there. For example, the Covenant with North Carolina's Children polled taxpayers regarding their priorities. The Fight Crime: Invest in Kids survey (2001) found that reducing child abuse and neglect, helping schools better educate disadvantaged students, and access to after-school programs and school readiness programs are more important to taxpayers than cutting taxes. Again, people want action; they only need the vehicle.

A strong partnership stands ready to provide that structure. It can, for example, develop its own funding streams to augment public funding for worthy, effective work. Effective interventions do not begin when a child enters kindergarten; they really begin at birth. With this focus, partnership by partnership, communities can change the emphasis from assuaging hurt (a child dropping out of school or into the courts) to never having the hurt in the first place. This is really a distinct change from the politically expedient needs-based programming.

BENEFITS OF TARGETING SERVICES TO YOUNG CHILDREN

The benefits of providing targeted services to young children are incalculable but must be considered to understand the impact of this intelligent way of disbursing the public effort. After the statistical or cost case is made, it is often the discussion of benefit, especially that which defies quantification, that makes the case and justifies the project at hand. Consider the winning

Innovations in American Government Award application for Smart Start: The stated expectation, which it is now realizing, is "a high return on its dollar in terms of improved quality of life for participants, and actual financial savings due to decreased rates of juvenile crime, welfare dependency, teenage pregnancy as well as increased high school graduation rates and enhanced tax revenues" (1998 Innovations in American Government Applications, p. 1). In fact, there is the happy circumstance of realizing that the well-working partnership achieved a core purpose of leveraging private funds. There is a significant dynamic of the multiplier effect on time, money, and resources invested. The initial years of Smart Start (1995–2001) alone produced more than $125 million in private funding and more than 1 million volunteer hours (Smart Start, 1999), and those numbers continue to grow. Furthermore, this demonstration of public-private collaboration is even more dramatic when we considers funding for programs other than Smart Start that funnel through the local partnerships.

Broader research has focused on a continuum of benefit. The Rand Corporation, a research and policy institute, set out to argue that "a balanced, thoughtful analysis of (such) programs, including illustrative economic analyses, that will be (a) useful resource for policy planners and early intervention researchers" (Karoly et al., 1998). Rand studied eleven projects that addressed the needs of children and observed benefits in four domains: cognitive emotional development, education, economic well-being, and health. They noticed improvements in areas such as IQ, behavior, achievement, special education, grades passed, graduation rates, crime/delinquency, employment, income, welfare participation, emergency room visits, and teen pregnancy (Karoly et al.,1998, p. xiv). The Rand study was followed by the High Scope Perry Preschool Study and The Abcedarian Project, both of which found that "of the children studied, those who attended high-quality, active learning preschool programs at ages three and four had half as many criminal arrests, higher earnings and property wealth, greater commitment to marriage , and higher graduation and college attendance rates" (Smart Start: *www.smartstart-nc.org,* 2001).

Conversely, the study investigators noted that "of those not in quality preschool programs, 35 percent had five or more arrests, only 13 percent owned a home, 80 percent received social service assistance, and only 54 percent graduated from high school (Smart Start: *www.smartstart-nc.org,* 2001). Various agencies of the public sector and especially the private sector not only agree with this broader research but are enthused about their experiences.

Clearly, Smart Start is a wise investment in North Carolina's future. Furthermore, 86 percent of police chiefs when surveyed nationally said the government could reduce youth crime by beefing up child care and after-school programs. Nearly nine of ten agreed that failing to do so will cost the nation more in the long run in crime, welfare, and other expenses, according to Fight Crime: Invest in Kids. A lack of reliable child care can cause workers to lose time and be less productive at work. What is most appealing to any group is that more than 95 percent of all funds contributed to Smart Start are being used directly at the community level on behalf of young children and their families (Smart Start brochure, "Building Brighter Futures"). That benefit alone attests to the efficiency and effectiveness of the local partnership and provides justification for the effort.

If anything, local partnerships working in conjunction with the state initiative in North Carolina are happily receiving an inordinate amount of helpful scrutiny. As we see throughout this model of the local partnership, understanding how well things work via a range of analytical methods is woven throughout the initiative. Take, for example, the results of a study sponsored by the Frank Porter Graham Child Development Center, University of North Carolina—Chapel Hill (Buysse, Bernier, Skinner, & Wesley, 2000). Parents and professionals reported that there were several benefits of high-quality inclusive child care. These benefits include the following:

- Enhanced development and well-being for children with special needs;
- Increased acceptance of children with disabilities by children without disabilities;
- Additional support for all parents, such as regular communication and opportunities for parent education and family social events; and
- A positive impact on all parents' expectations and beliefs about child development and disabilities (Buysse et al., 2000).

North Carolina's former Governor, James B. Hunt, Jr., also observed that during the initial start-up years of these partnerships, more families moved from welfare to work when they had support from the simple mechanism of accessible, affordable, quality child care.

The North Carolina Partnership for Children (NCPC) observes that a fully funded program to provide child care, preventive health care, and support for families will cost the state $330 million (NCPC, 2001). This works out to about $1,633 per child per year compared to over $6,300 per child per year for K–12 schooling. The Connecticut Commission on Children, by way of noting national implications, observes that "every dollar invested saves, on average, $5 later for the taxpayer (Zimmerman, 1994, p. 2). And this is saving just in social services not used. Just think about the return on this investment that produces a neighbor who is capable in the workplace, family, and community. Can we afford not to make this kind of investment? Compare the foregoing costs with the present cost of about $150 per day for detention and about $50,000 per year for training school (i.e., reform school) at the very least. And remember, those costs are incurred only after a chain of costly, damaging misbehavior and juvenile crime (Sweat, 2000). Even though most children fare well without expensive social interventions, the relatively few who need a little tactful support are well worth the cost, especially when it is offered early and consistently.

But programs represented by Smart Start, in a true continuum of community-based programming that addresses the developmental needs of children, do keep citizens off the dole, do reduce crime and delinquency, and really do enhance lifelong productivity. The benefits, which are sometimes characterized as unmeasurable are actually quite immense when counted collectively. The Smart Start Collaboration Study (February 2001) determined that staff became more efficient, there was less duplication of services, information sharing increased, services were more convenient, there was more awareness of services, and waiting lists for those services were reduced. There are also benefits to participating families beyond those to the children. We have seen an increase in total productivity from engaged citizens, savings from greatly reduced use of public services, and collective contentment from pursuing a career. The real benefit is in the cumulative return on investment of enhancing the successes and capabilities of all children with emphasis on the neediest.

RESULTS FROM TWO SMART START PARTNERSHIP SITES

Evidence in favor of partnering resource development and services compiles almost daily. What is most telling, though, is an overview of some of the initial accomplishments of only two of the early North Carolina partnership sites. From 1994–1999, the Down East Partnership for Children did the following:

- Reduced occurrence of lead poisoning in children by 52 percent;
- Reduced child care teacher turnover rate in targeted centers by 20 percent;
- Helped twenty-one child care centers achieve top state licensing and four child care homes and one child care center achieve national accreditation; number of top-rated centers up 666 percent (from three to twenty-three);
- Awarded 1,259 child-care scholarships to children of working and in-school parents;
- Assisted 1,261 children in getting immunizations for school enrollment;
- Worked with over 10,276 preschoolers in creative educational programs to enhance learning and preparation for school;
- Screened 6,050 preschool children for vision problems;
- Educated 6,719 families on current parenting issues and pertinent parenting information;
- Provided crisis care for an average of thirty-five children a month during family emergencies, preventing the possibility of child abuse or neglect; and

- Helped develop a network of family resource centers throughout Nash and Edgecombe counties.

The Forsyth Early Childhood Partnership (FECP) (Dean Clifford, Ph.D., Executive Director; *www.forsythchild.org*) from 1995–2000, working with fifty-six contracted services and thirty-four service providers had similar initial accomplishments:

- 10,119 children received scholarships for child care and other preschool experiences;
- 124,873 enrichment programs (were) offered to children;
- 25,352 early childhood teachers received education and training experiences;
- 29,159 direct health services were provided to children;
- 52,618 parents participated in parent education and parent support programs; and
- 41,432 children were served by quality improved early childhood programs.

These are just some of the overall numbers of people affected by early partnership work. Compound these numbers by the partnerships that have spread to all 100 North Carolina counties. There is more evidence of local effect demonstrated again by the FECP:

- *Kindergarten readiness.* Fifty percent of children enrolled in full-time pre-K scored average or above on the Learning Achievement Profile (LAP). When children were served by Smart Start Child Care Scholarships and Emergency Assistance, Jump Start, and Head Start Wrap-Around Child Care, 75 percent of them scored average or above average on the LAP.
- *Outreach.* From 1996–1998 there was a 72 percent increase in children and a 54 percent increase in parents served. Also, there was a 70 percent increase in early childhood professionals served, usually with appropriate training.
- *Educational level and compensation of child care workers and professionals.* College degreed home providers increased 17 percent. Child-care teachers without a high school diploma decreased 40 percent. Minimum hourly pay increased $.57 per hour, which increased staff qualification and decreased turnover.
- *Service quality.* National quality rating scales noted substantive improvements in child-care educational environments.

- *Health.* Dental care to targeted parents and children increased 300 percent during this period. Also, 789 more children gained access to primary care physicians through Medicaid or Health Choice.
- *International services.* Translation services reached 1,100 Hispanic parents and children per month.

The director of the FECP, Dean Clifford, noted the dramatic effect of just one of the sponsored preschool programs that served a low-income neighborhood. Experience showed that most children at the school were poorly prepared for public school. After one year of scholarships to a high-quality prekindergarten program, all fifteen students made the maximum possible score on their pre-K assessment. Imagine the possibilities of these results when multiplied by collaboratives that can be built in just about every county in any state.

The health arena shows us additional proof that a continuum of services, especially for the very young, pays greatly. Brain development is medically proven to be a matter of external influences. Doctors at Baylor College of Medicine studied twenty children who were raised in a globally understimulated environment; they were rarely touched or spoken to and were understimulated with, for example, toys. Brain imaging showed their brains to be 20–30 percent smaller than those of most children their age, and in more than half the cases, parts of their brains appeared to have wasted away (An Ounce of Prevention Fund, 1996).

Many early childhood services can be directly linked to substantial tax savings (*www.smartstart-nc.org/News/Newsletter/*).

- *Family planning.* Save $4.40 for every $1 spent on family planning.
- *Quality preschool.* Save $7.16 for every $1 spent on providing quality preschool services.
- *Home visits.* Save $5.63 for every $1 spent on home visitation programs.
- *School-based clinics.* Save $7 for every $1 spent on school-based services.

The case is compelling even with a casual survey of research; more evidence will be available as partnerships have more and wider effects on their respective communities.

Study after study reveals that targeting resources and effort via programs such as Smart Start, significantly improves language, cognitive, behavioral, and social skills of youngsters. As children are strengthened, communities grow stronger. Field interviews and on-site observations indicate that there have been substantial increases in both the number of inter-organizational relationships established since the inception of local activities, and in the productivity of existing relationships. Children are better prepared for school, child-care quality improves, teachers are better educated and their turnover reduces, children are healthier, and parents are better at being parents (Smart Start Website: *www.ncsmartstart.org/overview/results.htm*). The need for, benefit of, and evidence of working in the community with children are forceful and based on common sense. Still, there needs to be an understanding that the tasks are neither simple nor easy.

COUNTERING ARGUMENTS AGAINST LOCAL PARTNERSHIPS

Arguments against local partnerships are largely based on the difficulty in putting together productive, sustained partnerships and especially in the running of them. The effort is fraught with politics, competing/conflicting purposes, misunderstandings, expense, personal agendas, and more. We are reminded of the observation by Magda Baligh, director of the Halifax-Warren Smart Start Partnership for Children (*www.ncsmartstart.org*), who said during an interview, "It is tough to think of expansion! It took us (the Board and staff) several years just to have a common understanding of what we mean by a goal, an objective, a measure, and a target." Service provision, though it is performance based, has a hit-and-miss nature; certainly "proof" has to be pried from it. Partnership staff note it really takes at least four years of measuring effect before results are evident and these results just hint at measurable improvement in the people served.

Aside from these real problems for the local collaborative, state involvement requires oversight that is challenging to local leaders. There is the real problem of unfunded mandates, which looms large when a state considers child development. Local governments are constantly beset with difficulties providing basic services, let alone with assuming an expensive prevention program with a long-term purpose. The business of local service provision is urgent and does not need the state providing the daily "to do list." Most city managers are concerned, for example, with clean air, traffic flow, clean water, waste treatment, education, and public safety. Their attention span for a pitch to increase home visitations for the underprivileged is quite short. An understatement is that the effort is expensive. In truth, pockets are really very shallow. The long-term project has a nearly impossible time justifying limited tax dollars and developing other funds which are the life blood of these works. So, why jump into this fire?

The simple and compelling answer to many contrary arguments and competing issues that have plagued citizen action as long as there has been citizen involvement in local affairs is that *all are better for having tried.* The fact is, it can be done in spite of the obstacles. The loss, then, is not in the trying and failing; it is in not beginning at all. In fact, without exception, people at every site we visited encouraged those who follow by stating that planning is good but action is better. Plan but do not be timid. Get to work; progress will be made. Whenever we went to the field, every staffer, every service provider, every director was exuberant about his or her work. Even though they expressed and epitomized exhaustion, they radiated with the true glow of knowing they were doing something important, something meaningful, something lasting that truly improved the local community, its citizens, and, most important, the lives of its children. To get started with this important endeavor let us look at the life cycle of public programs.

USE THE LIFE CYCLE MODEL

The remaining chapters in Part II detail the project life cycle. This way of thinking about community development is to think in terms of doing a detailed job of building service infrastructure under services no matter what they may be. It also lends real perspective to the fact that effective delivery of services is a long-term prospect. It is almost futile to engage the talent, time, and money necessary for this work if the intention from the outset is to do a one-time, short-term project. If done at all, the driving motivation should be to stabilize and expand to the total population in need of a continuum of services. That is where the difference is made. This is long-range, tough, frustrating work. The life cycle is a way to keep people from getting distracted by the multitude of confusing, confounding, and competing variables in public service while keeping everyone thinking and acting for the generations to come.

Besides ordering a lengthy and complex process, the Project Life Cycle is laid out in the form of a checklist (see Exhibit 2.1), to facilitate assignment of duties and responsibilities and to monitor progress. Project staff and leadership can easily see when progress is or is not being made. Problems can be identified before they become crises. Each phase—planning, operating, and expanding the project—is followed by steps which are in turn followed by action items. Each action item is then followed by some of the most effective ways of accomplishing the item as proven by practitioners. Everything suggested works, but each item needs to be scrutinized for fit to the unique needs of a particular municipality.

If the life cycle is compressed to steps and action items it becomes a checklist of items to be done. The checklist format implies that the suggested tasking has to be done in sequence; in actuality, many activities are accomplished simultaneously. This format is to assist with essential project-building work and focus necessary attention to detail. It is quite easy to get distracted from the task at hand. The best way to use this suggestion for project building is to personalize it. Most suggestions will apply to one's effort, some will have to be tailored to one's needs, some will have to be augmented with steps and actions unique to a community, and some may not need to be done at all. The soul of the life cycle is that community infrastructure is possible because ordinary people in communities are doing it. This process is built on their knowledge and experience. Remember, the goal is to build permanent, productive, accessible, and quality services no matter the path we take.

Notes

[1] According to the Search Institute there are forty developmental assets, external and internal. There are four external groups and four internal groups. For example, the external support group has six assets: family support, positive family communication, other adult relationships, caring neighborhood, caring school climate, and parent involvement in schooling. Internal assets connected to a commitment to learning are achievement motivation, school engagement, homework, bonding to school, and reading for pleasure, for example.

References

An Ounce of Prevention Fund. (1996). *Starting smart: How early experiences affect brain development.*

Buysse, V., Bernier, K., Skinner, D., & Wesley, P. (2000). *Smart Start and quality inclusive child care in North Carolina: Study highlights.* Chapel Hill: University of North Carolina, Frank Porter Graham Child Development Center.

Dombro, A. M. (2001). *What is Smart Start* (Monograph for the North Carolina Partnership for Children) [On-line]. Available: *www.ncsmartstart.org/Information/publications.htm.*

Fight Crime: Invest in Kids. (2001, February 19). *More than 2/3 of public say boosting investments in kids is higher priority than tax cut* [Press release].

Karoly, L. A., Greenwood, P. W., Everingham, S. S., Hoube, J., Kilburn, R. M., Rydell, P. C., Sanders, M., & Chiesa, J. (1998). *Investing in our children: What we know and don't know about the costs and benefits of early childhood interventions.* Santa Monica: Rand.

Karr-Morse, R., & Wiley, M. S. (1997). *Ghosts from the nursery.* New York: Atlantic Monthly Press.

Loeber, F., & Farrington, D. (Chairs). (2000, November 14. Conference of Office of Juvenile Justice and Delinquency. *Child delinquency: Early intervention and prevention* [On-line]. Available: Juvenile Justice Teleconferencing Website: *wwwjuvenilenet.org/jjtap/young.*

Sampson, R. J., & Raudenbush, S. W. (2001). *Disorder in urban neighborhoods—Does it lead to crime?* National Institute of Justice Research Brief.

Sweat, G. L. (2000, December 15). [Speech given in Bladen County North Carolina, by Secretary, Department of Juvenile Justice and Delinquency Prevention].

Search Institute. (1999, May). What is healthy communities, healthy youth? (Report from the Lutheran Brotherhood). Minneapolis, MN: Author.

Sentencing Project. (2001). [Untitled letter.] Washington, DC: Author.

Zalkind, H. (2001). [Interview]. Down East Partnership for Children; P.O. Box 1245; 215 Lexington Street, Rocky Mount, NC 27802; 252-985-4300 [On-line]. Available: Smart Start Website: *www.smartstart-nc.org.*

Zimmerman, E. (1994). *School readiness Is one smart little investment* [On-line]. Available: *www.cga.state.ct.us/coc/school.htm.*

Zuckerman, M. (2001, February 12). The education paradox. *U.S. News and World Report,* p. 64.

Chapter 4

Planning a New Local Partnership

Everyone is ready. Everyone understands the need, benefits, and evidence. There is political will and perhaps even the wherewithal to devote to strategic planning. With a collective deep breath, it is time to begin. But how do we proceed? Again, we want to emphasize that the "how to" is not *the* way to do a local partnership, it is *a* way. Effective practices are "proven" by the individuals who have done and are doing the job. An individual's path will be just that, an individual path—the same road but traveled in a unique way. What is common to successful efforts in developing local partnerships is the process.

ASSEMBLE KEY LEADERSHIP

> "Leadership *is the art of accomplishing more than the science of management says is possible."*
>
> —Colin Powell

Establish a Working Relationship With Key Collaborators

There will be a struggle with this thing called leadership. Before the partnership comes the local champion or champions who decide something more must be done to make the community what it should be. We dwell on leadership because it is as misunderstood and difficult to arrange as it is vital to the very existence of the partnership. Leadership is the spark that ignites the community flame of meaningful collaboration, and it is the engine that pulls it through inevitable project-ending threats. A good place to begin a discussion of leadership is to understand the character and characteristics of a board member.

Leaders must lead especially by example if things are to succeed. At first glance, we are taken by the fact that all board members are there to work, to contribute to the common good, and to succeed. They are not there for business as usual or a fancy posting. They do not have a defeatist attitude; anything is possible. Least of all, they are not selfish. Some of the character traits of the ideal board member are as follows:

- *Spirit.* Each member seeks to really cooperate; this cooperation builds value.
- *Inspiration.* Each member is guided by the noble pursuit of helping young people reach their potential as good citizens.

- *Creativity.* Here creativity means the ability to do the scores of detailed activities in the building process just a little better, more efficiently, and more effectively.
- *Patience.* He or she must be willing to wait for the appropriate opportunity (then have the aggressiveness to act).
- *Energy.* Each member needs to bring an ample measure of pure steam to the table.
- *Persistence.* The good board member is not deterred by "no."
- *Sense of time.* This work is long term; each piece of work must be approached with that mind-set.
- *Passion.* Each member must believe in working with children.

These are ideals, but they are realistic, especially in the local partnership environment. In selecting board members one should look for these traits and "grow" each member to the task at hand. We should not expect to welcome the ideal board member; such a member evolves over time with the experience of working together, a thorough orientation, and appropriate training, such as classes on the operation of a non-profit. Members should be seated for one, two, or three years and appointments should be staggered to ensure a continuing core of corporate knowledge. It should be mentioned that the local Smart Start board in North Carolina is inundated by legislation, which is good and bad. Certainly there is plenty of direction, but, at the same time, it is confusing and at times stifling. A varied group has the greatest potential to provide leadership and garner resources (Exhibit 4.1 shows the composition of one partnership's board of directors). Of course, each partnership's board composition should reflect specific local needs. It is also most helpful to have an attorney on the board simply because of the volumes of legal issues in the nonprofit undertaking.

Establish Consensus of Purpose

Once in place, the board needs a sense of purpose. A good way to begin establishing consensus is to understand the values or beliefs that one's group wants to reflect. This is not a vision or mission. For example, following is the statement of purpose from Forsyth County, North Carolina:

- Appreciate **C**hildhood as a critical and vital state of the human cycle.
- Facilitate **H**igh impact services that are accessible, affordable, and of excellent quality.
- Directly **I**mpact the loving, stimulating, healthy, and safe environ-

ment of each child, birth through five, in the context of family, culture, and society.

- Be a Servant **L**eader, bringing professionalism and passion to all efforts, through partnership within the community.
- Respect the **D**ignity, worth, and uniqueness of each person in the early childhood system.

Developing a consensus of purpose is important in general, and specifically for a unique reason. Inevitably the project will face the precipice of demise or life; ideally, this process of ripening common purpose nurtures those partners who just will not let the project die.

DEVELOP A GOVERNANCE STRUCTURE

Organize Task Forces

From the first days the board comes together, members should organize into functional groups, better termed as task forces. We suggest that the first group organized be the Development and Fund Raising Task Force. Funding is and remains the overarching worry of the local partnership. The sooner a complete strategy to raise mone is in place, the sooner the board can focus on what it should be doing. If the reverse is done and the group first gets distracted by "important" committee work, then ignores the money issue (it is much more fun, and easier, to get services going), then the partnership dwindles away. Another important point to make is that the partnership must also demonstrate effective work and sound organization before meaningful fund raising can be achieved. Simply, people need to see that their money will be well spent even if it is for a good cause. A task force structure may have the following groupings:

- Development and Fund Raising
- Audit and Finance
- Bylaws
- Personnel
- Strategic and Long-Range Planning
- Program and Budget Planning
- Outreach/Awareness
- Projects and Activities
- Evaluation and Needs Assessment

Naturally, organization is only part of the battle. People have to know what to do when they get together.

Define Roles, Duties, and Responsibilities of Leadership

This initial leadership group, the primary initiators, needs to know the rules of the game. Here it helps to go through the process of understanding who does what before it becomes an issue or, worse, a damaging argument. For that, leadership needs to understand expected standards of conduct, as well as legal, ethical, and fiduciary obligations of the job. The board as an entity needs to understand what the members are to do (see, e.g., Exhibit 4.2, which details a job description for board members). Likewise, a personal understanding of duties and responsibilities of individual officers and committees is paramount (see Exhibit 4.3 for an example from the Halifax-Warren (North Carolina) Smart Start Partnership for Children[1]).

Set Up Administrative Support

A partnership should not even think of bringing together the board unless there is staff support. The board is there to work, yes, but to work on strategy, planning, policy, and direction, not to answer the phone and get out the mail. Once the core group has established its purpose and initial direction, an executive director and perhaps clerical support should be on hand. If administrative support cannot be funded locally, perhaps a start-up grant or a local foundation will be able to help the partnership get on its feet. The trick is to have staff in place before they are needed. It takes time to get people productive. A partnership may begin with one or two staff, but the mature partnership mirrors the small corporation in organization, specialization, and talent. Retirees are easily a partnership's "secret weapon," the board members or staffers who tirelessly do the bulk of the work for the partnership simply to have the opportunity to be involved and do good things for the community.

Establish an Operational Plan for Governance

This is deciding *how* to decide so that the governing board is happy with decisions. It comes from understanding duties and responsibilities and having the structure of task forces (subcommittees) to carry out the work. The board chair is responsible for governance and setting policy and is the keeper of the vision and mission. He or she understands and respects (enforces) the role and relationship of the board to the executive director. The executive director implements policy. This is more a tactical role, one of making selected services productive and operating the partnership. Committees implement strategy. They work out the details of recommendations. For example, if the board determines the partnership needs a competitive personnel policy, the committee works out the details for board approval.

Orient Working Groups

This is how one gets from "me" to "we." Having a professionally guided retreat with a primary purpose of learning to work together may be worth considering. Thus the retreat actually has workshops on team building, followed by actual work of the partnership, in teams to determine real commitment then action. This may seem elemental, but more than a few partnership staff reflected on some almost otherworldly initial meetings where screaming and yelling marked the struggle for a piece of the pie. Consider the following five-part orientation strategy from the Halifax-Warren Partnership:

- *Reference.* Build a professional orientation packet. In it include at least your vision, mission, beliefs, goals, and objectives. Also include duties and responsibilities, bylaws or charter, organizational chart, list of key people, and suggested board development, education, and training.
- *Meetings.* Develop a work plan according to what needs to be accomplished on a quarterly, an annual, or an ad hoc basis. Meet when there is something to do, not merely by the calendar. Time wasted at a meeting is a sure way to lose the most productive board members whose most valuable contribution is their time.
- *Education.* At the very least the board should have workshops and training on the strategic process, how to be a board member, and how a nonprofit works. Naturally, how much the member wants to do is an individual choice, but give board members minimum requirements, something material to do. The worst case is to let the new member flounder and to figure the job out for him- or herself.
- *Technical assistance.* Leadership comes to the board with all levels of expertise. There needs to be a common frame of reference. The parent's understanding of evaluation and outcome is much different from that of the bank president. "Peace of mind" is not an outcome. A class or a workshop can help define what the partnership needs for evaluation, analysis, and monitoring.
- *Consultants.* Experts are also a resource to help develop a common frame of reference and definitions that all understand. However, a word of caution on hiring consultants: Think twice. This route is expensive, sometimes with little result. Make sure the fit is right, there is a solid track record of delivering the promised expertise, and a written understanding of deliverables. Take the time, even if you think you don't have it, to check references.

All this is good, but nothing is as effective or motivating as a core of experienced board members setting the example for action and direction while being willing and able to take the new member under their wing. Consider assigning a mentor to new board members. Next, to begin the work of the partnership, the "think tank" should better understand what the community needs.

CONDUCT A NEEDS ASSESSMENT

Resources to Tap

There is so much information, expertise, and especially misconception about needs assessment that even the most resolute can be discouraged. However, we must not be daunted by something that sounds so technical and laborious as to be the special domain of a gifted few. It is as simple as asking, "What do we look like and what do our children need?" "What do we do well and what can we do better?" "What do we have versus what do we need to do the job." All the people who have been through a needs analysis speak of its necessity, and, going through it was not as bad as expected.

Needs assessment is a thoroughly discussed and documented managerial tool. There are entire series of college courses, many institutes, and frequent workshops on the topic. Thus there will be no want of prescribed procedures and experts to follow or assist in a local assessment. What matters is that everyone concerned with the project thoroughly understands specific needs according to the populations the project intends to serve and the resources it has and requires to satisfy those needs. It is a point of departure. If project staff and appropriate decision makers do not understand the environment of demands and ability to satisfy those demands, the project will flounder and eventually fail.

There are several choices to be made. A partnership can do its own assessment, contractors can do it for the partnership, or the partnership can have a combination of both. The best route is collaboration. First, a consultant will bring necessary expertise and, more important, sweat. Second, the partnership will learn from the process, which will be woven into the fabric of service. The local university or community college is a great source of help, usually at the right price. Also, the partnership should check to see who in the area has a proven track record of conducting successful assessment. Remember, no one can understand a partnership's needs and its wherewithal to address them better than the partnership. Proceeding without a needs assessment is traveling in darkness without a lantern.

Be creative with limited resources. Remember to appoint a board member who has been through or is responsible for needs assessment in his or her regular day job. Put that board member in charge of the task force for needs assessment. The Down East Partnership for Children[2] got quite creative with its needs assessment. It developed a corps of "Community Fellows"—a group of trained volunteers who simply wanted to do something for the community. They were trained in leadership for fifteen weeks via the local cooperative extension office. Then they were sent to professional development workshops to develop community development skills. And then they got individual training in necessary specialties such as needs assessment. A core group of these unpaid community fellows are full-time volunteers with a waiting list of individuals ready for training and subsequent task assignment. These people were "hired" just for the asking!

Considering the volumes of what is out there, we mention only a few points that are more relevant to a partnership building effort. Have a basic plan for assessing needs; some call this the methodology. This includes how to collect data, how to analyze it, how to use it, and who the audience will be. Again, utility is the guide; if it is not needed, don't bother with it.

Questions to Address

The World Bank Group suggests that the astute community assessment is designed to answer the following questions:

- *Readiness/political will.* Are the key design assumptions focusing on local organizational capacity and community-based management systems valid for the program and community's preparedness for increased responsibility for management and development and contributions (including resource transfer to the communities)?
- *Priorities.* What are the key priorities of (your) community in terms of focus and particularly those most vulnerable to the particular problem addressed?
- *Organizational infrastructure.* What are the different institutional arrangements possible and their relative performance and feasibility?
- *Resources.* What is the existing state of preparedness of the community for financial and organizational management (adapted from The World Bank Organization Field Guide, see Website: www.worldbank.org/participation/fieldguide.htm)?

Analyze Relevant Data

Include a variety of data collection techniques using existing data, self-generated data, surveys, interviews, focus groups, and direct observation. Also, consider household surveys, service provider surveys, key informant surveys, town meetings, and children's (key stakeholder) focus groups. A quick review of county-level statistics to get an overview of current issues may be a good place to start:

- Child and youth population (by age group);
- Child abuse/neglect rate;

- Children reported as abused/neglected;
- Child immunization rate;
- Children in custody of the Department of Social Services;
- Children on public assistance;
- Children using health departments;
- Children with untreated dental decay;
- Exceptional children;
- High school graduation rate;
- Student dropout rate;
- Infant mortality rate;
- Juvenile arrest rate;
- Low birthweight babies;
- Median family income;
- Population living in poverty;
- SAT scores;
- Teen pregnancy rates;
- Teen birth rate; and
- Unemployment rate.

Analysis of existing data on the county level is a good start even though the needs assessment may be contracted out. But whatever the partnership does, it should not abdicate complete responsibility. A partnership should be hands on. It must continually assess the moving target of its environment, its needs and resources, and especially the profile of those it serves. As with most effective practices, the best advice we have heard, over and over again, is, "Just get going with it." What matters is that a partnership attempt to understand who it is (as a community), what it has versus what it needs, and how to close the difference.

Once a partnership has an understanding of its needs (i.e., a complete picture of its community, who it wants to serve, the resources it has available, and an idea of the people and agencies that need to be involved), the rest of the needs analysis process remains, getting from information to action. Consider the following steps:

- *Define the problem.* Belabor this. The time spent defining what you want to correct is pivotal. From this definition and understanding come your measures, benchmarks, and, the golden goose, proof you are doing something.

- *Define the target population.* Know, intimately, who you intend to serve. Is it an entire age group? Or, is it a specifically profiled segment of a larger population, or a combination of both? The overall aim of the partnership is to define and address the needs of all children. Then address specific needs of specific populations with specialized programs/services and targeted resources as ability and willingness dictate.
- *Define the target area.* The need for targeting cannot be overstated. Once the community knows there is an effort to help with some of its most intractable difficulties, the floodgate of pleas for assistance opens; everyone wants access. You will find your resources, people, money, and time widely scattered and often wasted. Start small in a specific area to figure out what you are doing and most importantly to demonstrate results. You can't do that when you are blown by the wind here and there.
- *Research resources.* Every community has a wealth of programs, services, and infrastructure working on every difficulty identified. Line up what you have counterposed to what is needed to work on the problem in question. A word of caution here: don't entertain action simply because it is easy to do, or popular, or grantable, or what have you. What you fund must address an assessed need and contribute, quantitatively, to a stated goal.

The philosophy of needs assessment is to poke, prod, and investigate the nature of the environment until there is comfort with a core of knowledge that allows a sense of direction and focus. This does not mean the needs assessment is done quickly merely to satisfy the board, a grantor, or a prescription for project development. Nor does it mean that analysis should pursue excruciating detail or illusive (statistical) confidence in numbers. It does mean that a mix of techniques employed by staff and perhaps a team of academicians from the local community college should be used to develop a narrative of mutually agreed needs, a profile of target populations and focus area, appropriate programming suggestions, and benchmark standards to begin and guide the work. Needs assessment is not so much a vital part of making real differences in the community as it is a part of "building" real bricks-and-mortar solutions to maddening problems that took decades to manifest. While a well-structured performance-based delivery system cannot eradicate a problem, it remains a matter of essential importance to the community in its effort to produce viable citizens.

STATE VISION, MISSION, GOALS, AND OBJECTIVES

We recommend that the newly formed partnership go through a professionally facilitated retreat to work on vision and mission, organize itself, and dive into initial action. Again, there are any number of consultants and agencies capable of helping. But rather than rehash the strategic planning process, we suggest that the visioning retreat is a preferred time to consider a hierarchy of service characteristics, the reason being that an effective vision needs to be rooted in the reality and work of delivering effective services. We are talking about project stability, accessibility, and quality.

Stability

This means to establish permanent funding. Ideally the partnership needs to seek and get long-term funding service by service. Realistically, services will be sustained by a combination of funding streams, not the least of which is via the local development effort. A partnership should avoid the temptation to immediately jump into serving clients. A detailed understanding of monies helps prioritize what is done. It lets the partnership say no to projects; and the partnership will have to say no to many a good idea. It is better to say a kindly, justified "no" up front than, after spending a few years and a good bit of money and a chunk of hard-earned reputation, realizing the service cannot produce. This is where accountability begins.

Accessibility

Services have to reach those who need them. This means the service goes to the target group or the target client can come to the service, usually both. Many a good idea has failed for lack of transportation. Sometimes there is an enticement to connect the needy to the service. New parents need parenting skills, but how do we get the parents to training? One partnership has a family night out where, before training is offered, all who come know they will have fun, food, facts, and child care. The event responds to all objections the at-risk parent may have for getting necessary training. This accessibility is a product of a concerted effort of getting the word out and an intense networking effort. No single method of communication is spared in connecting with the target population. The event itself is an opportunity for exposure, referral, and networking. Everyone is made aware of what the partnership is doing; everyone, especially those served, is compelled to be a salesperson for the work. A partnership must make sure its vision is built on the vital need for accessibility.

Quality

Because there are so many definitions, and so many of them misleading, we need common ground. Quality for the partnership is experience and a history of service that change lives for the better. The reason quality is last in the hierarchy of stability accessibility, and quality is not to diminish its importance but to make sure it does not overwhelm the other priorities. The streets are littered with quality local projects that just did not work out. With quality anchoring the hierarchy of program characteristics, it defines productive service, stability, and accessibility. Quality then is defined in terms of stability and accessibility instead of overwhelming project stability and accessibility, which adds materially to the strength if not the very existence of the project—that way they work together, rather than being exclusionary. Quality also means that the partnership is constantly asking, "Are you getting what you paid for?" Constantly knowing what is working and what is not is serious business. If there is no tangible outcome, effort has to be redirected toward productivity or abandoned.

The Strategic Process

As with every recommended action in the planning phase, the danger is that strategic planning is not done with appropriate intensity and thought or not done at all. A partnership must spend time on the strategic process, defining what it is and what it would like to become. There are many good examples of appropriate visions and subsequent missions, goals, and objectives (see, e.g., Exhibit 4.4). The vision, distilled from a tough strategic planning process, communally agreed and inspiring, is well worth the effort and really imbues everything else that is done. It actually defines the successful endeavor. Via the vision/mission, success is defined before resources are committed. A sense of fairness and values permeates. Every action reflects a systematic construction, a kind of energizing theme flows through every aspect of the project. For example, every global initiative in a successful partnership is based on a vision-inspired need. Need helps determine service choices. And projects/services chosen must materially contribute to the vision. Likewise, the vision motivates. For example, it is a sense of vision that drives the pervasive, persistent work to develop funding streams. Staff and providers reflect the vision. There is a natural sincerity that exudes from people involved in meaningful, even noble work.

OUTLINE IMPACT ANALYSIS AND PROCESS EVALUATION PLAN

Of all the tasks necessary to grow the well-working, established service delivery system, the most productive, pound for pound of effort expended is evaluation. It is also frequently the first abandoned. For clarity, we differentiate "evaluation" and "analysis." Evaluation determines how well a partnership functions on a daily basis. Analysis determines results. The partnership needs both.

Evaluation: Ensuring Accountability

The purpose of evaluation is to make sure the right thing is done the right way; it is an action tool. Therefore, an evaluation plan must be persistent, matched to the need/maturity of the project, and, importantly, it must assign responsibility to ensure accountability. An evaluation/analysis is not worth beginning unless its purpose is to define goal-oriented action for a specific entity (preferably a specific person) and a target time for completion. Note also this is not meant to be a "Big Brother" machine for oppressive demands. It is a mutually agreed upon process to collectively move resources and people to a common result. The philosophy of evaluation and analysis is constructive, not a mechanism to find fault and punish: There are no problems, only opportunities for improvement. Read the previous sentence again and think about it. Evaluation and analysis are a coach's tools to keep the team sharp on a daily basis and productive for the long term.

One of the best descriptions of the local evaluation effort comes from the Smart Start Website (*www.smartstart-nc.org/information/publications.htm*); to order Tool Kit from North Carolina Partnership for Children staff). Here is the gist of it:

> Evaluation indicates whether individual activities are making a difference in the lives of children and families. Information that is gathered from any evaluation determines the worth of an activity. It is critical that all activities are tied to the mission, vision, and goals of the organization. Activities are clearly defined by set goals, objectives, measurable outcomes (quantitative and qualitative) and strategies. Determining the target population and required staffing and funding streams are key working components of the activity. These help local partnerships determine whether to continue, improve, or discontinue the activity (North Carolina Partnership for Children).
>
> - *Evaluation is a journey, not a destination.* Begin evaluation *before* activities start.
> - *Evaluation is a system by which management processes and procedures improve*. The evaluation effort makes partners of all necessary stakeholders.
> - *Evaluation is both quantitative and qualitative.* Success is by the numbers and by feedback from those getting the services.
> - *Evaluation is objective.* Evaluation must be objective to be valid; this is neither cheap nor easy, but it is vital.
> - *Evaluation is realistic.* Goals are a moving target; evaluation must be flexible and ingrained into the organization to move with goals, objectives, and the environment as they evolve with the maturing organization.

Essentially, evaluation is accountability. As we construct organizations that have an impact on the lives of children and families, it is imperative that measurable, quantitative, and qualitative changes have occurred as a result of the funded activity (North Carolina Partnership for Children).

Evaluation is dynamic and fluid as program improvements are made, evaluation adapts to assess change and growth. Let's take a close look at a well-working evaluation program at the community level. The Down East Partnership for Children has four key components in its evaluation process:

- *Data.* The collection, analysis, and reporting of results for program activities. Each funded program must provide program services designed to move the partnership toward achieving its vision, mission, and goals.
- *Performance-based programming.* The assessment of a program to determine if it is doing what it says it is going to do and meeting its outcomes. Annually, each funded program must write individual program outcomes and establish an evaluation plan. These outcomes must be client focused and program specific and must clearly link to the partnership's five-year benchmarks and objectives.
- *Long-term goal attainment.* The assessment of a program or organization to determine if it is meeting its long-term benchmarks and objectives. Quarterly, each funded program must collect and report results of its program activities.
- *Flexibility.* The assessment of a program or organization to determine if it is moving toward achieving its vision, mission, and goals. Annually, objectives and benchmarks are reviewed for appropriateness and to determine if the activities and outcomes of individual programs are moving the partnership toward the vision. Every five years the partnership reassesses its vision, mission, and goals and (re)establishes objectives and benchmarks.

Integrating Evaluations Into Routine Objectives

It is one thing to understand what makes a good evaluation; it is entirely another thing to make it work. For that, a local collaborative should consider the following mechanics of weaving evaluation into the fabric of daily operation.

- *Reporting.* Every program is required to report progress on a regular basis (i.e., monthly or quarterly). Each program is discussed in detail; progress from the last quarter is noted. Any anomalies or opportunities for improvement are noted to project staff at the earliest convenience.
- *Evaluation coordinator.* The evaluation coordinator ensures that evaluation is done properly. Here is the in-house technical assistance to make sure everyone knows what must be done and that it is reported. This person is also responsible for most of the evaluation meetings.
- *The quarterly meeting.* This meeting is conducted and attended by partnership staff. Reports and observations from the field are discussed to determine successes and problems. Of course, successes are perpetuated,

praised, and proliferated via the network of key stakeholders. The lessons learned are likewise recommended to all partnership players.

- *Program operations meeting.* This is a required quarterly meeting for service providers. Here they tell their own stories of how they are contributing to overall success. In turn, staff brief them on general information such as pertinent legislative action and current topics of interest. This is also an opportunity for training on, for example, how to write an objective, and perhaps there are team-building exercises also. Every minute of the meeting is well paced, organized, and productive by intention; this sends a powerful message to providers: "The partnership means business. Yes, we can have a lot of fun doing good things; but, produce or pack your bags."
- *The committee review.* Annually, board members review the annual reports of each service, adding another level of expertise and guidance to overall purposes.
- *Community public relations.* Every avenue for wide communication of successes is employed. The Down East Partnership uses the foregoing suggestions and newsletters, the web, and town meetings to get the word out.

There are also other noteworthy characteristics of good process evaluation. There are a series of targeted site visits. In particular, each provider can expect fiscal, programmatic, and evaluation visits from local staff. It is important to distinguish the difference and appropriately emphasize performance (evaluation) as separate from compliance (fiscal) issues. Furthermore, staff continually hone themselves on evaluation expertise and skill via retreats, two a year. One is a daylong affair at the central office; the other is an off-site, overnight retreat with more global purpose. Although there is physically a lot of pure work done, there is always an air of fun. Whenever there is a gathering, whether it is a brown-bag lunch and lecture or a board meeting, there are food, fun, facts, and child care. Everyone expects to work and enjoy!

Another key to program and process improvement is that the partnership service providers are used to seeing partnership staff on-site: participating, teaching, advising, discussing, leading. That is, partnership staff are there and they know what to do; they are a constant, able, and welcome presence. They lead by being capable, involved, and especially present. More than that, no staffer ever asks a provider to do anything the staffer is not willing nor able to do. This exhibits itself in several ways. Take, for example, program monitoring. While programs are intensely monitored, the partnership monitors itself even more closely. The local partnership subjects itself to two types of quarterly meetings. They analyze the overall progress to goals. They meet to work out internal operating procedures. Monthly, they have a brown-bag luncheon with a team-building purpose. There is regularly scheduled training on anything of significance and the twice-yearly retreats, all devoted to the continual process of becoming better.

Define Measure(s) of Success

Another key to being productive is a real understanding of common terms and clear definitions of where the partnership wants to go and how it will know when it gets there. There is no substitute for a clearly stated goal, subsequent objectives, and the mechanism to ensure success. Of the many examples, the best are the ones the partnership defines for its projects. Exhibit 4.5 is adapted from the Smart Start Website which takes example from the successes of the Down East Partnership for Children.

Notice how so little is left to chance. The who, what, when, where are all answered. The how then becomes much simpler, not easy, but simpler. Benchmarking is also a very practical effective practice.

Establish Benchmarks/Targets

This brings us to benchmarking, a highly recommended tool. It is the logical extension from goals and objectives which sometimes are too loosely defined and thus become unrealistic to attain, then result in poor performance or worse. But if we take the time to benchmark (i.e., establish specific, realistic intermediate targets), an objective has a real measuring stick. Sometimes the benchmark is simply a comparison to another, similar program's measure. Sometimes it is a realistic guess, a challenge for what your program must do.

First and foremost, such a comparison is motivating; there is nothing like competing against the numbers, against other programs. Needs are defined. Objectives are organized. Problems are discovered, accurately defined, and answered. Trouble is noted before it becomes disaster, when something can be done about it. People see and feel movement to stated purposes. There is evidence that lives are improving. Benchmarking, or targeting one's effort, is an important managerial tool that makes a strategic plan an organic document that grows as the partnership grows. This then is the hallmark of a benchmark; it is flexible, made to be adjusted. The elegance of having a benchmark is that it is clear when missed, which is often, especially when exuberant wishes face reality.

Definitions and Examples

A helpful document is the Government Performance Reporting Act's (GPRA) *Primer on Performance Measurement* (Office of Management and Budget, 1996). It should be mandatory reading. If the partnership plans to work with federal funds, and it will, the partnership must comply with the GPRA. On the positive side, the document is well written and is an excellent point of departure when a partnership works toward a common understanding of terms it will use to conduct business.

Evaluation really depends on leadership. Evaluation can be a powerful tool for service delivery or it can be a great bother, just another thing to be done and with no time to do it. The evaluation program really depends on the involvement of the people at the top, and to be clear, the board must be materially involved in being a performance-oriented operation. If the program director and board thrive on living, real-time data and reports that really tell a story, if they make meaningful decisions based on those reports, if people can see that statistics are used to strengthen and perpetuate a program, and, yes, to cancel nonperforming experiments, self-assessment, process evaluation, and outcome analysis will become part of the fabric of success.

Ideally, evaluation is layered, depending on the life-cycle phase and strategic purpose. Essentially, planning requires needs assessment and an evaluation plan. Operation focuses on process; it must be efficient. Therefore, processes need to evolve under daily scrutiny that determines if output is effective and has economized input. Finally, expansion requires outcome statistics and a reassessment of need. Overall strategy focuses on operation and mission accomplishment based largely on the numbers if it is to make a difference in community well-being. Likewise, mission accomplishment demands that today's effort leads inexorably to the betterment of the community by bettering the individual.

CREATE RESOURCE DEVELOPMENT AND FINANCIAL MANAGEMENT PLANS

Here, we are talking about money, the life blood of the partnership. Yes, there is a range of resources, material and human, that needs to be developed as well, but that steady stream of dollars is what the partnership is after. An, for further clarity, developing resources is different from the marketing plan that follows. But, as with each of these action steps in every phase of building the local partnership, they are interconnected. Resource development is based on many aspects. This section deals with the leadership and organization of resource development as well as some of the structural details for managing it, including the development campaign, board structure, and accounting systems. Remember, the partnership is still in the planning stage; it is only getting things set up. Each phase of the life cycle has a different take on resource development. Failure to plan this activity well has caused the demise of more than a few local endeavors.

Develop a Plan for Permanent Funding

The partnership executive directors we interviewed commented that developing a strategy for funding initially took a back seat to the torrent of start-up work, but they all wished the development plan was one of the early, most material investments of time. Partnerships are generally started by a person with a vision for an idea. This person is good with people skills, collaborating, and networking. Unfortunately, there can be a critical flaw with this early exuberance: Longevity is in the details of operation, not necessarily in the glow of an inspired idea. Most nonprofits that fail, fail within the first year or two because there is little or no accurate, appropriate, sanctioned record of the fiscal story. There is no fraud, just no proper record, and then no program. The money carelessly chases the idea, then is gone, sometimes in a matter of months. The answer to this bear trap is the dual development of strategy and procedure, not one to the exclusion of the other but both in tandem. We will consider leadership first.

The strategy of the board, especially the development committee (or task force), has to be "grown" through orientation and training. The partnership's board members may regularly change and come to the board with all levels of expertise, thus your board has to be "grown" through orientation and training. The message during orientation is that board members are responsible for setting and approving policy and leading development by example. Their example is that they contribute time and money to the work. Training is largely skills development. For example, board members should get instruction on how to read and interpret a financial report, what a budget represents, and the audit process with emphasis on the role of the board.

Strategic Planning for Funding. The Forsyth Early Childhood Partnership, Winston-Salem, North Carolina,[3] having just made grants for the first three years of its existence, did not have a plan for resource development or an overall plan for organization and development. Forsyth knew something was not right and approached a local foundation for advice. The answer was expensive, but it worked. Forsyth needed a development officer. The problem was that the successful ones command six-figure salaries and are tough to find. With help and funds from the foundation, Forsyth contracted with a consultant for six months to get a development program going. In its initial work to begin a development strategy, the partnership asked for six deliverables from its consultant:

- *Donor database.* The partnership needed an organized donor Rolodex of agencies and people that would be the envy of a Washington lobbyist.
- *Annual campaign.* Solicitation and giving are continual and need to be goaded by a series of mechanisms from presentations to Internet giving, which builds to an annual event, then starts all over again.
- *Granting.* The partnership wanted the consultant to submit at least two grants per month of the six-month contract in order to have grant funding in the pipeline and a granting process started. By the next year, the

partnership had developed a plan for grants to be submitted and matched to program needs and priorities.

- *Development committee organization and training.* The board as a whole and the development committee specifically need to be organized and "grown" with training and actual development activity to be competent fund developers.
- *Support.* The coherent case for giving to the partnership had to be documented. That case was the performance evidence from an evaluation and analysis program that made the argument that the partnership "pays," it does not cost.
- *Training.* The partnership needed a skilled in-house development person to carry on the process of hammering out the funding streams.

Organizing the Project to Focus on Funding. The Forsyth Partnership ended up with much more because it worked on what a development strategy should be. Even soft money (donations, grants, aid, fees, cost sharing) can be considered an essential funding stream when it is considered within the larger financial picture. Resource development is really programming development. Every aspect of the partnership is employed in the money development effort. And "every" is not an exaggeration. Let us take the partnership by its major elements and see how that is done:

- *The board.* The board sets strategy and leads by example. The Forsyth Partnership has created a canned presentation, complete with slides, that any member can give at any time to just about any group that needs to have a speaker or hear about the partnership. Also, each member is expected to donate money.
- *The development committee.* This committee designs the overall effort, sets goals for board approval, and is intensely involved in the campaign.
- *Executive director.* The lead staffer is also the lead developer. He or she is busy organizing the campaign, facilitating events, training, on the phone and Internet, and keeping partnership performance public.
- *Staff.* Every staffer is a salesperson for the effort. Staff members are selected because they are passionate about the work and exude the vision and mission.
- *Service providers.* Every contracted service is imbued with the vision and mission and the need to be performance based. It is clear that performance is the direct link to funding.
- *Clients.* Even those served become champions for the partnership. Their needs are not only taken care of during the process of getting services,

they are made to understand what the partnership means and does. The collective goodwill of satisfied service recipients throughout the community is immeasurable.

- *Facilities*. Even the facilities are a selling tool! When one enters the Down East Partnership for Children, he or she is presented with a professional reception and an engaging display of printed materials. The walls are tastefully covered with children's art and inspirational thoughts. Someone has even taken the time to close the stairwell balusters with plastic sheeting to keep them child safe. The building "says," "Welcome, come with me, be with me, help me be part of something good happening."

The Campaign Mentality for Funding. Then there is the campaign mentality. There are so many ways to give, whether it be a dollar or a fortune, that, with the message of progress in the community, most people are compelled to do so. Partnerships should consider putting a donors page on their Websites. A good idea is to outline what each level of giving does for the community. Make a denomination small enough for any contributor and large enough to be a challenge. There is a return on even a $20 investment; the implication is that anyone can give and be part of something special. The Forsyth Partnership's campaign has five elements that seek to "help people think differently, let them know who and where the partnership is, and create some passion."

- *The annual banquet.* This is a celebration of collective accomplishment and awards with the emphasis on food and fun.
- *Conferences.* Noted professionals teach and inform on any relevant topic (e.g., kindergarten readiness).
- *Brown-bag lunch.* Nationally noted experts and authors come to these well-attended noontime affairs. They are not only educational and fun, they accomplish business outreach and build community "assets." Lunch is free if they come. Rarely does a "free lunch" have such a handsome return.
- *Business outreach.* This is a minicampaign in itself. The partnership targets businesses in an effort to educate management and employees on the real benefits of family-friendly practices, such as work-life benefits and flex time. Partnership staff consult at the business, and there is an annual luncheon, highlighting success testimonials. There are presentations, an awards ceremony, and a "Toil for Tots" program in which businesses sanction employee time for volunteer work with children.
- *Formal solicitation.* This is full-scale, multifaceted, direct request for dollars which employs the phone and mail.

Developing Formal Giving. The formal giving aspect needs elaboration. First, it cannot be mounted until the partnership proves money is being well spent. A partnership should not even think of asking for large donations until it has a record of performance based on fiscal discipline and procedures, intense project monitoring, and tight operations. Here is where the partnership wants to be a mirror of a foundation, very businesslike, very intent on earning monetary support. With documented efficiency and effectiveness in place, the partnership can put its tools for the "give" in action:

- *The "package."* Send a solicitation package of materials to appropriate potential donors, corporate and private, from the Rolodex. This is done about two weeks in advance of the visit. There is also a mass mailing of a brochure to solicit the smaller donation.
- *The visit.* The purpose here is direct. Usually a board member, handpicked for the donor, and the executive director tell the host about the partnership, request suggestions on how the partnership can help, and suggest how an appropriately large gift from the donor can help the partnership and community.
- *The follow-up.* Donors are always informed of the progress of their contribution because there will be a next time.

This large thrust for money is not random. Every source of dollars is first "critically" examined in relation to the vision, mission, and goals, as well as in relation to the ability to provide quality services to meet the needs of the community. As painful as it may be, if a certain pot of money has strings or requirements that do not contribute to stated purposes, it is not sought or is even turned down if offered. Leadership and fiscal discipline require independence. This is an important distinction in fund development. Merely going for available funds by, for example, writing a proposal that parrots the grantor's wishes will not assist in achieving the partnership's mission. Producing funding streams that contribute to overall, mutually agreed purposes will. These ends then stand a better chance of being effective (measurable), which then provides further justification for additional funding. But the fact remains, even pots of money with strings can adjust those requirements to be part of the partnership's success. The trick is for the partnership to know who it is, to know what it wants, and to have a plan for getting there; many will want to follow.

Establish Fiscal Procedures and a Budget

There are two aspects to budgeting for the partnership: financial policy and procedures and accounting. The former is how money is handled by staff and the latter can be considered the chief financial officer functions. This is a simple statement of a detailed and vital endeavor for the partnership. Brevity here is meant only to get the partnership functioning immediately on what will be a major and continuous expenditure of time and effort. The main concern is having staff knowledgeable in standard accounting and budgetary procedures and the fiscal processes demanded by the nature of a public nonprofit corporation. The Smart Start Website overview of budgeting quotes Genevieve Megginson from the Chatham Partnership for Children,[4] who says it best: "The key to fiscal success . . . is creating a record of information that tells a good story. A good story conveys all pertinent information in a logical, easy-to-understand manner, has continuity and consistency of plot; and leads to a logical conclusion."

Fiscal Standard Operating Procedures

Let us start with standard operating procedures. Exhibit 4.6 presents a list of items to be addressed in specific financial policy and procedures; the suggested items, developed over time by the Chatham County Partnership for Children,2 are for illustration only. These are the fiscal policies and procedures that work for the Chatham Partnership. Any partnership's list should be similar yet may reflect a few different topics the particular partnership feels should be covered by the formality of a documented statement and outlining of process. These fiscal regulations should address internal and external stakeholders. There should be a specific policy for each major area requiring fiscal discipline and clarity (see Exhibit 4.7 for a sample policy/procedure document). Remember, there has never been and never will be a set of rules that cover every contingency confronted in the hurly-burly of getting the job done. The written policy should, therefore, be simple; outline what is expected, what needs to be done, and who is to do it. Above all, staff must understand what fiscal discipline is and exercise it correctly and diligently whether or not there is a "rule" covering the question at hand.

Accounting: The Chief Financial Officer's Duties

Many people will be interested in the partnership's operational financial/fiscal discipline. The sooner each level of authority, including the board, the chief financial officer (CFO) (which can be the executive director), and the staff understand their duties and responsibilities, the better. Simply put, the partnership is looking to establish internal controls with third-party approval of expenditures. For example, the service provider makes the request, the chief executive officer (CEO) approves it, and the CFO writes the check. In other words, the board does not have to approve every expenditure. The board sets policy that is within its oversight responsibility. Still, the key person to fiscal quietude and a better night's sleep is the CFO. One of the first and most important duties of the board is to recruit a well-qualified person with accounting experience, preferably a certified public accountant. The board will want to discuss and document a detailed job description (see Exhibit 4.8 for an example) to guide the hiring process.

Automation for Finances

A partnership should not skimp, though it may be tempted, on its automation. This includes hardware, software, and training. There are many quality software packages available for nonprofits. There are also recommended modules to the basic software package: Accounts Payable, Bank Reconciliation, Budgeting, General Ledger, and Cash Receipts.

Establish Lines and Modes of Communication for Project Fiscal Matters

Having tight fiscal control and accounting procedures by the book is not enough. Once set up, the toughest part of the fiscal/accounting job is not done. Take the next logical step and make sure people know the good story the partnership has documented. Consider the following suggestions for fiscal reporting:

- *Grant reporting.* These are summary reports on progress/performance for the partnership's grantors.
- *Organizational reports.* These are essentially for the board, the finance committee, and for IRS requirements pertinent to tax-exempt status.
- *Reports on private funds.* These reports are for major private donors such as State Employees Combined Campaign, for example.
- *Financial report.* We mention the financial report here as it fills so many purposes, not the least of which is as a marketing tool in an annual report (see Exhibit 4.9 for a sample list of financial statement categories).

Monthly reporting is recommended to ensure that expenditures are allowable, allocable, and fundable using the terminology of federal funding. When everyone is informed, especially about how the money is performing in the community, the partnership just seems to function better, and in fact is.

The vital importance of financial stewardship via skilled leadership and disciplined fiscal processes cannot be overstated. The planning project team must prioritize its allocation of time to designing accountability systems that are part of the fabric of the operation. Internal, external, corporate and noncorporate partnership stakeholders, as well as clients, must know that public funds do have a return on investment. Early on, the partnership needs to consult standard accounting and operational practices and necessary technical assistance when designing financial systems. An oversight in planning the proper financial systems will at least disrupt the delivery of services and has the potential to do irreparable harm to the effort.

Getting the Most Money for the Effort

The partnership's effort needs to maximize funding streams (Mitchell, Stoney, & Ditcher, 2001). Exhibit 4.10 lists possible sources of funding for local partnerships. Any and every formal source of funding should be pursued to augment the solicitation of the community at large for donations (Mitchell et al., 2001). The partnership needs to coordinate funds to build capacity. Its service plan targets a specific population for aid and services, funds the professional development of staff and service providers, builds organizational production capacity, and contracts performance-based services. Funding is essential to that process. It is essential that the partnership develop new streams via granting, taxing, and fee options, and, of course, charitable giving, which includes estate planning. Finally, the partnership should invite the large potential of in-kind support via volunteerism and donated resources. This then becomes a major bulwark of the healthy partnership. The partnership should consider all these aspects of the comprehensive development effort, start small, be practical and realistic, and grow.

DEVELOP A MARKETING COLLABORATION PLAN FOR ESSENTIAL SUPPORT AND PARTNERSHIPS

People need to know who the partnership is, what it does, how it does it, how they can participate, and where partnership staff can be reached before the partnership can expect them to help. This strikes at the core purpose of a local partnership: to assemble and leverage resources, especially the human kind. And with the people enlisted, the partnership wants their most valuable gift: time. The Smart Start Tool Kit on Planning observes: "To successfully leverage [these] existing resources, your Partnership must ensure that institutions from these sectors (public, private, private non-profit) participate fully in the development and implementation of your strategic plan, and that together they help the entire community embrace the needs of children and families as an action priority."

The Tool Kit also observes that "broad-based participation is a critical first step . . . members and staff must learn how to share information, vision, resources, power, and accountability . . ." (as mentioned earlier, the Tool Kit can be ordered from North Carolina Partnership for Children staff at *www.smartstart-nc.org/information/publications.htm*). Marketing the partnership is essentially a plan for inclusion and collaboration; people have to be included in productive ways and they need to be taught how to collaborate before they can be full partners. This is deceptively simple but not easy.

Describe the Collaboration

It is good to review what makes collaboration work. There are important factors for defining characteristics and principals of the successful collaborative effort. As described by Mattessich and Monsey (undated) in their research, the Principles of Collaboration are:

- *Commitment and participation.* Key people agree to participate, commit their resources, and are involved in the design process.
- *Process of collaboration.* These key participants understand and respect the ongoing process of change and are well educated on the issues which result in agreement regarding the problems to be addressed.
- *Legitimacy.* The collaboration is open and has demonstrated successes for all to see.
- *Planning.* Planning is sequential where consensus is periodically reaffirmed.
- *Meetings.* Meetings are essential, thus have to be productive and may have to be facilitated by a third party.

These descriptors of the successful collaboration were observed in every well-working partnership we visited. Mattessich and Monsey (undated) further their description of the healthy collaboration by observing key factors. The following is an adaptation of their summary:

- *Environment.* There is a history of successful collaboration in the community where the collaborative body is seen as a leader and the political/social climate is favorable to the purposes of the partnership.
- *Membership characteristics.* Members respect, understand, and trust each other. There is appropriate representation of stakeholders who demonstrate a willingness to compromise and who see collaboration as beneficial. Leadership is skilled and competent if not, on occasion, inspirational.
- *Process/structure.* Each member has a stake in the successful outcome. The process is marked by layered decision making, flexibility, clear roles and policy directives, and adaptability.
- *Communication.* The flow of information is open and frequent, formal and informal.
- *Purpose.* Goals and objectives are realistic yet challenging. There is shared vision and unique purpose.
- *Resources.* There is a financial base to support ideas.

Notice how each of the action steps in this planning phase weave together. While each step can be described as distinct, one actually moves seamlessly to the other, and most times, all work simultaneously and synchronously. Note also that there is no escape from the need for money and how the push for it pervades all work. The trick is not to let the concern overwhelm, or exclude other, essential work and there is none more basic than cementing one's partners.

Outline the Partnering Process

Research into and questioning regarding this topic will reveal plenty of advice on how to get the local group of "movers and shakers" together. We found a good point of departure for bringing together the right people is the ideas suggested by the Child Care Resource and Referral (CCR&R) service offered at the partnerships we visited. The following is adapted from Chapter 8 of the *CCR&R Planning and Startup Manual*[5]:

- *Identify key players.* Identify who in the community can help the partnership get its message out (advisory committee, funders, local partnership, professional fund raisers, other nonprofit directors, media, parents) and how they can help.
- *Make contacts.* Get out and about. Attend individual meetings and business breakfasts, speak to groups, and join local professional and business groups (such as the Chamber of Commerce) and statewide groups.
- *Spread the message.* Talk about the partnership's role and services at provider training events. Communicate in every medium, spoken, written, and electronic.
- *Develop relationships.* Get to know (and have them get to know you) the local media, radio, and television.
- *Share data.* Wherever you go, have plenty of communication ammunition that relays essential messages. A good strategy is to have a range of informational material from the one-page fact sheet to complete descriptive reports, each tailored to any audience of opportunity. And do not forget to build a Website as soon as possible.

Child-care professionals point out an important marketing target, the service providers. When a partnership is initially focused on getting its key stakeholders together, the people on whom it will depend for success are easy to overlook. The partnership should prepare, as they suggest, for a relationship with its providers with training, recruitment, and policies and procedures for working with them.

Involve Key Stakeholders: Corporate and Noncorporate, Internal and External Clients

The individuals who are successfully marketing and partnering should think about the various client groups they represent. Their marketing plans call together all groups and people who may be affected. Instead of immediately jumping into what everyone was "supposed" to do, begin with general information and the offer of support. Generally, talk about possibilities, how things could work, roles and duties, and, most important, set expectations. In other words, begin the collaboration with a spirit of sharing and inclusion. The partnership's stakeholders are internal and external, corporate and noncorporate, public, private for profit and nonprofit, and community leaders. Contemplate and value them all.

Internal Clients. Regard staff. They are some of the first people the partnership needs to cultivate, from recruitment to retirement.

Noncorporate/Agency Clients. The partnership's external key players may be considered all those agencies that help the partnership deliver its key services (more on that to follow). Here the partnership would have, for example, the Department of Social Services, the local Board of Education, criminal justice professionals, and the Health Department. Network by putting a representative from each on the partnership's board. Make sure they understand what constitutes conflict of interest and how to handle it to avoid the possibility of that problem. Connect by channeling resources to mutually beneficial services, and deliver the overt message of collaboration by demonstrating that the partnership aims to further mutual goals and objectives. These are largely public and private nonprofit agencies including a real champion of the neighborhood, the faith community.

Corporate Clients. These people are distinguished as a group as they are not direct service providers but they do bring monetary, technical, and in-kind expertise to the table. Think of this group by sector, including banks, pharmaceutical companies, grocery chains, communications, and utilities, for example.

The Community/The Client. Consider target areas and populations. Have a campaign of outreach to children, families, and the community. The Down East Partnership has been known to go door-to-door with flyers and brochures in targeted neighborhoods.

When so many diverse people get together there is conflict of interest, not the fraudulent type, just differing perspectives on the world of the partnership and how to proceed. The partnership must expect it. It must work to ameliorate the result from the outset. First of all, everyone has to know that business is conducted fairly and there is equitable treatment of all. Get input from all parties. Focus on performance; do not focus on personalities. All services must have a return on investment; thus even "friends" of the partnership must produce measurable results. And nothing focuses energies more than a clear bead on their vision and mission. A noble purpose raises perspectives above personalities and ulterior motives.

What is most helpful is to have key players hash out and agree on stated values and document them in a Code of Conduct and a Statement of Ethics. Finally, the partnership must make sure there is a written policy on conflict of interest. Make sure board members know to recuse themselves from business that may be conflictual. The partnership must be aware that people differ passionately about their public duty and help them deal constructively with it early in the endeavor and get on with the business of building.

What we are discussing is the coming together of resources to create value via leverage. It is the process of partnering, sharing resources, accepting accountability and responsibility, and sharing authority. It is done via mutual trust, respect, and understanding among a necessary cross-section of community leaders and service providers. The process has to be marked by frequent and open communication. The value created is the manifestation of the well-oiled, communal organization delivering specific services to those who can benefit most from them.

DEVELOP A LONG-RANGE PLAN FOR ESSENTIAL SERVICES

Here we are talking about strategy, what the partnership wants to achieve and how it intends to get there. Basically, it is taking what the partnership knows and making a strategy that leads to the specific actions necessary to make it happen. Again, the partnership will find a wealth of resources and consultants on the process of strategy. Thus, in keeping with the practical theme of this volume, we mention some of the more helpful practices found in the field. It is good to begin thoughts on strategic planning by reiterating a point: The process of strategy, which begins with visioning, is continuous. Still, it has a distinctness and specific purpose depending on the phase of development and the maturity of the partnership. In this initial planning phase, the partnership states its vision, mission, goals, and beliefs. During the operational phase, which is discussed in Chapter 5, the concern is performanc, "Is the partnership achieving what it said it would?" Finally, when the partnership expands, it reassesses everything again with the aim of closing the service-to-needs gap.

Developing and adjusting strategy is a process that never stops. In fact, each executive director commented similarly that strategy is very much an "organic, living, breathing thing," meaning it is fluid and evolving as the people, politics, environment, and landscape with which the partnership must contend inevitably change. Aside from going through the laborious and necessary process of deciding who and what the partnership wishes to be, an inordinate amount of time must be spent arguing definitions.

Define Basic Terms

When considering strategy, partnership staff's first suggestion is to decide on the meaning of the terms of the business of building a local partnership (for a helpful elaboration of key terms, see Exhibit 4.11). This is important work because more than a few planning bodies get quite distracted, going on and on about what a goal is and how it is different from an objective, for example. Do this early on because the partnership will revisit the need for common understanding of terms again and again when board members rotate, when services are contracted, and when staff come on board. The partnership just does not need to have the same discussions every time there is a personnel or service change.

Detail the Planning Process: Short, Mid-Range, and Long-Term Objectives

If the partnership can afford it, it should hire a skilled strategic planning consultant. The partnership must make sure it is specific about what it expects from the services offered. All the standard cautions of selecting a consultant should be employed. Again, if the partnership can afford it, it should arrange the service at appropriate intervals, say every other year for five years, to make sure the process is embedded in operations and that it reflects the partnership's inevitable growth. This way the consultant has more than a passing interest in an initial contract for help with the partnership's strategic planning. An effective mechanism is a planning retreat. Be aware as well that strategic planning in the public sector is different in kind and character from strategic planning in the private sector. Hire a person who knows this. The local university is a good place to begin the search. The partnership may also contact other local partnerships in its state for names.

The initial retreat needs to settle vision, mission, goals, objectives, beliefs, and program philosophy. Have a good understanding and necessarily brief discussion on essential definitions such as needs, benchmarks, measures, and outcomes. Besides a common strategic planning lexicon, have for the planning process short-term goals (one year), mid-range goals (three to five years), and long-term goals (five plus years). As was observed, the "trick" is to nurture people. This especially means the board, whose members must "walk the talk" of organizational purpose. This begins with asking the basic questions inherent in the visioning/strategy process. The partnership embarks on this journey with a passionate, inspired, intelligent leader. That initial spark must translate, in turn, to capable board members, staff, and service providers. This is key. Note also that it takes time and patience.

Plan for Performance

It is inevitable that the partnership will apply for and receive federal funds whether it be directly or via the state's pass-through agency. Thus the partnership must be ready to comply with the GPRA (Office of Management and Budget, 1996). The GPRA (5 U.S.C., adding § 306, Public Law 103-62) simply formalizes the business sense of getting a return on an investment. Actually, the printed material is quite helpful as it is chock full of examples and practical advice. It is useful to understand the federal definition of terms so that they can be considered as the partnership plans (adapted from Management Concepts, 2001):

- *Strategic plan.* An agency's plan for achieving its general goals over a period of five or more years. GPRA requires that agencies consult their stakeholders when developing their strategic plan. For a federal grant program, stakeholders could include partners, potential applicants/recipients, beneficiaries, cooperating agencies, members of Congress, contractors, and the public, among others.
- *Performance plan.* An agency's plan for one fiscal year which includes measurable goals to specify how it will progress toward the general objectives outlined in the strategic plan. Required by GPRA.
- *Performance monitoring plan.* A detailed plan for managing the collection of data to monitor performance. It identifies the indicators to be tracked; specifies the source, method of collection, and collection schedule for each piece of datum required, and assigns responsibility for collection to a specific office, team, or individual. This is not required by GPRA, but generally considered necessary for adequate stewardship of federal funds. Agencies employ such plans to keep track of recipients' progress and results.
- *Project performance plan.* This is another term for a performance-based grant application. It should show how the proposed project contributes to agency objectives by tying project activities and measures to those objectives.

Structure Continuous Planning

Experience suggests that strategic planning for a partnership should have several foci. There are three distinct areas that need strategic development: programs and service, organizational structure, and resource development. Goals cover partnership services, internal operations, and global goals (these are goals assumed by agreeing to the state's goals for school readiness, for example). They are made distinct to place proper emphasis on each; otherwise effort would be distracted from essential organizational/partnership building and concomitant service delivery. They have an external and internal character. If service goals are external, then organizational development is internal; to ignore one is detrimental to the other. Internally, the partnership has to "grow" its people. This is a goal-oriented endeavor. Then there is the ubiquitous question of money.

Strategically planning fund development pervades all planning. It is the essential starting point. Services cannot be provided without money. Staff cannot be hired or trained without money. The community cannot be engaged without money. Hence, there is the need to have distinct goals for funding. An effective model explores strengths, weaknesses, opportunities, and plans, but with a focus on strengthening allies. Again the focus is on strong collaboration via strong people.

Planning at a successful partnership is continuous, alive, and organic. It is alive in that it causes action and it is organic in that it "grows" ideas. This, as much as anything, captures the character of the well-working planning process for local community development. These are the attributes to which the partnership's efforts should aspire. So what process is it that causes this organism to come into being and grow? For this we turn to the Smart Start Tool Kit on Planning (Smart Start: *www.smartstart-nc.org*). The following is how successful local partnerships interpret these essential strategic planning steps:

- *Build the group.* These are the individuals who need to be at the table to get things going. They bring resources and expertise. A first order of business is to name a Strategic Planning Committee.
- *Develop the vision/mission.* This is a statement of the desire or dream for the future of the community. Make sure it also includes internal and external purposes mentioned above.
- *Assess current reality.* This is a statement of need with attending resources and the collective will to commit those resources.
- *Define priority results.* These are specific goals, subsequent objectives, and associated benchmarks. Some partnerships take this a recommended step further by defining measurable targets for each benchmark for the short, mid, and long ranges; Exhibit 4.12 provides a good example of necessary detail of performance tracking. See how a measurable goal translates through objective and need to the benchmark. Actual outcomes are counterposed to projected outcomes, and from that, "refinements" suggest improvements, even the possibility of program discontinuation if certain mutually agreed-upon targets are not met. The table in Exhibit 4.12 establishes accountability and responsibility, and thus becomes an instrument of performance.
- *Develop feedback system.* This communication system is the mechanism that tells the story of outcome/impact. It is also the network of communication channels and media it takes to get the word of project performance to every nook and cranny of the community.
- *Conduct stakeholder analysis.* This is the vitally important continual assessment of your collaboration and its willingness/capability to trudge on with the stated work.

- *Develop high-leverage strategies.* These are the overall activities that make goals happen. Remember that this is not a case of deciding what is nice to do; it is deciding what is essential to do as each decision represents a trade-off of what cannot be done.
- *Detail action plan.* This is the who, what, when, where, and how of the activity. It assigns the all-important responsibility for results.
- *Get feedback and begin again.* This reassessment is quintessentially necessary to develop the organic nature of growth and idea development the partnership wants in its strategy. The partnership wants to sustain performance and the bettering of targeted lives.

The Forsyth Early Childhood Partnership structured a committee for each of six major goals it wanted to achieve. Essentially, each committee asked if the partnership was accomplishing what it said it would and "fixed" things if it was not. The committees identified possible gaps in services, evaluated necessary new services, and kept an eye to the horizon. That is, the committees always took the time to look for what tomorrow might bring in terms of problems and opportunities. Any recommendations were then proposed to the strategic planning committee for discussion, prioritizing, and recommendation for implementation. The executive board made the final decision to commit to a suggestion.

The "organic, living" quality was nurtured by *how* the process was done. The formal strategic plan was shown to all stakeholders, such as the Mental Health Department, the Health Department, and the Department of Social Services for buy-in and comment. It was referred to partnership funding agencies for review and in some cases suggestions. External evaluators used it as part of their analysis. And it continues to serve as a guide to assess proposals and rank-order them for action when support, will, and money line up to actually put an idea into action. While the multilayered nature of board operation may seem oppressively bureaucratic, and it does create work at each level, it forces people to get their heads together and agree on what is best for the partnership. Action directed toward the true population of need is then communal and consensual.

Conceptualize Essential Services

Each goal suggests services. It is good to discuss what may fit the final bill of offerings. This discussion is not to decide what services to support; it is to discuss their nature and characteristics. This guides the acquisition and shaping of services so they have the best chance of contributing to the vision and mission. Another wise suggestion, besides that goals should be performance based, is that there be an attempt to have services answer a developmental need for targeted clients. This will lessen the chance that services are developed just because they are handy or fill a "shopping list" of a particular interest or person. Not only that, an array of services for each stated purpose addresses the fact that problems are multidimensional and complex. Progress is made when multiple agencies and interests employ a range of strategies and programs over time. Several services, perhaps even a dozen or so, each working on the same long-term goal, will eventually have a noticeable effect on the community. This noticeable effect then translates to further support (see Exhibit 4.13).

Plan the Character of Services

Stability. The sooner the partnership imprints the need for partnership stability, accessibility, and quality of services, the better. Stability for the Forsyth Early Childhood Partnership is appropriately based on the stability of the nonprofit service organization. For planning expertise, the people in Forsyth County turned to local foundations. These organizations, such as the local Z. Smith Reynolds and K.B. Reynolds foundations, recognized that if the nonprofit collapses, the vision, no matter the energy it generates, dissolves. Thus various foundations awarded grants to build capacity. They established working groups and suggested appropriate staff. Standards of operational excellence were written and adopted. Events celebrated achievement and offered training. The Forsyth Partnership is also exploring the possibility of establishing a resource center for nonprofits. Forsyth saw early on that noble intentions built on wishes are, in their failure, devastating to the people who need and deserve things better. Forsyth also recognized that stability needs to be defined in terms of accessibility and quality.

Accessibility. The Forsyth Partnership offered a unique case for addressing accessibility. It needed to get child care to as many needy families as possible. As always, the neediest are the toughest to reach. And further complicating the issue is that there were different measures of outcome by some of the providers. For example, the Department of Social Services (DSS) was in the business of "subsidizing" child care; getting the maximum number of mothers to work was the goal. However, the Forsyth Partnership has additional goals: increasing quality of care for the children and making services user-friendly, with less stigma and fewer gaps. Thus, in addition to subsidies, scholarships were offered with a collaborative committee directing monies to the best source of help. Simply by asking the right questions and devising a rather clever solution, everyone realized real improvement in their lives. The partnership was then fully invested and could affect child-care quality and accessibility. DSS was able to record more needy mothers who were reached, and difficult-to-reach mothers got their children to good child care. The whole was made much better than the sum of the parts. Quality was also handled in a pleasantly unique fashion.

Quality. Though the term "quality" has been on stage for decades and has lost much of its meaning by familiarity and overuse, the topic must still be considered. Again, when we talk about public service quality, it is the experience and history of delivering services that better lives. If the intent is to make life better, quality then, depends on performance. Performance depends on measurement. Because we have devoted a section to evaluation (see "Outline Impact Analysis and Process Evaluation," p. 4-13), we need make only a point or two relevant to planning and quality as an essential character of service. The Forsyth Partnership designed a micro/macro approach. The micro focus is program specific. The intention is for each service to demonstrate performance via separate site visits formatted for technical assistance, monitoring, and fiscal compliance. Each project is required to prepare a series of reports covering daily operations which culminate in an annual summative report. The macro, or partnershipwide, focus on service performance was accomplished by periodic, third-party impact analyses. Together, micro and macro assessment tools help define and shape services, especially service quality.

The partnership must differentiate the essentials of planning. It must identify the issues, resources, and functionality, then plan accordingly. The partnership should have two categories of goals: to maintain organizational strength and to foster service performance. The advantage here is that these categories are interdependent, which permits a dual yet mutual focus on providing feedback on essential, goal-specific results. This is a different approach from merely marching toward the mission. By defining two mutually supportive sets of measures, process travels more smoothly to strategic assessment. It proceeds daily, if not minute by minute, to awareness of the need to be frugal with effort. The effort must then lead to mutually agreed results. Moreover, by having two sets of measures, internal and external, staff and stakeholders will not be distracted by overemphasis on one at the expense of the other. That is, blindly striving for mission only sacrifices the productive processes that get us there, and vice versa. Likewise, awareness of the intricacies of daily work allows the partnership's people and the organization to understand what needs to be done when demands change, and most important, it allows them to understand how to build a stable project. Staff must be aware of necessary details that need to be in place, over time, to support the experience of service delivery that changes lives for the better.

ESTABLISH AN IMPLEMENTATION PLAN ACCORDING TO YOUR VISION AND MISSION

Notice how much "work" the partnership has done to this point without having done the "work" of delivering services. Yet this is some of the most productive endeavor the partnership will undertake. The trick is to know when enough is enough. The partnership can plan to do things nearly forever; there comes a time to begin the march. It starts with the implementation plan. In keeping with practicality, the implementation scheme should be neither elaborate nor sketchy; it further defines direction such that well-meditated, prioritized action finally takes place. It is rooted in the ultimate purpose of just about any local partnership, that of building for the future.

Reaffirm the belief that there is some basic purpose to pooling resources and talent. With Smart Start it is the belief that investment in children is an investment in our neighborhoods of tomorrow. It bears repeating that strength as a nation is not top down; it is bottom up and begins very early, by developing and involved, capable, mature young neighbor. A capable citizen, one who is thriving to the best of his capacity *and* contributing to the community, does not "just happen." The individual becomes capable by being motivated to be a competent part of the work force in a career; an educated, involved neighbor; and an informed citizen. Certain, perhaps elevated abilities are not the question; each person is prepared to contribute in his or her own way. This process does not begin when the child fails in school, gets a juvenile record, or is out of control at home; it begins at birth. These beliefs, stated in terms suited for your partnership, are what lay the philosophy of your implementation plan. Reaffirm them then commit the plan to paper.

Write the Performance-Based Implementation Plan

We received a wealth of good suggestions from federal sources. Many of their project managers hail from local experience and possess years of watching the good, the bad, and the not so pretty happen in project development. The Government Accounting Office has a few tips on developing results-oriented plans that were adapted in a Management Concepts (2001) Grants and GPRA course and are summarized in the checklist that follows.

☐ *Make the case for the cause:*

- *Set out performance goals and measures.* Create a set of prioritized, major performance goals and measures counterposed to competing priorities (e.g., timeliness, service quality, customer satisfaction, project cost, and concerns of other stakeholders).
- *Show progress.* Establish intermediate goals and measures to show progress or contribution toward intended results.
- *Explain yourself.* Include explanatory information on your goals and measures. For example, how and why were they chosen? Why are they the most appropriate? If it is not clear, what is the relationship between goals and measures? When the project will measure processes or outputs, an explanation for the need to measure these, rather than outcomes, is important to justify the resources required.
- *Develop goals for the organization.* Develop performance goals to address mission-critical management problems. These are the partnership's capacity-building aims.

- *Consider external factors.* Describe the partnership's approaches to attack the degrading effect of external factors. Consider, for example, economic, social, and technological dynamics. Here point to the strength of the partnership's collaborative network.

☐ *Establish the yardstick for measuring the partnership's results:*

- *Show past performance.* Detail the baseline and trend data for past performance.
- *Set targets.* Identify projected target levels of performance for multiyear goals.

☐ *Make connections clear:*

- *Link goals.* Connect the goals of operational units to the partnership's organizational strategic goals.
- *Link activities.* Connect strategies and project activities to specific performance goals and describe how they will contribute to achievement of those goals. Clearly connect where the partnership wants to go (goal), how it is going to get there (activity), and what it will cost (budget).
- *Show budget sense.* Demonstrate how budgetary resources relate to achievement of performance goals.

☐ *Detail the partnership's data collection plan:*

- *Identify data sources.* Identify internal and external sources of data. People must have faith in the numbers; thus, a plan to acquire reliable data is crucial.
- *Verify and validate data.* Data collection procedures should be "credible and specific to ensure that performance information is sufficiently complete, accurate, valid, and consistent to document performance and support decisions on how best to manage" the project. Include scope, methodology, and timing of reporting in the plan.
- *Consider unavailable or low-quality data.* Perfect data do not exist. The best data also command the best price. When data collection, or the expense of it, hinders mission accomplishment, compromise and explain.

Whereas the checklist implies a rigid procedure for planning implementation, practicality overrides rigidity. The plan can be as simple as an expanded "to do" list or an elaborate, desktop-published booklet. What matters is that it works for the partnership.

Develop a Practical Board Skilled in Implementation

Implementation is a process of necessity. When helping the board move from ideas to action to service to change to benefit, it is important to keep several things in mind. The board needs to be comfortable with the vision and mission. "Comfortable" means that enough is mutually agreed on to promote effective action and avoid internal strife that leads to the possible destruction of the partnership. The board needs to constantly ask, "Is this the right thing to do?" In fact, that question is at the root of implementation, especially for the small partnership that may need to take action based on necessity rather than optimal structure. This is an important point to planning. Adequate planning nurtures the ability to know when something is right and when the time is right for action rather than merely jumping at a supposed opportunity.

This leads to another point: Board preparation and training are needed to guide implementation, but there are many ways to fulfill training needs, and not all of them cost money. For example, members of the board of the Halifax-Warren Smart Start Partnership for Children were trained on implementation by the North Carolina Blue Cross and Blue Shield, for free. The board learned about structure, function, fund raising, and strategic planning, just to mention a few topics taught. They also got valuable insight into proper board attitude and philosophy, not the least of which is that the purpose of the board is to raise money not to spend it. This insight alone put much more gravity into board action as it came at a personal price. Board members also learned that goals are really the plan of how to plan and that documenting a plan, especially an implementation plan, puts an end to interminable discussion. Resources for free or low-cost training are available. Local universities, junior colleges, foundations, and professional associations are just a few places the partnership can look for needed instruction.

Implementation is building on practices proven effective in similar situations, not the analytically proven product or template from some place a world away in distance and comparison. Interagency coordination is most important. Halifax-Warren Smart Start found it difficult to adopt "peace of mind for parents" as an agency goal. This kind of goal is common; however, it is impossible to measure. Still, the Halifax-Warren needed to partner with the agency that defined it, so it had to find common ground to accommodate its "goal." A compromise was found by defining peace of mind as having money for child care and a car for work.

Another key part of board leadership is seeing weakness and mustering or directing appropriate talent and resources to address that shortcoming. For example, the Halifax-Warren Smart Start did not have a skilled grant writer early on, so it formed a grant-writing team for that implementation plan action item. The art of the plan is to stay true to the vision and mission yet comply with mandates and bureaucracy in an environment of limited means. The goal of the implementation plan is to stabilize and institutionalize a successful service so that a new one can be initiated and, in turn, be institutionalized. Again, we must strive for whatever is practical for our partnership, with these few things in mind, then do it.

PROFILE KEY STAFF

The argument can be made that the partnership's ideas will live or die on the quality of the people it puts on staff and in charge of its services. The question is, "When does the partnership start building a team of qualified and motivated, even passionate, people and service providers?" Furthermore, how does the partnership go about building its team? And, how much does it invest in the undertaking? We suggest that during the planning phase the partnership think in terms of a process of human capital development, which considers people in concert with vision and mission, from hiring to retirement. This is important because effective staffing goes way beyond just plugging someone in a position. The next section discusses this issue in more detail. We do suggest that in the planning phase there be enough discussion to form an idea of what kind of people are wanted in key areas, such as the program director, key operations staff, and service provision. We begin with the program executive director as this is the first person to hire; this person has to be a gem.

Describe the Project Executive Director

The education, talent, and characteristics a partnership wants in its lead person are similar to what it wants in its operational staff and service providers. But be realistic. Can a partnership find the perfect person to head up its effort? No. Can a partnership find a person probably better than it expected, considering the genuinely difficult challenges? Yes. Consider some of the qualifications of the executive directors of some of the partnerships we visited. One is a corporate lawyer, one has a doctoral degree, another has extensive experience running nonprofits, and another has a master's degree in public health; all are passionate about their work. All of them, though eminently qualified, said they learned most when on the job. The process is not magic, but it bears some contemplation and discussion. One partnership went through two executive directors before it found the right person. But it helps to have some expectations to minimize the real tragedy of making a bad match. There are some things to look for when considering qualifications and character.

When considering qualifications, one should contemplate tangibles such as background, education, and experience. The lead staffer should have proven experience in running a nonprofit and working knowledge of how the local community functions. Perhaps the leader may have had experience in running a company or managing a large operation. A graduate degree in an appropriate area is good. But do not overlook passion for plaques on the wall. Passion will overcome where degrees may not. Training is important. Ideally, the candidates have had courses in project management, time management, team building, and contracting for example. Look for professional development such as formal training in funds development. One should be a bit of a guru in automation so that he or she is comfortable with the technology to back up the need to be a superior communicator with the spoken, written, and electronic word. Actually, these tangible qualifications are easy to consider, easy in comparison to the intangible talents the successful partnership professional needs.

The executive directors who were interviewed spent considerable time ruminating about all the intrinsic, intangible qualities that make up a person who succeeds against the formidable odds. We heard such descriptors as "innovator," "risk taker," "visionary," "negotiator," "people person," "values people," "open to criticism," "role model," "willing to learn," "flexible," "honest," "great communicator," "treats change as a constant," and, of course, "passionate." This person sounds nearly other worldly, but he or she is out there and worth the search.

Describe Staff and Service Providers

The education, experience, and character dynamics of the executive director reflect in what the partnership is also looking for in leadership, operational staff, and service providers. When speaking of operational staff in particular, instead of the general, tangible qualifications sought in the executive director, the partnership is looking for expertise in a specific area such as human resources, budget, and evaluation. The large, mature partnership can have a full range of staff. For example, the Down East Partnership has the following functional areas: executive director, fiscal, administrative assistant, human resources, evaluation/analysis, public information, contracts management, facilities management, and reception. A small partnership may have only two or possibly three staff people, requiring skills in multiple areas. This brings up an overlooked point, staff in a partnership need to expect and be trained for multitasking. When hiring, a partnership must be sure this expectation is understood and that the prospective employee is multitalented relative to the needs of a start-up public service operation.

Because it is so important, and stressed by those interviewed, here are some of the intangible character traits a partnership may wish to have in the people who comprise its team. At the top of the list, assess passion for the task at hand, for working with the target clients in their environment. See if they have a history of helping people succeed (i.e., that they are natural and good coaches). Are they good "keepers" and communicators of the vision? Especially, a partnership should look for someone who has had successful experience working on a team. We could go on describing these ideal qualities. Ultimately, the partnership must choose. Be aware that there is no perfect choice, just degrees of good.

Also expect that every staffer has much to learn. A partnership must look for as many of these qualifications and qualities as it dares hope for, then hire! The partnership is looking for the raw material to build the team that makes the vision happen. It takes time, some mistakes, and understanding.

OUTLINE KEY PROJECT STAFF ROLES, DUTIES, AND RESPONSIBILITIES AND PROFESSIONAL HUMAN CAPITAL DEVELOPMENT PROCESS

Treat staff like the project depends on them; it does. So much has been written and said about the importance of staff. Everyone knows qualified staff are vital, yet relatively few organizations get the process of developing staff right. View the partnership as an opportunity to get "the people thing" correct when it comes to staff development. These are the people who will spend as much time with each other as they do family, the people who make the vision possible. We were impressed at every successful, thriving site visited that the staff had jelled into a team, that, though everyone talked about the long hours and really crushing work, all were suited and happy in their work. They did not get that way by magic; they are well led, well selected, well trained, suited to their jobs, and supported. We review here some of the better effective practices that partnerships employ to get their staff to be productive and "rowing in the same direction." It is best to approach staff development in terms of the concept of human capital development.

Consider Key Positions

In considering key staff positions, a partnership should start small and grow with a predetermined sense of the skills it would like in critical positions. Practically, the partnership may begin with only a lead staffer and an assistant. If the partnership is lucky enough to have considerable support and funding, it may start with all the key positions filled, but this is unusual. Mature organizations have an executive director working with human resources, fiscal, development, communications, and program directors. Support for these key positions is in direct proportion to the workload. Also, it pays to have staff cross-trained in an area or two as, especially early in the life of the partnership, most staffers do a little bit of everything. Have them ready to accept, even willing to volunteer for, and be productive with multitasking. Also consider minimum duties and responsibilities—in other words, the essentials of what must be done by the position. The partnership should take a little more time to develop performance-based job descriptions that have a quantitative basis for essential functions; it is well worth the effort. Here we mean that the better job description has a narrative description of job requirements and, wherever possible, a numerical statement of productivity. It is then a natural progression to draw periodic evaluations from a job description that has quantitative and qualitative elements that make it that much easier to tie performance to reward, monetary and intrinsic.

Outline Human Capital Development Process

Building a team is a series of tasks in a commonsense process that considers the needs of the organization while respecting the needs of the individual team member. Thus a partnership should think in terms of the seamless progression of recruiting, retention, and retirement. It should outline a process of hiring, orienting, professional development, training, personal evaluation, and benefits (see Exhibit 4.14, which demonstrates a range of possibilities for compensation beyond money, which is a major concern for a not-for-profit organizaton). As we might expect, just about every major organization-building task begins with the vision and mission—hence the paramount importance of having the vision and mission firmly stated. The inspiring vision and mission weave in and out of every pebble, every stone that builds a partnership castle. From the vision comes the job description that produces the job posting that develops a pool of qualified and motivated people from whom to choose. People are interviewed using a predetermined list of questions designed to determine both qualifications and the desire to do the job. A board of several people can interview, but the executive director should have sole hiring and firing responsibility. The new hire is carefully oriented by all key staff and given a plan for professional development and the best benefits package possible (see Exhibit 4.15 for a sample performance-oriented job description). A performance-oriented evaluation system, mutually agreed upon by staffer and supervisor, keeps the team member on track and results oriented. Is this perhaps a little too much effort considering the remarkable pounding of daily work in a nonprofit? Not at all. The process pays many times over in effort that succeeds.

PREPARE THE PROJECT SITE

It is nice to be able to design and have a hospitable, functional facility. In reality, this home away from home evolves. Initially a partnership takes what it can get. Still, it is good to have a few things in mind when finding a place from which to conduct business.

Decide Location

The partnership's operational base answers one of the primary service objectives, that of accessibility. A partnership should try to locate within its client base. Clients should not be burdened with having to come to the partnership; at least, the partnership should have bus access and perhaps even be within walking distance. The Down East Partnership in Rocky Mount, North Carolina, for example, was most fortunate to be able to purchase a "condemned" YWCA building for a token amount. The necessary rehabilitation was an opportunity to design offices and facilities suited to the task at hand, including meeting/training areas (former basketball court), a media/lending library, and a model child-care operation/laboratory combination. The Forsyth Partnership in Winston-Salem, North Carolina began in downtown rental space, added more space as it became vacant, and now has moved into space large enough to share with a major service provider.

Describe the Facility

Whether the partnership begins with a lovely YWCA in need of "a little paint" or grows as opportunity presents, it may want to have some of the following physical plant attributes. In addition to staff and support personnel space, a family resource center is primary. Here the partnership will have its files of resources, contacts, training materials, lending library, and such for families. Of course, the partnership will need space for large and small gatherings and possibly a speaker system and audiovisual equipment. And how can a partnership have "food, fun, and facts" without a kitchen? It should have an ice machine. It needs a workshop for the copier, posting, storage, and a work area for miscellaneous jobs such as assembling brochures. The reception area should be welcoming and the building must be secure. Parking should be ample and adjacent. An outdoor play area is great if the partnership can afford it, if the partnership is insured for it, and if it fits with the services the partnership delivers. Ideally, a partnership may want to have a research and development play space that is a working lab that displays the current thinking and techniques for developing clients. Again, necessity will be the first determining factor, but it also pays to have a vision for the home base.

Plan for Automation and Well-Equipped Office Space

Staff and providers, the partnership, and its existence depend on information, free flowing and accessible. The partnership must not skimp on automation. A good investment is to have an automation systems analysis. The partnership should seek a good computer consultant rather than a discount store salesperson. The partnership wants someone to analyze what it does and how it would be most efficiently and effectively done. It may also want more than one opinion. The partnership should get the latest and most powerful hardware it can afford. Off-the-shelf software is preferred (let others worry about the bugs). The partnership will probably need a general office suite, communications packages, and specialized packages such as accounting software. For communications, a local area network, perhaps a wide area network, and Internet access are indispensable. Because this is a topic with volumes of readily available information, we leave it at that. Likewise, when setting up office space, the vendor also provides consulting, usually as a service of the purchase. Consider correct layout, sturdy furniture and appointments, communications, support, maintenance contracts, and recordkeeping. What is important is that the partnership anticipate office and automation needs rather than rush down to Sam's when the start-up grant is awarded.

PLAN WELL, THEN ACT

The effort expended in planning is returned many times over. All successful campaigns are based on diligent, if not extensive, planning. Mistakes are largely avoided or minimized. With a suggested process, when a partnership make mistakes, ideally they will be novel, having learned from those who have gone before it. More important, critical errors that can end a project are anticipated. A lengthy planning process also allows consensus to be built. Without consensus there is little chance for progress, let alone meaningful success. Limited resources are focused, which allows a demonstration of impact early on so that the partnership knows it is on the right track plus where and when it should adjust. Also, building a partnership is a learning process that happens only by doing the work. The process we have just taken our readers through should also be seen as an opportunity to learn. There is nothing special about getting a partnership up and running once the "how to" is figured out. It is a matter of a lot of work by a lot of people. The planning process suggested gets things started in some sort of orderly fashion. It is a transition vehicle for that initial burst of enthusiasm that needs direction, not dissipation. But now the planning is finished. Although it may be tempting to plan a little more, discuss a few fine points a little more, make sure of a few more data, nothing is going to change without action. The planning is over; it is time for the partnership to get going.

Notes

1. Halifax-Warren Smart Start Partnership for Children, Magda Baligh, Executive Director, P.O. Box 402 24 King Street, Halifax, NC 27839; tel.: (252) 583-1304; or via the North Carolina Smart Start Website: *www.smartstart-nc.org*.
2. Down East Partnership for Children, Henrietta Zalkind, Executive Director, P.O. Box 1245; 215 Lexington Street, Rocky Mount, NC 27802; tel.: (252) 985-4300; or via the North Carolina Smart Start Website: *www.smartstart-nc.org*.
3. Forsyth Early Childhood Partnership, Dr. Dean Clifford, Ph.D., Executive Director, 7820 N. Point Blvd., Winston-Salem, NC 27106; tel.: (336) 725-6011; *www.forsythchild.org*.
4. Chatham County Partnership for Children, Genevieve Megginsion, Executive Director, 200 Sanford Highway, Suite #4; Pittsboro, NC 27312; tel.: (919) 542-7449; *chatchld@emji.net*; *www.chathamkids.org*.
5. The CC&RR manual can be obtained by contacting staff at the North Carolina Partnership for Children, *www.smartstart-nc.org*.

References

Management Concepts. (2001). *Grants & GPRA: A performance-based approach to federal assistance.* Vienna, VA: Author . (Available from Management Concepts Inc., 8230

Leesburg Pike, Ste. 800, Vienna VA 22182; tel.: (703) 790-9595; *www.strategicplan.org*)

Mattessich, P. W, Monsey, B. R. (undated). Collaboration: What Makes It Work. St. Paul, MN: Amherst H. Wilder Foundation.

Mitchell, A., Stoney, L., & Ditcher, H. (2001). *Financing child care in the United States.* Kansas City: MO: Ewing Marion Kaufman Foundation.

Office of Management and Budget. (1996, June). *Primer on GPRA performance management* [On-line]. Available: *www.npr.gov/library.resource.gpraprmr.html.*

Powell, C. (2001). *A leadership primer* [On-line]. Available: *www.freepages.military rootsweb.com/-rootsrus/powell.html.*

Exhibit 4.1
Down East Partnership for Children: Composition of Board of Directors

The Board of Directors shall include representation from the following categories:

- County commissioner
- County manager, director of the county department of social services
- Director of the local area mental health agency
- Director of the local health department
- Superintendent of public schools
- President of the community college
- Chair of the local cooperative extension agency
- Director of the local public library
- Two business leaders
- Two family members
- Child-care provider
- Head Start representative
- Nonprofit organization related to child care
- Representative of the religious community
- Representative of the local Interagency Coordinating Council or parent of a disabled child
- Representative of a local foundation

Exhibit 4.2
Forsyth Early Childhood Partnership: Job Description for Board Members

All board members should . . .

General Expectations

1. Know and support FECP's mission, vision, purposes, goals, objectives, policies, programs, services, and strengths;
2. Perform duties of board membership responsibly, conforming to the level of competence expected from board members as they apply to nonprofit board members;
3. Participate in decision-making with careful consideration of all available and pertinent information and in light of what seems best for the optimal development of children and the accomplishing of the mission and goals of the organization; declare any conflict of interest that may exist in decision-making;
4. Seek information on research, best practices, and emerging developments in the field of interest;
5. Be willing to serve in leadership positions and to undertake special assignments willingly and enthusiastically;
6. Suggest possible nominees to the board who are persons who can make significant contributions to the work of the board and the progress of FECP and its efforts;
7. Bring commitment, good will, energy, enthusiasm, and a sense of humor to the board's deliberations.

Meetings

8. Be an advocate for the organizations and for young children; promote FECP and its efforts in ways appropriate to your profession and contacts;
9. Regularly attend board meetings every other month and the meetings of at least one committee and actively participate in decision making and the work involved;
10. Read written materials in preparation for board and committee meetings;
11. Ask timely and substantive questions at board and committee meetings consistent with your conscience and convictions, but support the majority decisions on issues decided by the board;
12. Share your particular areas of expertise with the board and staff;
13. Suggest agenda items periodically for board and committee meetings to ensure that significant, policy-related matters are addressed.

Financial Development and Fiduciary Responsibilities

14. Give an annual gift according to personal means;
15. Assist the development committee and staff in implementing fund-raising strategies;
16. Be willing to suggest potential sources of gifts, and/or to participate in the solicitation of funds, and/or to express appreciation to donors on behalf of the organization;
17. Exercise prudence with the board in the control and use of funds;
18. Faithfully read and understand the organization's financial statements;
19. Help the board fulfill its fiduciary responsibilities.

Maintaining the Integrity of the Organization

20. Council the chief executive as appropriate and support him or her in relationships with groups or individuals;
21. Ask staff only to complete tasks pertinent to the work of the organization;
22. Respect the need for Board to avoid involvement in day-to-day management of staff;

22. Respect the need for Board to avoid involvement in day-to-day management of staff;
23. Serve the organization as a whole rather than any special interest group or constituency;
24. Disclose any possible conflicts of interest to the board in a timely fashion;
25. Urge those with grievances to follow established polices and procedures; bring any matters of potential significance to the attention of the board's elected leader and the chief executive;
26. Maintain independence and objectivity;
27. Support the decisions and work of the organization.

Exhibit 4.3
Sample Duties and Responsibilities Statement: Treasurer of the Corporation

Purpose:

To help ensure the fiscal integrity of the Partnership by providing oversight of its financial activities and ensuring the accuracy of all financial records.

Duties and Responsibilities:

1. Attend as member Board, Executive Committee, and Audit/Finance Committee meetings.
2. Using the proper chain of command, work with staff to review and submit full and accurate financial data to the rest of the Board.
3. Work to ensure that the Board's financial policies are being followed.
4. Meet with staff regularly to review financial records and prepare reports for the board.
5. Give reports to the Board as to the financial health of the Partnership.
6. Review the partnership's annual audit and answer any questions other Board members may have about it.
7. Serve as ex officio member and Executive Committee Liaison to the Audit/Finance Committee.
8. Assist that Executive Director in preparing the organization's annual budget and in meeting audit requirements.
9. Provide signature when necessary on Partnership checks and other documents.

Rationale:

The role of the Board Treasurer is to ensure the financial integrity of the partnership. S/he accomplishes this through oversight of adherence to the Accounting Policies and Procedures adopted by the Board.

Under no circumstances should the Board Treasurer become involved in the day-to-day management of the Partnership's finances. S/he should not approach staff who have been delegated the responsibility without being directed to do so by the Executive Director.

The Executive Director will keep the Board Treasures informed regularly of the Partnership's financial condition on a regular basis.

The Board Treasurer should never give his or her opinion about a Board decision to the public or the news media.

Source: Halifax-Warren Smart Start Partnership for Children.

Exhibit 4.4
Halifax-Warren Smart Start Partnership for Children Vision Statement

Our Vision

All young children and their families will have the same opportunities for social, physical, emotional, and intellectual development. Our vision is that children will enter school healthy in all aspects and ready to learn. Our hope is that these opportunities will help ensure lifelong success and improve the quality of life for the citizens of Halifax and Warren Counties.

Our Mission in the Halifax-Warren Community

Through collaborative efforts, opportunities will be made available for county citizens to create nurturing and supportive environments in which young children can develop physically, socially emotionally and intellectually to their fullest potential. The primary emphasis will be on children ages 0–5 and their families. We will strive to ensure that comprehensive services are available to those who need them. These services will be provided in a way that empowers families, protects their dignity, fosters self-sufficiency, and encourages them to be productive citizens.

Our Goals and Objectives

Goal 1.

Halifax and Warren County children ages 0–5 will be provided the opportunity to be healthy and prepared to succeed when they enter schools.

Goal 2.

Halifax and Warren County families will be provided the support they need to effectively fulfill their roles as primary providers, nurturers, and teachers helping children reach their full potential.

Goal 3.

Halifax and Warren County families with children ages 0–5 will be provided access to high-quality, affordable services, including early childhood education, services for children with special needs, and other services that support families.

Goal 4.

Halifax and Warren County will provide resources and encourage collaboration to help children and families reach their potential.

Exhibit 4.5
Program Standard: Every Child Has Access to a High-Quality Early Childhood Program

Teacher Education

Objective: All teachers working in early childhood programs have an associate or bachelor's degree in early childhood education or child development or they are enrolled in a degree program leading toward the attainment of such a degree.

Example benchmark: By June 30, 1999, the percentage of early childhood teachers possessing a bachelor's degree in early childhood or child development will be increased from 10 percent (10 of 100) to 25 percent (25 of 100).

Example benchmark: By June 30, 1999, the percentage of early childhood teachers with a one-year diploma in early childhood or child development will be increased from 40% (40 of 100) to 65 percent (65 of 100).

Example benchmark: By June 30, 1999, the percentage of family childcare providers completing an associate's degree in early childhood will be increased from 17 percent (17 of 100) to 35 percent (35 of 100).

Example benchmark: By June 30, 1999, the percentage of early childhood teachers completing or enrolled in a Childhood Development Associate, CDA, program in early childhood or child development will be increased from 40 percent (40 of 100) to 65 percent (65 of 100).

Data sources: Workforce Study; T.E.A.C.H.

Data collector: Direct service provider (NC Partnership for Children)

Exhibit 4.6
Sample Topics to Be Covered by Financial Policies and Procedures

Part A—Internal Policies and Procedures

I. General Policy
II. Segregation of Duties
III. Cash Management
IV. Bank Account Signatories
V. Budgets
VI. Allocation of Joint Costs
VII. Computer Accounting Package
VIII. Cash Receipts
IX. Purchasing
X. Cash Disbursements—Nonpayroll
XI. Cash Disbursements—Payroll
XII. Tax Compliance
XIII. Fixed Assets
XIV. Financial Programs and Grants
XV. Donations of Materials, Facilities, and Services
XVI. Cash Basis Reporting
XVII. Close Out
XVIII. Sales and Use Tax Paid
XIX. Audit Preparation

Part B—Subcontractor Policies and Procedures

I. Procurement Policies and procedures
II. Budget Revision Policy
III. Financial Reporting Policies and Procedures
IV. Cash Match Donations
V. Contract Monitoring

Source: Chatham County Partnership for Children

Exhibit 4.7
Sample Policy and Procedure Document—Cash Disbursements, Nonpayroll

Policy

It is the policy of the Chatham County Partnership for Children, CCPC, to ensure a system of checks and balances which will allow for the timely and accurate payment of all disbursements while minimizing the possibility of errors and maximizing the earning potential of funds. Compliance with the following procedures and duties, as detailed in the section on segregation of duties, is essential to achieve this goal.

Procedures

The following procedures are necessary to ensure proper cash disbursements:

10. Prenumbered checks will be used for all disbursements.
11. The unused check supply will be adequately controlled and safeguarded.
12. Adequate controls will be established to ensure accountability for all voided checks.
13. Adequate controls will be established to ensure no duplication of payments.
14. Adequate controls will be made from an original invoice. *Photocopied or faxed invoices or statements should not be paid.*
15. Duplicate copies of invoices will be destroyed to prevent duplicate payments.
16. No blank checks will be signed in advance.
17. No check will be made payable to cash. Instead, the check may be made payable to the organization (as in the case of checks for petty cash).
18. Proper approval of all expenditures prior to payment will be performed by an authorized individual.
19. Control over mailing and distribution of checks will be maintained.
20. Supporting documentation will accompany all disbursements.
21. Procurement will be conducted following the Purchasing Policy.
22. All disbursements will be made as close to the due date as possible without incurring late fees.

Duties

To carry out the procedures to ensure proper cash disbursements the following duties must be performed:

1. A purchase order will be received and authorized for each purchase.
2. Approved purchase orders and recurring obligations will be received and maintained in an accounts payable file.
3. The completed documentation will be reviewed to ensure availability of funds and to review account coding.
4. Accounts payable folder will be checked weekly to determine if any payments are due.
5. Checks will be prepared weekly and delivered with documentation to the authorized financial official.
6. Review supporting documentation for all checks, sign check, and deliver all information to a second authorized financial official.
7. Mail check to vendor and stamp PAID on the invoice and all accompanying documentation to prevent repayment.
8. Information will be filed by the vendor.
9. Voided checks will be retained, never thrown away, and never torn into pieces. The signature space on the voided check will be cut off. VOID will be stamped across the face of the check and the voided check will be filed in numerical order with the canceled checks. All voided checks are entered in the accounting system as void items also.

10. Control and safeguarding of check supply will be maintained.

Segregation of Duties

To assist in performing these procedures with adequate segregation of duties, a breakdown of duties is provided. The number next to each position refers to the number of the duty that should be carried out.

Administrative Assistant: 2, 4, 7, 8

Executive Board Director Designated: 1, 6

Officers and other Board members: 6

Finance Director: 3, 5, 9, 10

Source: Chatham County Partnership for Children.

Exhibit 4.8
Sample Finance Director Duties and Responsibilities

General Statement of Duties

Perform complex professional and responsible managerial and administrative work in planning, organizing, and executing the financial, purchasing, and personnel activities of the Partnership.

Distinguishing Features of the Class

An employee in this class plans, organizes and administers the activities of the finance department involving the process for receiving, disbursing, and accounting of revenues and expenditures. Work involves supervision of the budget, purchasing, accounting, contracts administration, and payroll operations. Employee performs professional specialized accountant level work in the preparation and analysis of financial reports, investment of funds, and posting revenues. The employee must exercise considerable independent judgment and initiative in planning and directing the fiscal control systems. Work is performed in accordance with established nonprofit finance procedures, and State Childhood Partnership policies, procedures and regulations. Work is performed under the general administrative supervision of the Executive Director, and is evaluated through conferences, reports, and an independent audit of financial records.

Duties and Responsibilities

Essential Duties and Tasks

Plans, organizes, and supervises the operations of the finance department, including disbursement and accounting for Partnership funds, preparation of payroll, and maintenance of payroll and time records.

Tracks and analyzes expenditures, cash contributions, and in-kind support; prepares monthly, quarterly and annual financial reports; prepares reports of trends with recommendations for policy, procedures and practice changes, and improvements; submits fiscal reports required by funding sources and NCPC; prepares and presents Treasurer's Report for the Board and Finance Committee.

Supervises staff responsible for fiscal process including clerical accounting activities involved with maintenance of financial records and audit preparation, and contracts management.

Coordinates and develops annual budget; works with Executive Director and other staff to project revenue and expenditures; assures accuracy and compliance with State Partnership requirements; works closely with the Director in directing formation of financial policies and final preparation of the budget; serves as liaison to the Board Finance Committee, accountants, State auditors, NCPFC and NCDHHS; and may assist in presenting to the Finance and Executive Committees and Board.

Makes hiring decisions, trains, counsels, conducts performance evaluations, and takes disciplinary action; recommends discipline and dismissal action.

Manages and supports office technical systems; acts as liaison with State Partnership and software company on implementing computer accounting system; defines software needs; monitors system performance; assists employees in using applications; makes recommendations for system changes and enhancements.

Performs professional accounting activities; completes chart of accounts; makes journal entries, transfers funds; reviews contract disbursements monthly; balances bank accounts; and prepares year end journal entries and various state and federal reports.

Schedules independent auditors; assists auditors during the audit process; prepares audit papers; and takes action in response to findings to improve financial systems.

Assists staff with solving difficult technical problems.

Manages purchasing and payroll processes and procedures; issues pay checks and purchase orders, and maintains related records.

Oversees personnel policies and benefits; orients employees and assures employees complete necessary forms; interprets policies and may draft new or revised policies and procedures.

Additional Job Duties

Performs related duties as required.

Recruitment and Selection Guidelines

Knowledge, Skill, and Abilities

Thorough knowledge of North Carolina General Statutes and administrative policies governing governmental financial practices and procedures.

Thorough knowledge of the principles and practices of public finance administration including accounting, budgeting and payroll in government, including fund accounting.

Thorough knowledge of the field of accounting, principles, and practices.

Skill in operation of computers with underlying knowledge of accounting software, spreadsheets, and word processing, and technology support for efficient management.

Ability to evaluate complex financial systems and efficiently formulate and install accounting methods, procedures, forms and records.

Ability to prepare informative financial reports.

Ability to exercise sound judgment and discretion in decision making.

Ability to plan, organize, direct and evaluate the work of subordinate employees in the specialized field of accounting.

Ability to establish and maintain effective working relationships with department heads, government officials, subordinates, and the public.

Ability to work effectively in collaborative teams.

Ability to conduct long range fiscal planning.

Ability to communicate effectively in oral and written forms.

Physical Requirements

Must be able to perform the basic life operational skills of fingering, grasping, talking, hearing, and repetitive motions.

Must be able to perform sedentary work; exerting up to 10 pounds of force occasionally and/or a negligible amount of force frequently or constantly to move object.

Must possess the visual acuity to prepare and analyze data and figures, to perform accounting work, to operate a computer terminal, and extensive reading.

Desirable Education and Experience

Graduation from a four-year college or university with a degree in accounting, finance, or business, preferably with certification as a Certified Public Accountant and considerable experience in public finance administration, including some supervisory experience; or an equivalent combination of education and experience.

Source: Forsyth Early Childhood Partnership.

Exhibit 4.9
Sample Financial Statement Categories

Early Childhood Partnership
Financial Statement
July 1, 200X to June 30, 200X

Educational/Care Programs

Subsidies/Scholarships for Children/Transportation
Teacher Education/Training/Support
Enhancement Grants for Child Care
Inclusion Program for Special Needs
Enrichment Programs for Children
Resource and Referral Services

Family Support Services

Family Education and Support Services
Family Resource Centers/Community Support Services
Group Parenting Experiences
Informational Material for Parents/Care Providers

Health Services

Dental Clinic/Screenings
Screenings/Immunizations
Mental Health Services
Health Education/Other Health Services
Prenatal Services

Other Expenses Relating to Child and Family Services

Systems Change/Community Education
Shared Facility
Evaluation/Program Coordination
Special Events/Conferences

Partnership Administrative Expenses

TOTAL SMART START FUNDING EXPENSES:

Total Income Sources:

Smart Start Funds for 200X/200X
Other Funds and Grants

Source: Forsyth Early Childhood Partnership

Exhibit 4.10
Sources of Funding for Local Partnerships

Public

1. Local property taxes
2. Sales and excise taxes
3. State income taxes
4. Tax credits, deductions, and exemptions
5. Fees
6. Lotteries and gaming

Private-Sector Revenue

7. Employers
8. Unions
9. Philanthropy

Public-Private Partnerships

10. Employer and public-sector partnerships
11. Community and public-sector partnerships
12. Capital investment partnerships

Source: Mitchell et al., 2001.

Exhibit 4.11
Strategic Planning Definition of Terms

- *Values.* The beliefs or principles we hold precious. Our internal guidelines for distinguishing what is right from what is wrong and what is just from what is unjust. Beliefs are held tightly. They are not changed or swayed by external forces.
- *Vision.* The futuristic or ideal picture of the community.
- *Mission.* A statement of purpose that defines the responsibility of (the partnership) in achieving the larger vision.
- *Goals.* Ambitious statements of a desired end—what needs to be achieved in order to reach the vision the partnership has for the community. Measures the progress toward achieving our vision and mission.
- *Objectives.* More specific statements of what (the partnership) hopes to achieve. May focus on 2–5-year results. Are countywide in scope and are necessary steps toward achieving our goals.
- *Benchmarks.* Specific, measurable statements of progress toward achieving county-level objectives. Benchmarks focus on 3–5-year results.
- *Program/strategies.* Program refers to the services funded by (the partnership) and offered to children, families, child-care providers, professionals, etc. Strategies are plans, methods, or sequences of steps used to implement a program.
- *Outcomes.* Yearly, specific, measurable results of each program. Outcomes answer the question: "what has changed for the recipient as a result of participating in this program this year?" Outcomes are directly related to the recipient's need.
- Evaluation:
  - — *On a yearly basis.* Evaluation is the process of collecting, analyzing and reporting the result of the program (the outcomes). Evaluation assesses whether or not each program is:
    doing what it says it is doing and meeting individual outcomes.
  - — *Over time.* The evaluation assesses whether or not (the partnership) is meeting its 3–5-year benchmarks and objectives.
- *Ultimately.* Evaluation ultimately assesses whether or not (the partnership) is moving toward achieving its vision, mission, and goals.
- *Needs.* While needs are constantly assessed, in the process of strategic planning, the needs of the community are reassessed to determine if change is necessary. The reassessment is based on the yearly results of each program's evaluation and the cumulative results of the evaluation of the short-term benchmarks and objectives. The needs assessment may indicate that the needs of the community are met, not met, or changed.
- *Partnership Values (an example).* Collaboration, tenacity, flexibility, accountability, quality, unity, respect, caring, community, creativity, inclusivity, diversity, acceptance, tolerance, empowerment, planning, vision, hearing others, evaluation, local control, optimism, public-private partnerships.
- *Partnership Vision (an example).* We believe that all children and their families, when surrounded by a united and supportive community, can reach their full potential.
- *Partnership Mission Statement (an example).* To improve the quality of life for children and families in Nash and Edgecombe Counties through advocating and supporting quality, lifelong education and facilitating a trusted and coordinated system of community services.

Source: Adapted from the Down East Partnership for Children hand out on Strategic Planning

Exhibit 4.12
Table of Evaluation Outcomes by Goals and Objectives

Goal I. To ensure a system of quality early childhood educational opportunities which are available, accessible, and affordable for all children.

Objective A. Improve the educational level and competency of early childhood teachers and care providers.

Identified Need: Less than one-third of all teachers in child-care centers have Associate degree or higher and slightly less than one-half of family child-care providers and directors have an Associate degree or higher.

Benchmark: By June 200X, the number of teachers, directors, and in-home providers with Associate degrees or higher will increase by 1% for each group.

General Services	Activities	Outcomes		Refinements	
General Information	**Numbers Served**	**Projected Outcomes**	**Actual Outcomes**	**Major Obstacles/Needs**	**Recommendations for Future Evaluations**
Agency: TAC Work Group FECP Activity: Journey to the Stars Started: Jan 200X $ Allocated: 696,671 $ Actual Spent: 696,671	Projected: n/a Actual: 134 Children 26 FCCH 25 Centers	By June 2001: 25% of licensed programs will have a3 star rating; Children demonstrating a lack of kindergarten readiness will drop from 30% (1994) to 15%; Teachers will receive a monthly stipend for being enrolled in classes beyond the NCCCC. The number of teachers enrolled in classes will increase.	**Measured by WFRC database and TAC database** 26 FCCH providers are participating in the journey to the Stars. Among these participants: 21 have applied for a related license. 2 have received 5 stars. 25 centers participated in the program through TAC. Among thee participants 16 have received stars. 5 have applied for their ratings. 8 programs have 3 stars. 7 have 4 stars. 1has 1 star. 4 centers have not reported their status.	It is possible this program will be discontinued depending on outcomes of subsidy program changes. The market rates for subsidies are increasing based on star ratings. Centers and homes will have to increase their rates for private paying parents to qualify for the higher subsidy rates. This may cause money to be reallocated to the subsidy program to serve children currently in the program, as well as additional children who may qualify due to the increase in rates.	Program is new and complete data is not yet available. Collect baseline data as of June 20, 2000 on star ratings, and teachers enrolled education classes for comparison in 2001. Continue monitoring during 2000–01 and include results of star ratings in year and summary.
Agency: Forsyth Tech Activity: ECE Instructor Started July 1999 $ Allocated: 43,025 $ Actual Spent 27,616 $Reversion: 15,409	Projected: 220 additional class spaces will be added as a result of 11 additional classes Actual: 14 Classes were added, and 124 new students enrolled	By June 30, 2000, an additional 7 evening and weekend classes will be offered. 4 new sections will be offered in the Summer of 2000. By June 30, 2000 a minimum of 35 new ECE graduates will qualify for salary supplements. By June 30, 2000, a minimum of 20 early childhood educators will earn a certificate or Associate degree in ECE.	**Measured by FTCC class schedules, attendance records, and degrees completed** Between Fall '99 and summer '00. 14 additional classes were offered nights and weekends to accommodate work schedules of childcare providers. 124 new students enrolled in the program; 76 students enrolled in the Associate program and 48 students enrolled in the Certificate program. 47 ECE graduates qualified for salary supplements. The number of Early Childhood Education graduates increased by 88% over last year, from 25 to 47.		Monitor retention of new students this year and increases in number of students in the coming year. Continue to report number of graduates and include the number for each type of degree. Number of additional classes exceeded original estimate. 11 classes were projected. 14 classes were added.

Source: Forsyth Early Childhood Partnership.

Exhibit 4.13
Sample School-Readiness Services by Category

Child Care

Subsidized Child Care
Pre-Kindergarten
Child Care Resource and Referral Services
Quality Improvement Project
Salary Supplements for Child Care Teachers

Family Support

Parenting Education Support and Training
White Oak Parent Child Center
Parent Resource Guide
Mini-Grants

Health Care and Immunizations

Perinatal Health Education and Coordination
Health Screening for Preschool Children
Nutrition Education
In-Home Breastfeeding Support
Children with Special Needs

Source: Halifax-Warren Partnership for Children.

Exhibit 4.14
Sample Benefits Summary

- *Benefits*: Base pay plus 15% used for the following benefits if elected:
  - — Medical
  - — Dental
  - — Retirement
- *Flex plan*
- *Short-term and long-term disability*: paid by employer
- *Life insurance*: paid by employer ($15,000)
- *Employee assistance plan*
- *Exempt employees*: hour-for-hour time
- *Flexible work schedule*
- *After-school care*: for school-age children
- *Paid lunch time*
- *Child-care reimbursement*: while parent is away from home on travel, $750 per year for child care
- *YMCA*: no sign-up fee to be paid by employee
- *Leave time*: up to 5 years, employees earn 2 days per month; over 6 years earn 2½ days per month
- *Mileage reimbursement*: business travel reimbursed at $0.31 per mile
- *Longevity plan*: begins at 5 years
- *Staff development*
- *Holidays*: 11 holidays

Source: Down East Partnership for Children.

Exhibit 4.15
Sample Performance-Oriented Job Description

JOB TITLE:	Program Coordinator—Early Childhood Development
JOBS SUPERVISED:	None
JOB PURPOSE:	Optimizes development of children by monitoring, improving, and advocating for childhood education programs.

ESSENTIAL FUNCTIONS:

% time

20% 1. Develops programs to improve early childhood education in Forsyth County by: planning, organizing, and managing improvement efforts; identifying and facilitating collaborations.

10% 2. Improves quality of early childhood teachers and caregivers by: planning, organizing, and managing efforts to increase compensation and benefits.

10% 3. Increases awareness of early childhood issues by: contributing information to advocacy programs, early childhood educators, parents and the community at large on issues related to early childhood education.

20% 4. Monitors program results by: visiting contracting early childhood education partner agencies; observing and evaluating early childhood education approaches and methods; providing technical assistance.

10% 5. Maintains early childhood development program standards by: enforcing compliance with state requirements and FECP contract expectations.

20% 6. Develops contracting partner staff by: planning and conducting training programs; providing information at monthly meetings, providing individual technical assistance.

5% 7. Maintains professional knowledge by: participating in educational opportunities; reading professional publications; maintaining personal networks; participating in professional organizations.

5% 8. Accomplishes FECP goals by: accepting ownership for accomplishing new and different requests; exploring opportunities to add value to job accomplishments.

Job qualifications are already stated as Essential Functions in the job description. The Essential Functions are what an employee must be able to accomplish in order to be competent in the job.

Source: Forsyth Early Childhood Partnership.

Chapter 5

Operating Your Service Delivery System

It may seem that preparation is never ending, but there comes a time when the group senses that it is time to get going. Now the partnership commits time, resources, and especially money in earnest; plans turn to activity. Though it has picked its way through the suggested process, the partnership is well prepared to begin appropriately, probably slowly and relatively small, but with great dreams for the future. It will continue to pick and choose its way through the operations phase. What remains is the organizing effect of a process that causes necessary attention to detail without people being overwhelmed to a standstill by the bulk of work. Planning, though vitally necessary and good, can never take the place of action. Every successful person understands this. Colin Powell (2001) says it best: "You don't know what you can get away with until you try" (p. 5).

DEVELOP AN ORGANIZATIONAL STRUCTURE AND HUMAN CAPITAL

When the organization is being developed, the infrastructure to get things done is being created; the partnership is developing the capacity to do work. This is the support for the partnership's services. The partnership may want to consider logistics: the things, supplies, and equipment needed to get the job done. Naturally, the partnership will need policy on how it wants to work with contractors, its partners, and its collaborators. Evaluation needs to begin on the first day of operation. Most important, the partnership needs to consider how it will develop its key internal stakeholders, its staff, and its board. In keeping with the brevity of these effective practices we will address a few of the more important things to do to organize operations, beginning with organizational structure.

Design a Functional Organizational Structure

Practically speaking, the partnership begins small. At the outset the executive director will be the lead for all functions, with "marching orders" coming from the board of directors through board committees. The executive director then directs contractors, consultants, fiscal matters, administration, and programs.

As success demands more support, a partnerhsip may want to pattern its organizational diagram after larger operations. In keeping with promoting a collegial working atmosphere, the Forsyth Partnership is organized functionally and in teams (see Figure 5.1). In fact Forsyth displays a link to the governor, to the North Carolina Legislature, the North Carolina Partnership, and then its board of directors. The board in turn directs internal committees, program committees, contracts, and the executive director. Note the internal and program committees. This is a superior way to provide oversight and involvement of leadership. Here the board is subdivided into the following committees: Executive, Personnel, Allocations, Finance, Strategic Planning, Leadership Development, and Fund Development. All critical tasking is headed by a committee. Programs, the services provided, likewise get the committee treatment:

Figure 5.1
Organizational Team Chart

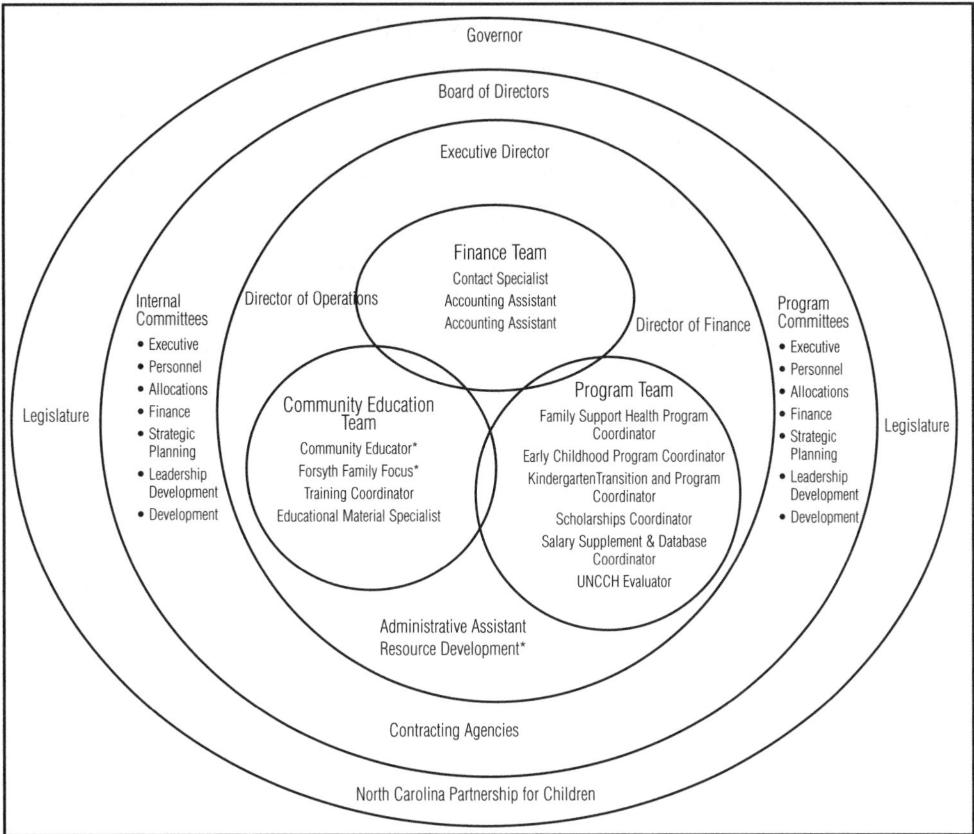

Early Childhood Education, Family Support, Health, Community Involvement, Strategic Planning (not the same as the organizationally focused committee), and Facility Development. The executive director is supported by department directors and teams. The executive director has a director of operations in charge of the program and community information teams and a finance director in charge of the finance team. Every key service has just enough oversight and support to direct, nurture, and deliver performance-based services to the greatest need.

Develop Human Capital

Human capital is valuable capital. Although there is a personal, personable element to successful staff building, there is a process to lead, recruit, train, retain, and develop a first-class cadre of staff. As with all parts of successful project building, human resources development is a continual process that begins with the vision statement, long before the first advertisement for help is posted.

Job Posting; First Interview. In the planning stage, the partnership began putting staff together by describing essential staff positions, outlining duties and responsibilities, and agreeing on a pay and benefits package that is as competitive as possible, as discussed and illustrated in in Chapter 4, Exhibit 4.14 (in this volume). At this stage the job search begins, with a job posting that reflects the education, experience, knowledge, and skills required to realize the partnership's vision. Ideally, a good pool of qualified applicants respond. The first interview, conducted by a team of stakeholders, verifies strengths, weaknesses, qualifications, and assesses the desire to tackle a tough but rewarding "career." Note here that *career* is emphasized as the team building begins from the first contact with the prospective team member; working with the partnership is a long-term opportunity to do good. Much will be demanded from everyone on staff, but only in direct proportion to what one earns in satisfaction from the work. It is important to note that in most nonprofits, a committee of the board interviews for the executive director position and makes recommendations to the board. For staff, the executive director has sole hiring and firing responsibility. It generally works better that way.

The Second Interview. The second interview, again conducted by a team that includes the executive director, looks at the finalists, who have passed background and reference checks. The selected candidate is not only the most qualified for the job but has the qualities demanded by the position and can fit into the culture of the partnership. More than that, this person overwhelmingly demonstrates the "fire" necessary to succeed as a part of a real team effort with real consequences for the community. Getting to the accepted offer is only the first step of staffing.

New-Hire Orientation. In keeping with the concept of human capital development, a new hire is "treated like an adult" from the first day. The first day is usually spent with the human resources (HR) director (or executive director if there is no HR director on staff, as in a small partnership), who provides an orientation checklist of items that includes a visit with key staff to go over corporate values, the vision, and mission. Orientation lets new hires know where they fit into the scheme of things and how to navigate the nuts and bolts of organizational bureaucracy; orientation kick-starts the new hire's acclimatization to the environment and culture of the partnership in its unique position in the community. The new hire is also given an orientation binder of policies, standard operating procedures, and pertinent information and a schedule of events that ensures that the new hire has complete understanding of how things operate.

The First Year. During the first year, the new hire is taken under the wing of a formal, detailed personnel development process, with formal, written follow-up based on the policies of the partnership and the agreed individual performance measures for each staffer. This is often on a ninety-day, six-month, and one-year sequence. Employee and supervisor mutually agree on tasking, performance measures, goals, and personal/professional development, which, after the first year is done on an annual basis. Specifically, a self-review evaluation instrument can be used. The Down East Partnership, for example, has one that covers the following:

- *Accomplishments.* The three most outstanding accomplishments or strengths of the past three months;
- *Areas of improvement.* The three areas in which the employee could improve to increase overall effectiveness;
- *Professional goals.* Three professional goals for the next three months with a list of objectives to achieve each goal; and
- *Desired training.* A list of training needed to accomplish goals.

During the first year, a career progression and professional development plan can be written. After the first year, the employee can have a chance to suggest how the job description can be revised to reflect what he or she discovered about getting the job done in the dynamic of an environment in flux. While this may seem like a commonsense thing to do, it is rarely done even though it is one of the marks of a successful human capital development plan and a successful operation.

Adopt a Philosophy of Continuous Human Capital Development. Every aspect of people management is an opportunity to improve production and expansion for the organization and the individual. People are given a remarkable amount of necessary oversight and freedom to do their jobs and to grow.

There are as many ways to design a wholesome staffing program as there are partnerships; yours will be unique, fashioned as dictated by unique resources, individual personalities, and local environment. Still, it is helpful to learn from a mature program. For that we suggest some of the personnel development tools used by the Down East Partnership. It is good to observe that much of a partnership's evolution is dictated by circumstance. For example, the Down East Partnership had to completely restaff and add ten people when they were asked to help a massive recovery effort after a major natural disaster. Note also the versatility this represents on the part of a well-run partnership. Just think where the community might be without a partnership in place to help handle initial disaster relief and years of recovery. Thus, a partnership should begin with the hiring process as outlined previously and then consider the following:

- *Retention.* Keeping staff is constant work. Aside from significant input from the employee about job design, decent benefits, and training, time must be spent on development. The partnership has two staff development retreats per year: one on-site and one off-site. Each is devoted to skills and professional training, and, of course, a hefty dose of fun.
- *Staff training development teams.* The partnership should put together a team, including the HR director, the community fellows coordinator, and the program development specialist, whose sole purpose is to devise, lead, and conduct staff development events. Their goal is to improve providers, volunteers, and partnership staff according to a career development "map" for each specialty. They solicit employees for suggestions; hence there may be training topics such as "Machine of the Month," where all learn how to use a new postage machine.
- *Training events.* Aside from more formal retreats, there could be brown-bag lunches twice monthly where everyone pulls facilitator duty and each member gives updates on his or her progress or lack thereof in his or her particular sphere of responsibility. Such lunches are a remarkable team-building tool that also builds esprit de corps.
- *Internal self management.* If it can be afforded, a consultant can be a great help in getting the organization on track. The Down Ease Partnership worked with a consultant on Program Review for Internal Self-Management (PRISM), which put the team on the path to continuous improvement, performance orientation, and goal attainment.

Relative to staffing, it will be apparent when a partnership has the right mix. There is a real sense of energy at the well-working partnership; staff are always in a constant state of agitation about "all the stuff" they have to do.

There is never a spare moment, because all are gainfully employed, productive, and enjoying their labors.

HIRE STAFF COLLABORATIVELY

"Good leaders stack the deck in their favor right in the recruitment phase" (Powell, 2001, p. 10). Colin Powell goes on to comment on the goal of picking the right people: "Look for intelligence and judgment, and most critically, a capacity to anticipate, to see around corners. Also look for loyalty, integrity, a high energy drive, a balanced ego, and the drive to get things done" (p. 10).

Does such a person really exist? Yes. And the hiring process will bring this person to the team. During the planning phase, staffing has been anticipated from developing a pool of qualified applicants to retirement. Now the plan is put to work. It is a good idea to have initial interviews done by a team of at least two people. Consider carefully a list of questions that determines minimum qualifications and, more important, the "desire" spoken of by Powell. Avoid the first mistake of the screening interview: do not talk too much. This is the prospect's moment. The interviewer has very little time, sometimes little more than a half hour, to determine whether this person is the kind of person with whom the partnership wants to spend a considerable part of its life! Give the prospect an overview of the duties and responsibilities expected and the courtesy of knowing when a hiring decision will be made.

At the Halifax-Warren Partnership, the executive director looks for the following in a prospective teammate:

- *"Complementary" personality.* This is a person who complements the multiple personality of the partnership. Note also that, especially in a smaller operation, the addition of one more person actually changes the personality of the whole operation.
- *Look for individual "personality."* You want a person who is professional, interesting, engaging, and works hard at doing the right thing, yet knows when to compromise in the best interest of the team, with respect to the vision.
- *Independent thought.* Creativity is most helpful because many components of the job and the process for handling each job element will have to be "invented" by the staffer.
- *Multitalented.* Staffers will be required to do more than their assigned duties; they have to be willing and able to do so.
- *Image.* Can this person promote the "image" of the organization? Does this individual personify the image you need?
- *High standards.* A job well done is as simple as good timing with a well done memo; is the candidate up to this subtlety?

- *Humility.* You don't want someone who constantly needs kudos and recognition.
- *Appreciation of the diverse.* The partnership is one of the most diverse environments in the public sector; the new hire must appreciate this.
- *Professionalism.* All of the above help to describe the level of professional the partnership needs.

Everyone in the partnership has to feel comfortable with staff choices. It is important to take time to select people without being afraid to begin the solicitation again until there is a choice or two whom the interviewer is quite sure will become a productive part of the team. Note that there is never a perfect choice, but there are usually good choices. Again Colin Powell (2001) says it best: "Organization doesn't really accomplish anything. Plans don't accomplish anything, either. Theories of management don't much matter. Endeavors succeed or fail because of the people involved. Only by attracting the best people will you accomplish great deeds" (p. 6).

So much is implied by this insight. At every successful partnership studied, we observed an executive director who was immersed in the work of the staff. It is fair to say that this was a large priority for these directors, if not the main priority of daily operation. They always had a moment to recognize, assist, work with, or otherwise be materially involved with their people. For example, at an impromptu pot-luck at the Halifax-Warren Partnership offices, the executive director brought and served the perfect homemade chicken salad. It was a simple thing, one among many dishes, but just imagine the building of esprit de corps, the strengthening of purpose, that happened that day.

The people who do the everyday work, no matter how talented, must have early, close, and relentless attention. It is a sweaty art. How does the leadership of the partnership ensure that people get the work done without smothering them? How will the partnership have necessary attention to detail without burning out the fire of inspiration that brings staffers to public work in the first place? How does the partnership ensure compliance with myriad rules and regulations and allow autonomy? Enough has been written and said about leadership, management, and administration of staff to fill libraries; thus no more can be added here. Those who define this process as beginning with the first interview will succeed. Those who do not will have a tough time of it.

ORIENT AND TRAIN KEY STAFF; CONCENTRATE ON CAREER PROFESSIONAL DEVELOPMENT

Molding individuals, as different as can be, into a single-minded purpose is not passively applying the latest personnel management fad. It is an intense process that is seamless and continuous. Next in the flow of process is how the new hire is welcomed. Aside from having the work space ready for production, new staff must be thoroughly oriented for a warm and efficient nestling into the pattern of daily operations and into a mutually agreed on career development plan as quickly as possible.

Orient Thoroughly

A thorough orientation exposes, as quickly as necessary, the new person to how he or she contributes to the vision and mission and fits in the organization and what information he or she needs to get through the day. Put yourself in the newcomer's shoes, take time with the jargon and acronyms, and allow time to assimilate to space and pace. Use a checklist so that it orientation is done thoroughly. Also, as with most things that are documented, the checklist will be edited over time to reflect the growth and dynamics of the operation. Orientation is the time when new staffers meet all coworkers and locate the break room, the restroom, and the parking spot. It is a great way to demonstrate the "people place" mentioned during the interview. Simply, it gets the new person off on the right foot.

Specify a Plan for Career/Professional Development

Have a career development plan ready for implementation. Everyone needs additional skills training, classroom education, and professional experiences. One way to do this is to chart your staff, discuss expectations, and actually schedule the first one or two training or development experiences; this demonstrates eagerness for and support of personal development for that individual. This chart may be delineated into initial, intermediate, and advanced training; recommended education (college courses); and professional development (workshops and conferences). Initial training may be a local community overview of how the community functions, who is who, and the role of the partnership within the communities it serves. For initial training, public speaking, how to do a site visit, computer skills, and perhaps conflict resolution can also be considered. Clearly, recommended initial training depends on the job and skill requirements. Education and professional training topics suggested include early childhood development and perhaps a certification in nonprofit management. Certainly it can include training on community development and grant writing and perhaps a workshop on funds development. A great place to look for superior training and education is the local university or community college, which may have a continuing education department.

What matters is that staff are not left to wonder about how to get the job done. Be explicit about expectations and give them the tools to meet them. Orientation and training are not enough; staff need regular, formal feedback on how they are doing and how to improve.

Begin Performance-Based Personal Evaluation

It is tough to say one personnel action is more important than the next, but right at the top of things to do for staff is the personal evaluation process (as introduced in section "Develop Human Capital"). The best evaluation processes do a regular review, every ninety days within the first year, using an instrument that has a combination of quantitative and qualitative components. Have a list of desired behaviors that have a numeric score. Emphasize certain goals that the individual is to accomplish, that in turn aid mission accomplishment. Include a few mutually agreed on goals for personal development. The evaluation should then paint a picture of how that person works within the bureaucracy and contributes to overall purposes. At the same time, the personnel evaluation instrument is a tool to promote personal growth.

Once a personal evaluation instrument has been designed, the lessons learned and pattern can be applied to each specialty. It is laborious, and certainly more time is involved than simply invoking a "standard" evaluation. Make *personnel* policies and procedures *personal.*

JUSTIFY RESOURCES AND EMPHASIZE PERMANENT FUNDING VIA A DEVELOPMENT CAMPAIGN

We return inevitably and continually to money. Now is when the partnership puts its development plan to work and work it must. We never had an on-site interview with anyone connected with a partnership who did not have a comment on the pervasiveness and vital need for steady funding and support. No matter the size of the organization there are a few fundamentals of conducting funds development that apply universally.

Conduct Organized, Comprehensive Fund Raising

As mentioned previously, the first activity is to get the board materially involved by their giving and soliciting funds. Board members may want to begin early in the planning phase. The partnership may be the largest nonprofit in the county; still, that does not absolve leadership from giving and getting. Board members must be encouraged to give and to be ready to make fund-raising presentations on behalf of the effort, no matter how uncomfortable it may be for the member. If the partnership can afford it, it should contract the services of a development consultant. If it cannot afford it, the partnership should do the things a consultant would do, such as devising an annual campaign, getting worthy grant applications in the pipeline, training stakeholders on development, and developing donors. Make sure that every stakeholder group knows its role and that it must also work at getting funding. Schedule regular, frequent events designed to put money in the bank while promoting partnership goals. For example, an annual banquet is a great time, a culmination of the year, when successes can be celebrated, the vision and mission reaffirmed, goals reset, and targets for funding streams set.

Be aggressive and realistic. Be comprehensive but start with small and realistic goals, then grow to meet requirements. Remember, this is an activity that has to be approached as if the partnership's survival depends on the outcome, because it does.

Develop a Research-Based Project Performance Presentation

The basis of a successful funds development strategy is performance. There is no way around it. Partnership supporters and citizenry at large need and demand to know what their money and effort produce. More and more, simply reporting numbers is met with skepticism, even disdain. The partnership owes it to the project to demonstrate how people are affected, how and why they are bettered by all the expense and work. Here is where evaluation effort pays. Now, early on, it is impossible to demonstrate effect (i.e., how lives are being changed for the better). Nevertheless, the partnerhsip can and must show initial progress that will lead to changes which are felt in the community. Thus, initial evaluation results about numbers generated should be linked to goals and the vision. As quickly as possible, also show that these initial measures have rates of change and growth in positive directions. As the project matures the partnership will be able to present numbers on real improvements in the community (e.g., how children, especially those at risk, are doing in school and beyond). Notes should be peppered with the many vignettes about individual successes and triumphs that happen simply by being in the business of a partnership. Just don't make the whole presentation on these warm stories or solely on lists and charts of numbers.

Note that we are purposely avoiding a prescription for what a presentation should relate. This is an individual endeavor. One partnership's measures of success are indeed only that partnership's measures, which derive from the partnership's strategic planning process and self-evaluation program. A partnership has to tell its story and one of the best ways is to have a ready, current presentation that can be tailored to any audience for any presenter at a moment's notice.

Also remember that one of the most effective ways to tell a story is through the media.

DEVELOP KEY SERVICES ACCORDING TO NEED, STABILITY, ACCESSIBILITY, AND QUALITY

Services are the instruments of goal accomplishment. This is where vision and mission are realized, or not. The pool of available choices for services does not appear ready and able to be a viable, continuing part of the overall effort. This then is an important nuance of success: service projects are not chosen on past success alone. Their selection and continuation are based on mutually defined and agreed on multiple measures that demonstrate positive evolution and the "bottom line" issue of bettering the community. They must address an assessed need (which is discussed in more detail later). Still, service providers do not begin their collaboration with the partnership focused on a specified purpose and with the proper skills and orientation.

Projects begin their association with the partnership oriented primarily to the service in which they specialize. That is, they are geared and motivated to focus nearly all attention on getting their service on the street. This is not bad, but that focus alone, to the exclusion of focus on overall purposes, is at least distracting and is often debilitating. Via a process of selection, collaboration, and evolution, ideally, the service takes on a subtle but paramount change. It becomes a performance-based service. Each service has to produce change, by the numbers, that contributes materially to the partnership's vision and mission. It is a matter of understanding the basic characteristics of a well-working service, the philosophy of communal benefit, and the process that helps services become part of and contribute to the overall effort.

Define Characteristics of Key Services

When deciding essential services, there are three primary characteristics that guide selection: experience, performance, and targeting. Experience is the organizational infrastructure and qualified people to deliver a product over time. The lesson here is, be careful when considering a start-up service that the partnership may want to contract. Be prepared to give it a greater start-up effort and support to become what it should be, effective. It must produce results that are meaningful to targeted clients. In addition, it must focus on a certain group of recipients for its service. That focus should emphasize a developmental need. The Search Institute has research on developmental assets for children at various ages. These assets covering "opportunities, skills, relationships, values and self-perceptions" are most helpful in designing or contracting services (Search Institute, 1999). Thus the service recognizes that, for example, child care is different for the 0- to 4-year-old who needs good nutrition and health care than it is for the 4–5-year-old who needs preschool and extended child care, among other things, of course. Certainly needs vary as the child grows. The elementary school child has much different developmental needs than does the middle schooler. The at-risk child presents different needs than the child with disabilities and so on. Experience also suggests that the earlier a developmental need is addressed, the more long-term benefits it realizes. Note that the example of addressing developmental, age-specific needs of children also applies to the organization and the community. The earlier we address important or key issues the better; whether early in the maturation of the organization or early in the development of a social problem. Public services need to recognize that it is preferable to address services ahead of a problem with ability and resources defined by the maturational level of the organization addressing the concern. Just be aware there is no "cure-all," but there is the better strategy of a network, a continuum of projects which focus on age-specific needs.

Keep these things in mind as the partnership outlines essential services. Every service contracted must produce results. If it does not, it should be discontinued so another deserving project or projects can be done in its stead. A most wrenching part of operating a successful partnership is a matter of making difficult trade-offs. But the ability and courage to make those decisions is one of the hallmarks of successful community collaboration.

Generate Performance-Based Key Services

Now the partnership has a good idea of what services it would like according to a specific need in the community and what, generally, comprises a good service. From that, the partnership should generate a pool of possibilities. This is done with a Request for Proposals (RFP), which begins the granting process. The Forsyth Early Childhood Partnership has a superior RFP process and document. Before a discussion of the request details, one notices that the instrument specifies that demonstrated performance is an expectation of every service contracted. This written requirement teaches the prospective provider how to contribute to the overall goal; this is an example of the execution of the philosophy of results. Note also that the philosophy of results is then imbued in everything associated with the effort. No one has to repeat the fact that participants must be dedicated to developing children and must demonstrate their work is changing lives; everyone knows it. Now let's look at some noteworthy effective practices in a well-constructed RFP.

- *Cover sheet.* Right off, the cover sheet specifies the funding cycle and ironclad due date.
- *Overview page.* The first page is a hard-hitting fact sheet stating vision, mission, goals, and objectives. The prospect knows his or her idea for service must satisfy one or more of the stated purposes to have a chance of being awarded.
- *Core services.* The next page summarizes, in bullet format, core services, eligibility, restrictions, preferences, and monitoring requirements. Again, more prospects are filtered out of the pool, or if they continue in the process, they know the expectations and criteria with which they must comply.
- *Evaluation.* There is no mistaking expectations for performance as the next page stresses the importance of measurement and gives examples of progress for each area of focus.
- *Application form.* The form guides the prospect through required narrative and documentation to include suggestions for formatting and word limits. Even required attachments are listed. Program expectations are

outlined in bullet format and the project description is prompted by specific questions. The budget is simple and direct; every line item is explained and requires justification.

- *Application checklist.* The final page is a checklist to help the applicant through the process in a timely and complete manner.

Everything about the results-oriented RFP has explicit and implicit purpose. The form itself is an exercise in completeness and efficiency. When completed it paints an accurate picture of what the service is, how it contributes, and what it will cost. Efficiency here is paramount as someone, usually several people, have to read and consider every word in what is usually a large stack of completed proposals. Still, accurate decisions, with true impact, must be made from this brief snapshot of the heart of a project. But beyond what meets the eye, the RFP begins the shaping of service providers. The first contact prospects have with the partnership is via a piece of documentation that is at once demanding yet respectful. The prospect knows what is expected and thus realizes that it is an honor to be part of an operation that is doing good and vital things in the community.

Another way to ensure that service providers are doing what they need to do is via an external examination. In addition to getting academics and consultants to help with outlining and conducting evaluation and strategy, there are groups that accredit services, that is, apply standards and assistance or recommendations for achieving them. For example, the North Carolina Child Care Resource and Referral Network (NCCCRRN) offers such a service. Note that a quick search on the Internet using "Child Care Resource and Referral" (CRCR&R) yields the latest and pertinent information in child care. The partnership can link to such organizations as the National Association of Child Care Resource and Referral Agencies, the National Child Care Information Center, and the Child Care Bureau. Such agencies can link a partnership to the local service providers it may need. When a CCR&R service is accredited by an agency, as the NCCCRRN is, the process provides another avenue for promoting organizational growth: clients have additional assurance that services are as good as can be, that data are collected well and are meaningful, and that the agency has a long-range plan for growth. Your partnership may also want to consider having selected services accredited. The National Association of Child Care Resource and Referral agencies, easily found on the Internet, is a good way to link to your appropriate accrediting agency. Just enter your state for a complete listing.

Ensure That Each Service Contributes to Stability, Accessibility, and Quality

The Stable Service. Public services must have stability, accessibility, and quality. There needs to be a true shift in thinking when it comes to acquiring services. Initially exuberant community members just want to get going; their philosophy is that the money will come if the initiative starts. Hence, these individuals tend to want new projects nearly every year in the beginning of a collaboration. That mind-set has to change quickly. Having constantly changing projects needs to give way to focusing on core services and organizational stability. *This quite rightly puts project development ahead of project implementation.* This is an important point; let it sink in. Here are three tips to consider when developing a service with stability in mind:

- *Stability.* Look for a stable organization to implement the service, a group or individuals with a track record of successes, the more successes the better;
- *Reliability.* Look for reliable partners, partners with whom you have a productive working relationship and with demonstrated community commitment because their services will be your services for the long haul; and
- *Value.* Look for the best buy (get value for your dollar), look for partners who have established infrastructure to support your service requirements.

This philosophy leads to careful consideration of the implications of actions, especially related to acquisition of services. It also ensures necessary relationships with service providers that are essential for the often tedious process of growing the project. The focus is changed from short-term view, with all its attendant difficulties, to long-range vision, which is a much healthier perspective for the endeavor.

The Accessible Service. Another essential characteristic of a good service is access. Practically speaking, accessibility means taking the service to those who need it, not the other way around. First, the partnership needs to find out where its target groups are and who they are, via appropriate analysis and observation. Yes, it is nice to have scads of professionally analyzed data, but few communities have the luxury of time and resources to get expensive help for the needs assessment. It is good to have some well-done assessment of need which combines with "street" needs assessment, that which comes from experience and being aware of what one's community is saying. The Chatham County Partnership tracked demographics and used informal research methods to analyze where to place services. For example, staff looked at health department utilization rates. This is unorthodox but effective. Staff discovered a rapid rise in demand for public health services by the exploding Hispanic community. This initial insight led Smart Start to develop an array of outreach based programs that takes specialized services to the Hispanic population. These services are focused primarily on offerings in one city that has the largest growth and development. Limited resources were targeted for the best and most effect.

In another case Chatham Partnership staff plotted the source of requests for child care. Clusters of requests became obvious. At one such location a private party offered to develop a facility for child care. At first blush this would seem like great luck. But by understanding what makes a good service Chatham turned the offer down, as the potential child-care operator was uncommitted and unqualified. The local school was then successful in developing the needed child care. Children were provided accessible, quality early childhood education just by understanding who was most qualified to support the needed service. The needs analysis, ideally, will employ some methodologically sound data analysis and similar practical, quick, and effective techniques. What matters is getting a performance-based service where and when it is needed most.

The Quality Service. We have discussed quality and the history and experience of delivering a service that changes lives at various steps of the partnership-building process and why it is the final program characteristic in the hierarchy. By considering quality last, it is defined in terms of stability and accessibility, not the other way around. Experience bears out the wisdom of doing this. From the beginning, a partnership must have a clear expectation of deliverables and outcomes; with close attention to impact and process, quality will then be the result. Expect an iterative process as some goals will be met and others missed. The misses will suggest needed change and improvement. Be patient and vigilant, "keep your eyes on the prize," experienced staffers counsel.

The foregoing suggested process will help a partnership, over time, build a full complement of viable services. For an example of what can be achieved let us examine the Forsyth Early Childhood Partnership. From its inception in 1995 through 2000 it worked with 50 partners and 250 child-care and preschool programs to promote early childhood education, family support, health, transportation, and related services (Forsyth Early Childhood Partnership, 1999–2000). As Dean Clifford, executive director of Forsyth says, "Working together—parents, educators, political and business leaders, members of the community of faith, and all citizens—we can become successful in building a brighter future for both our children and our community."

INCORPORATE ANALYSIS AND EVALUATION—FOCUS ON PROCESS IMPROVEMENT AND RESULTS

Volumes have been printed and said about analysis and evaluation to the point of confusion. In essence, analysis is concerned with results, it is as simple as asking, "How am I doing?" or "What is changing?" The trick then is to listen carefully to the responses to the question and then, as important to listening well, act on the best suggestions. Evaluation is concerned with improving how work is done. It is as simple as asking, "How can we do better?" again with intent listening and inevitable action. There is one more question to ask, "How much is enough?" In any project, especially a local, community project, there is a tendency to work in a crisis mode, people come to work to put out fires and do what seems most urgent. Essential infrastructure building, like analysis and evaluation programs, is glossed over in the cacophony of getting through the day. Conversely, if this is a priority, there tends to be overkill. As with all things there needs to be balance. If we weave a tight and hard-hitting evaluation component into daily operations, it will get done. The return on investment of time and expense in this activity is repaid tenfold.

Promote Performance and Improvement

Understand also that results in the community are achieved over time and by resolute movement toward an array of meaningful goals. Work improves not by the overall management dictate. The material improvement is accomplished by doing every task just a little better at every opportunity. Both happen when leadership, staff, and providers hear the mantra of performance and improvement. Also in keeping with the theme of balance, understand the levels of investigation needed to get results and improve how things work.

The well-working program has internal and external analysis and evaluation. Internally, goal progress is analyzed, personnel have performance evaluations, and processes are regularly and perpetually questioned. Externally, performance standards are set and ensured with a schedule of monitoring visits and regular reporting. Actually, this part of operating the partnership is simple, if not relatively easy to do, if all are determined to have an evaluation program and have it part of daily work for everyone. Remember, the partnership needs analysis and evaluation, but just enough to ensure that it is efficient and effective, in other words, that the partnership succeeds overall. Learn to ask throughout the day, "How much is enough?" and "Is this thing I am doing now the most productive use of my time?"

The Chatham Partnership for Children is fortunate enough to have a full-time evaluator. The essential duties and responsibilities of this position are as follows:

- *Analysis*. Take the lead in preparing and writing local objectives and benchmarks for performance standards. Conduct data collection and analysis for statewide and local indicators. Facilitate data gathering for outside research projects and studies.
- *Evaluation*. Measure the impact of programs in the community in terms of numbers served and services received. We would like to point out that the local partnership frequently interprets "impact" in terms of numbers served and services received which just begins to tell the story of success. This suffices for reporting, resources allocation, and programming development which are primary concerns. External support and expertise

are needed to sponsor a long-term impact analysis which determines appropriate measures of success, how to document those data, if stated goals have been reached, and that there has been material benefit to targeted populations.

- *Reporting*. Submit quarterly program reports to the state. Prepare annual reports for the local board.
- *Program monitoring.* Conduct site visits to contracted programs and agencies. Ensure program deliverables are met.
- *Technical assistance.* Provide technical assistance to contracted programs to facilitate accurate program data collection. Share expertise with other evaluators as needed.
- *Needs assessment.* Conduct or assist with needs assessment by program area.
- *Auditing*. Ensure documentation for annual external audits.
- *Staffing*. Serve as staff representative for local partnership committees.

Make sure analysis, especially self-analysis, is promoted. Programs must report output (e.g., units or things produced) as well as outcome (desired behavioral change) data. When considering, for example, efforts to educate parents, the numbers served and the changes in those numbers over time, give an idea of output. Also, a sample of parents are given pre- and posttests to get feedback on program effects. Furthermore, they are given interviews to get an in-depth feel for how the program is helping.

Next, multipurpose and frequent site visits help ensure ongoing relationships. Checklists guide each visit whether it is for program performance monitoring or for fiscal purposes. The last program evaluation component of the Chatham Partnership is the countywide trend analysis (refer to the Smart Start Tool Kit: Evaluation, for an example of performance variables). The trend analysis graphically depicts where services exist and especially where they are needed.

Implement Performance Analysis

Make sure you are ready for evaluation. According to the Smart Start Evaluability Assessment Questionnaire (to order the Smart Start Tool Kit: Evaluation from the North Carolina Partnership for Children, check the Website, *www.ncsmart.org/Information/publications.htm*), you must first make sure you have gone through the following steps:

- Gain and hold support of your managers;
- Clarify partnership intent;
- Explore activity feasibility;

- Reach agreement on any needed changes in activity design;
- Explore alternative evaluation designs;
- Document policy and management decisions; and
- Proceed with evaluation activities.

Spend time fine-tuning measures for your organization and each program. Document baseline numbers for each and begin the continuous process of watching each one. Your evaluation program is under way.

Implement Process Improvement

The importance of improving daily work cannot be overstated. The operation simply must get better and better at what it does or it gets stuck in the consuming routine of unproductive busy work, the beginning of the end. Here we are talking about monitoring organizational operations and projects. We observed that the successful monitoring program is itself a continuous process. Program consultants are in constant touch with their respective projects. They are at their events, observing service delivery, and offering technical assistance. There are quarterly meetings to review performance measures for every project, goal by goal. If a project is not tracking well, remedial actions are discussed and the appropriate action is taken almost immediately.

For better or worse, the unspoken but possible reality is that a project can be abandoned if it does not contribute, materially, to the overall effort. In other words, if any effort does not contribute in quantity and quality to the vision, it either adjusts until it does or the partnership moves to a program that will.

The Monitoring Visit Project. This simple management tool, the monitoring visit, belies its sophistication, the work required to set it up and execute it, and the patience it takes for the pieces to bear fruit. It takes an expert understanding of management technique, automation, statistics, and the dynamic of working with a team of people. When it works well, everyone understands the goals to which they are tasked and how they are to strive toward them. Projects are designed and committed to making benchmarks happen. Reports are organized by every objective, detailed with commensurate benchmarks, and documented with the history, or lack thereof, of the progress made. No item is left to chance. More than that, all concerned can pull the latest progress report off the real-time database and tell the story of what is happening. That is project monitoring: hard-hitting teamwork that marches effort, resources, and money toward the vision.

The site visit should be conducted in an organized way to make sure all necessary details are covered and time is not wasted. The visit should communicate the message of efficiency and effectiveness by the way business is done. The Down East Partnership for Children has some of the following required entries on its site visit checklist:

- *Identifying information.* This is basic information that identifies the program, who is contacted, and the date.
- *Program activities.* This is a demonstration of what the program is doing such as handouts, brochures, records, and so on.
- *Fiscal.* Document the process for tracking funds. Look also for the process of collecting and tracking in-kind contributions.
- *Program successes and failures.* Note greatest strengths and weaknesses, what works, what does not, what changes are needed, and barriers to improvement. You may want to share stories and highlights.
- *Evaluation.* Note the actual tools used to measure the program. Collect evidence of process improvement and performance.
- *Issues/patterns/concerns.* Comment on what the future holds for the program, any concerns, and other pertinent observations.
- *Other questions.* This is an area for miscellaneous documentation and comment.

Additional Monitoring Components. Naturally, a partnership's checklist should reflect the partnership's needs. It is also an effective practice to have a form ready for the impromptu contact, say a phone call or an e-mail, where the staffer may want to document current activities, assets, and deficiencies; recommended actions; and when the next meeting is scheduled. Monitoring is necessarily interpersonal and needs the structure of process and one or two checklists to guide relationship building.

The process monitoring program, by way of example, done by Chatham County has the following additional components:

- *Technical assistance conferences.* Twice per year the partnership calls all stakeholders together to talk about performance. There is no conjecture about progress; hard numbers are presented for all to see and critique.
- *Audits.* State and private auditors investigate every aspect of function, not to find things wrong but to offer suggestions for how things can be made better. This is an important point not commonly understood by "inspectors." Make sure your project monitors, especially outsiders contracted to help with audits, understand that their task is one of construction not destruction. The philosophy of inspection is that there are no "problems," only opportunities for improvement.
- *Checklist for continuing activities.* This checklist specifies, program by program, item by item, the road to process improvement and results.

Why go through all this work? Because this is how a partnership justifies the worth of its work to its most important stakeholders—its beneficiaries. And its most important recipients are its youngsters. Note that the tendency for most analysis is to "demonstrate" productive activity to the adults that surround a project. While this is important, because adults do provide the fuel for the partnership to do business, adults will be more than satisfied and willing to support when children demonstrate positive development. Therefore, analyzing performance should, above all, determine if young lives are kept on the path to productive adulthood.

INTEGRATE INTO EXISTING ENVIRONMENT

By the time a partnership has gone through a rigorous planning process there will be much said in the community about what it is trying to do. Many people won't understand what the partnership is doing,; some will be extremely confused. Expect that all those who need to know about the partnership's efforts will not have even heard the first word about the partnership; yet it behooves the partnership to have a certain number of people and certain segments of the community-at-large aware of the work it is doing.

Develop and Execute a Plan to Integrate Into the Existing Environment

Consider, then, who absolutely needs to know about the partnership. Go sector by sector, public, private, and private nonprofit. Include in deliberation the media, faith community, citizen groups, philanthropies, businesses, and public service agencies. It is not necessary to be exhaustive at this stage, the partnership's work and successes over time will help get the word out. But without this initial effort at connecting, some key person, group, agency, or resource may be uninformed and may thus feel excluded and possibly present a future difficulty. Once a strategy for getting the word out is set, it is helpful to have a canned presentation, preferably electronic, ready to go. With a ready electronic presentation, obviously, every opportunity, scheduled or unscheduled, to talk about the partnership can be taken by just about any staff member from the board chair to the administrative assistant. Remember, if it is there, it will be used.

Orient Key Stakeholder Groups

Careful attention needs to be given to orienting key stakeholder groups. And a key stakeholder here is any entity that either provides or assists some way in the delivery of the services. Consider what was done in Chatham County when its partnership began. The Chatham County Partnership logged over 11,000 people hours of meetings in its first year. Each meeting was organized with an agenda and goals to be accomplished, making clear Chatham County's purpose and desired ends. Each new project had a collaborative of stakeholders who, aside from the business of developing services, got training and technical assistance workshops on, for example, how to write measurable objectives. The partnership board, which oversaw all the planning, participated in seminars on how the applicable state offices are organized and function. As many people as possible got leadership training because everyone was considered a leader. Furthermore, the successful partnership needs to work diligently to ensure that key stakeholders learn what is happening. It needs to emphasize working together by having professionally facilitated retreats where action items are written, assigned to a responsible party, and made to happen. There has to be reason to get along; too much is at stake.

Integrating into the partnership environment is an easily missed detail. The time and attention devoted, early on, to building strong relationships is key to defining a place in the community for the partnership. Once set up and readied, an orientation program is actually quite easy to do. After all, it is much better to build bridges from the outset than try to mend fences later.

ESTABLISH MECHANICS OF COMMUNICATION

A partnership is all about communication. It is easy to gloss over the need to establish formal structure to make sure information goes out and comes back. Partnership staff need communication tools in place to get and give vital information to fellow staff and the community at large. For example, if regular meetings are not set up that are pertinent, organized, and purposeful, things break down, the service suffers, or worse.

Design and Use Internal Communication Mechanisms

It is important to devote a little time to formalizing the mechanisms for information flow such that information moves freely down the chain of command and especially back. Develop a schedule that suits the partnership's purposes. Weekly and monthly staff meetings, quarterly board meetings, regular training meetings, retreats twice per year (one on-site, one off-site), memos, and e-mail are all useful communication tools. Beyond that, for example, some partnerships have bimonthly brown-bag lunches just to talk about more personal happenings, team meetings, or a staff newsletter. Naturally, each meeting should be formatted so there are the essential "facts, food, and fun." A meeting can be fun, but it must be organized or it dissembles. One partnership observed to us that a meeting should not be held just because it is scheduled. If the business does not materialize, cancel. There must be no excuse to waste even a moment. Moreover, the efficiency and effectiveness of each communication tool help set the tone for the workplace.

Design Minimal Reporting

There has to be daily data gathering, as discussed previously. But the partnership should ake time to produce professional looking, meaningful reports.

At the very least there should be monthly, quarterly, and annual reports. Note also that the good report begins with purpose and evolves to suit the needs and dynamic of the operation. There are numerous examples of superior reports that compel good business and progress. Just make sure yours does the same.

Design and Use External Communication Mechanisms

The same applies when the partnership takes its message to the street. Every partnership should have a series of communication mechanisms that are formatted and organized for efficiency and effectiveness and then use them. In addition to the foregoing, your partnership may want to consider the following:

- Newsletter;
- Website;
- Tour packet;
- Brochures;
- Regularly scheduled community education forums;
- Membership to the local speakers bureau;
- Designating a community spokesperson;
- Assigning a staff person to a specific market/segment of the community;
- News articles and media interviews; and
- Stakeholder coordinators.

WRITE OPERATIONAL GUIDELINES

The well-working partnership documents procedures. This saves a remarkable amount of time as those things that are standard do not have to be revisited. Once documented, they can be edited and streamlined to suit the purposes and reality of operating the partnership. Established partnerships have a series of standard operating procedures in the following areas:

- Human resources;
- Board development;
- Contractor development;
- Constituency development;
- Evaluation;
- Fiscal management;
- Contracts management; and

- Facility and equipment needs/management.

The partnership should begin its procedures manual by getting examples, pro forma, from a similar organization, usually an established nonprofit organization. Decide on an overall format. Some of the best ones state purpose, assign responsibility, and then detail the procedures in as few words as possible. A good idea from the field is to assign the drafting responsibility to the appropriate board subcommittee and staff. Keep in mind here that it is impossible to have a rule and regulation to cover every contingency. Good staffers make the right decisions when the complexities of environment and the human condition present the unique situation. To sum up the partnership perspective, it does not matter how good a service provider the partnership is; if it is not a good businessperson first, it does not matter. In other words, if the partnership does not know its business, it is out of business.

BUILD YOUR PARTNERHIP TO LAST

Even the extensiveness of this suggested community-building process merely alludes to the amount of work and commitment such a project demands. But if the partnership has followed a process, it has come from inspiration via perspiration to being an accepted and viable part of community infrastructure that provides needed services. Yet the work is still not done. The partnership's work thus far gives the partnership a unique view and understanding of what the neighborhood requires to be adequately served. It is a view that comes only from this type of work and not before. Thus it is incumbent on the partnership to look at community needs and continue the building process to address them. The next chapter addresses closing the gap between needs and services that exists in all communities.

References

Forsyth Early Childhood Partnership. (1999–2000). *Anuual report* [On-line]. Available: *www.forsythchild.org.*

Powell, C. (2001). *A leadership primer* [On-line]. Available: *www.freepages.military.rootsweb.com/-rootsrus/powell.html.*

Search Institute. (1999). *Developmental assets* [On-line]. Available: *www.search-institute.org.*

Chapter 6

Expanding Your Service Delivery System

The expansion stage of developing and offering public services is the state of operational maturation to which vital projects should strive and few attain. When an idea is fortunate enough to be realized, it is only after a huge expenditure of time, resources, and reputation. The people who bring a partnership to fruition are justified by any measure to continue at their initial operational level. Much more gets done than ever before simply by the partnership's survival to the second or third year. But, in fact, this expansion phase is the stage of development to which the partnership has been working, where the partnership as community leadership wants to be. The brutal planning phase has yielded a good operational plan. The actual operation of the plan, improved by the fire of daily reality, has resulted in a range of targeted services being delivered to the neediest in the community. While the partnership is still demanding to operate and funding is a constant nemesis, but old services must evolve, new services must be developed, and the staff and the board are in a constant state of evolution. The organization is now uniquely positioned to make a palpable, overall difference in the community by reaching, as capability permits, increasing numbers of the neediest families and their children.

From the vantage point of an operational service delivery system, the partnership can now identify and, most important, address the gap between service needs and available services and resolutely address more and more of the assessed needs of the community as a whole. This is the stage at which the partnership evolves from being a revered part of the community to being a significant leader for the community. As with each previous stage, process is important. How the partnership is expanded will be unique to the environment; what matters is that that the partnership does expand in a logical and determined fashion.

STABILIZE THE INITIAL EFFORT

Initial operation is largely the work of figuring things out for the first time. In other words, the business is developed. This is a far cry from addressing the assessed need of a local community. Until now, the partnership has only scratched the surface of answering the questions of how much of what should be delivered to whom. This is not the time to acquire additional services for the sake of just offering more. Hard-won expertise and networking are brought to bear on identifying true needs, and then those needs are answered with a permanent solution as slowly, methodically, yet resolutely as is needed to continue the process of building solid infrastructure under the services offered. First the partnership must be stabilized; what follows are a few of the essentials.

Ensure Performance Orientation and Narrow the Scope

It is fair to say that the entire partnership, thus far, has been built on performance. Every effort has to have a return on investment. When it comes to expansion, performance orientation needs to be reaffirmed to ensure that this basic element continues philosophically and practically. Take time to make sure that indeed every aspect of operation has a performance perspective. Does the human capital development program have performance as part of hiring, training, development, and retention? Is the board comfortable with performance and the expectation for it in services acquisition and development? Are contractors and constituents likewise versed in the partnership expectations for performance? Are budgets and contracts designed to reflect a return on the funds spent? The partnership must also be realistic about expectations for what a performance orientation should and can do for the all-around effort.

It is important to revisit the place performance has in overall development because it represents a real change in thinking for all key stakeholders. Whether it be a staff member, a board member, an agency official, or a service provider, all have been accustomed to reading lists of numbers to determine whether a public project is doing well; the more numbers the better it goes (or so this wrong-headed mentality may lead us). In the past, few stakeholders, if any, ever expected to be looking for behavior to measurably change as a result of their efforts. In a well-designed activity, outcomes (changes in behavior of clients) are much more important than outputs (numbers served). It is a critical stage of development that all stakeholders grasp the meaning of these two terms, understand the difference, and begin to emphasize the expected outcomes. And to be perfectly clear here, the goal is citizenship via improved lives, preferably measurable improvement in the lives of our young neighbors.

In other words, when thinking has changed from output to outcome, the partnership is on the right track. Performance is dynamic and its measures change as the endeavor matures; therefore, expectations for performance need to be realistic. Too much academic input confuses the issue of performance. It is valuable and should be sought, but only to clarify policy and procedure. Thus, it is best to strike a middle-of-the-road understanding about what results the partnership wants. For example, a service may start by tallying numbers as long as there is a view to reaching those in need and making certain aspects of their lives better. The partnership should not be too ambitious; for some programs, simply doing what they said they would do is a satisfactory initial result. It is enough to help these programs evolve into true performance orientation over time.

Ensure Client Focus

Policy, procedures, rules, and regulations often determine what can be done. Dictates can be quite restrictive. Thus, a partnership must understand its clients: partnership collaborators and partners, service providers, agency clients, the community, parents, and children. Just ask if the partnership is really satisfying their needs. A good point of departure is for the partnership to try to do what is right for the common good with an understanding of the needs of each group. Then the partnership must do what can be realistically accomplished. Some progress is better than no progress no matter how noble the goal may be. The move to institutionalize client focus is gradual and ongoing. It is a basic business tenet that client orientation needs to be considered as an ongoing process that should be reflected in every aspect of partnership operation.

Ensure Efficient/Effective Operational Procedures, Especially Human Capital Development

Review all operating procedures for efficiency and effectiveness, especially regarding staff. We previously remarked that the success of the partnership effort rests on many things but primarily on staff. With that in mind, the partnership should revisit how it develops that vital capital. The partnership may want to have an annual review of all personnel procedures. It may want to achieve an atmosphere of cooperation and collaboration for personal and professional growth. Again, this takes time and vigilance for it to happen. Likewise, when considering expanding the operation, money and its steady acquisition are paramount.

SECURE PERMANENT FUNDING

Simply put, the partnership cannot expand without funding streams as steady and reliable as possible. But, as with the previous two phases of the Project Life Cycle, funds development evolves as the partnership seeks to expand programming. In this phase the partnership should try to have as many permanent sources of funding as possible. A motivating goal is to try to wean the partnership from federal and state grant funds even though the partnership will never, nor should it ever, completely shun those sources. The point is, if the partnership is completely dependent on grant funds it is subject to remarkable bureaucracy, requirements, and, worst of all, the uncertainty of continuation. Most grants are awarded for only a year or two; just enough to begin a project, not to stabilize it. It is just good business to have alternative sources of money in place. The point is clear here: The partnership should use grants; it simply should try not to depend on grants entirely.

Before expanding the partnership base, the partnership has been through planning a development strategy and starting that plan. During planning the partnership outlined a funding campaign mentality that involves every stakeholder and stakeholder group, especially leadership. The partnership planned to tap a range of sources with a range of solicitation techniques. And, just as important, the partnership has an automated financial accounting system to keep track and report on every dollar that funnels through the operation. When the partnership began operations, it put the plan to work and based the campaign on performance, accomplishment, and successes, knowing that achievement in the community meant success in the bank. Now as the partnership expands, it is time for us to review a mature campaign to suggest how the partnership might improve its solicitation process.

Review Solicitation Process

Working "the money issue" never gets easier. In fact, as an operation matures, so do money problems. In a small community, especially one dependent on state or federal funding, we often find the attitude that money does not have to be developed. This is a critical negative attitude as (nearly inevitably) funding fluctuates with the economy and elections. Every aspect of the grant-dependent partnership can be threatened with reduction or elimination. Just think of all the promises disappointed because services collapse. Another problematic attitude arises from many recipients of state funds: They often feel they are "entitled" to the largess. Consequently, their outlook reflects the expectation of easy money; there is no hunger to perform and return effort to the community. Even the people responsible for applying for a grant reflect a risky bent.

Initially, the attitude toward grants is often that a grant is something to be "gamed"—a grant is seen as an end in itself. People assume grantsmanship is just "getting a grant" whereas the attitude really needs to be one of developing an idea where earning a grant or source of funding is just part of the much larger process of infrastructure building and performance-oriented service delivery. This idea should always be preeminent; the grant is only part of the larger body of work to make an idea reality. As mentioned earlier, local leadership often persists in promoting and committing to new programs before the contracted services are stabilized. With this mentality, it becomes nearly impossible to get additional contributions for justified staff and support. Some people are turned off to the whole process of granting as those dollars are designated as "start-up" funds. Such people have difficulty facing the real work of putting services on individual funding streams and they abandon or minimize work in granting and project nurturing. These problems have an insidious nature of which every partnership needs to be aware. Their resolution lies in leadership and the well-organized solicitation campaign.

Strengthen Funds Development Campaign

Simply, revenue sources need to be diversified. Grants are temporary. Local dollars help keep decisions local. And prudent financial management calls for a general operating fund. Alternative funding is then used for funding gaps in grant cycles and payments, a contingency fund for emergencies that threaten the financial health of the partnership, and further operational and financial development. There are many sources to be plumbed to get dollar depth beyond a grant. The Vancouver Citizen's Committee (2002), for example, offers the following new ways to address old sources and a few additional possibilities your partnership may not have considered:

- *Individual contributions.* Money can come from memberships, voluntary subscriptions to a newsletter, collections at meetings, door-to-door canvassing, planned giving, memorial giving, and direct mail.
- *In-kind donations.* Only usefulness guides this source. Such giving includes donations of printing, equipment, furniture, space, services, food, and especially time—volunteer time.
- *Auctions.* At a big community party, the auctioneer sells some really creative things; how about ice cream for four at the local soda shop.

- *Grants from foundations.* Philanthropy is alive and well. Look on the web or subscribe to a philanthropy magazine for all manner of charitable organizations.
- *Charging fees.* Consider charging targeted fees.

Another partnership added to this list with real creativity. The Ashe County Partnership for Children started an endowment with the help of local banks, which also lent expertise and services (Smart Start Tool Kit: Planning: *www.ncsmart.org/Information/publications.htm*). The point is to put together what is doable for your community and your situation.

It all comes together in the campaign. The Forsyth Early Childhood Partnership[1] has "Journey to the Stars" and the Down East Partnership[2] has "Building Brighter Futures." Both evolved over five years of experimentation; both are effective. They have an aggressive grant production system, that is a given. What is interesting is how they work on those alternative sources of support:

- *Strategic plan.* This document projects five years into the future. It specifies an annual review and revision to clarify the view of partnership work. There is a reassessment of needs, a resetting of priorities, and refinement of objectives and benchmarks. Needed services are prioritized for acquisition at various funding levels. It is a document that communicates challenge and optimism on every page.
- *Development committee.* Leadership is institutionalized in the organization by designating a standing committee to concentrate on fund raising.
- *Community solicitation.* An annual mass mailout, including a refrigerator magnet, targets various levels of giving. In keeping with the "Journey to the Stars" theme, contributors can participate in a "constellation" of gifts from "Twinkle Twinkle" (children's campaign for less than $25) to the "Big Dipper" ($25,000 and above). Furthermore, each level is put in terms of what the money accomplishes for the partnership in the community, not as an expense to the donor.
- *Web site.* The Internet is mandatory as web site engineering is nearly elemental and a small price to pay to have such a large payoff of access to markets and participants. The best are professional, fun, and engaging and keep with the theme of opportunity for all to feel good about doing something good for their community.
- *Corporate giving.* Here a face-to-face meeting gets to the "give" in terms business understands. Board designees and staff present facts on contribution to community, how business can be involved, the business sense of doing so, and the "profit" realized from various levels of giving. Every corporate benefactor remains informed as to how its "investment" is doing because there will be another visit and another request to give.

- *In-kind and volunteerism.* Specific needs, from hanging files to stackable trays for lunches, are specified for every program, as is the donor of the item. There is no question as to what the needed item is and its purpose.
- *Communication tools.* Every media (oral, written, and electronic) is professionally employed. In addition to the web, flyers, electronic and slide presentations, annual reports, and staff are primed to stand at the ready.
- *Anniversary celebration.* To cap it all off, Forsyth had a gala five-year anniversary celebration. The program, which was very upbeat with most memorable quotes and pictures of children, is still used as an historical document of accomplishment, recognition, and possibilities.

Again this is what works for two locations in North Carolina. A variation will work for your partnership. Note also that there is an additional reason for this obsession with funding. Money means possibilities. When there is a range of resources coming in, there is a palpable lift to the pulse of operations. It is not only exciting to work with others doing good things, but it is mutually motivating. Furthermore, although your partnership may focus on anything from hurricane relief to juvenile delinquency, there is nothing as universally uplifting as focusing on the youngest of children. Be encouraged; there is money out there. We heard at one time, "If money is a problem, there is no problem." Now, that is optimism, and success is not far behind.

ESTABLISH A LONG-RANGE PLANNING/GUIDANCE BODY

Maintain a Stable Board

As with most key partnership action, the obvious evades attention with less than happy consequences. Therefore, we revisit leadership for a good reason: The board tends to lose its edge; the excitement of the new gives way to the work of maintaining a presence. At this stage of coalition growth, the executive director, chair, and committee chairs have to work to keep the board engaged and involved. In some cases, board members should be asked to relinquish their seats if they cannot make the transition from start-up to maintenance. The board, with the help of the executive director, has to guard against those who want to continue the excitement of doing novel things at the expense of doing well with what has been started. That is, the focus is more and more on stability and quality of service in the mature collaborative. The high-functioning board should include people with each of three important personality types:

- *Idea person.* There still needs to be an infusion of ways to achieve the mission.
- *Resource person.* Board members still need to have connections.

- *Worker bee/maintainer.* The business of leadership is not all meetings and dictates. Board members have to do a certain amount of work. These individuals understand how to stabilize operations to the dual whips of efficiency and effectiveness.

The insight here is that the board is never completely mature. It is in a constant state of beginning because term limits and normal turnover are always factors. The pitfalls of this inevitability can be mitigated with planning and education.

Orient, Train, and Develop the Board for Expansion

Leadership also needs a plan that anticipates this "mood swing" of the board as leaders have to change their mind-set from one of planning the new to maintaining the old. First of all, the executive director has to be ready and able to work with whoever shows up for a meeting. The composition of nearly every board meeting is different as these busy people have a difficult time with all their obligations. The point here is that business cannot back up to catch up the irregular attendee. The board chair can help manage the board by participating in orientation and assigning senior members as mentors and sponsors of the new members. The chair can also meet with individual members between meetings to keep them informed and intent on the business at hand. The executive director can facilitate the board's "self-policing" nature by enforcing bylaws, having a thorough orientation of new members, and endorsing appropriate development (especially self-prescribed professional development), when pertinent. They should each have a core of knowledge:

- *Roles, responsibilities, and operation of the nonprofit.* Board members need to understand that they are not to micromanage the operation; they are the keepers of the vision and mission and work with policy.
- *Legal aspects of the nonprofit.* Code determines much of what can be done; board members must master the basics of the law and understand their legal status as board members, including fiduciary responsibilities.
- *Partnership collaboration.* Partnership is collaboration; it is the art and science of it that take time and study.
- *Program operation.* Key leadership must know how to build service infrastructure and what makes a good service.
- *Strategic planning.* Planning for the long haul is a major function of the board. Training is a must, because planning that works has complexities.

A Shift in the Board's Role. These few ideas will help leadership understand and cope with maturation from a start-up to an operational, expanding corporation. At this stage, the board has moved from writing policy to managing and revising it; from making recommendations to passing judgment on staff suggestions. Each board member must understand this real and necessary role shift.

Any senior executive or community leader worth his or her regular paycheck is expert at laying out a course of action by establishing a hierarchy of action, whether it be in a five-year plan or by a daily to-do list. But in the most exemplary collaborations, essential functions have what appear to be equal emphasis. How can ordered items be equal? It happens with the elegant distribution of resources, especially time, toward each of these essential operational and planning tasks.

This equalization of essential priorities evolves, as does the well-working organization, over time. Thus we see real, productive energy devoted to targeting clientele, cementing relationships with selected partners, focusing on communities of need, building leadership, and making money happen. This kind of service agency intimately knows the clients it serves, especially collaboratives that serve children. It is obsessed with making a difference right down to the full-length dressing mirror in the restroom which is positioned at floor level so the little ones can check their look. Now that is attention to appropriate detail; it sends the message of client orientation and consideration to service that is loud and clear.

"Governing" the Board. The effective community collaborative does not merely court movers and shakers for their help, resources, and time; it "grows" them. Position in a company is not a ticket to the board. Board members begin perhaps as committee participants. They build up to their positions after demonstrating passion, commitment, and will on the job. They are constantly challenged to do more, and they respond. There are no titular assignments. Again, an equal share of oversight energy is devoted to this critical organization leadership-building task. Some organizational development pundits put people, staff development, at the head of the to-do list at the expense of other work. Somehow the exemplary local organization also elevates the nurturing of its leadership team to the top of its to-do list also. This equalizing of priorities is neither art nor science; it is a product of patient, deliberate work.

Many communities need the sanity of a central organization and distribution point for key services. Only those in need and with a will to help themselves are courted. It is not enough to merely want to improv. A community must want to build itself up, then the partnership assists in the community's efforts to become well and wholesome, as a collaborative team; this is leadership.

DETERMINE SERVICE-TO-NEEDS GAP

More and more we hear of the desire that services in the public sector be research based, yet, when we attempt even a small survey or investigation of available data, we are confronted with the difficulties, problems, and inadequacies of analysis, not to mention the political obstructionism to an intimate and potential embarrassing investigation. Still, we must base decisions on a rational process. It is incumbent upon the partnership to review and analyze available data, especially the data on needs. Over and over again, partnership staff talked about the difficulty of getting reliable data, accessible data, usable data. Staff also related the necessity of study, in spite of weaknesses in the numbers and real bother getting them.

A partnership needs good analytical information for three main reasons. Credible data and subsequent information are vital communication and education tools. Certainly the partnership wants to know if its clients are satisfied with the partnership's services and if the partnership was addressing the true need of the community. Second, analyses help monitor internal and external environments, both of which have an impact on operations and goal accomplishment. Third, analyses help measure managerial action in critical areas (Waldersee, 1999, p. 2). All senior partnership staff further observe that experience, judgment, and intuition are ultimately the main tools of decision making. Nothing takes the place, nor should it, of wisdom. Good analysis is a necessary part of the decision-making process, not the final word. The dynamic partnership recognizes when it needs research, how to do it, and when, with an educated discussion, it is time to decide and act. When the partnership as a collaborative decides to do an investigation, it must determine right away that the results of the work will be used. There are few things as tragic as a good analysis that is relegated to the bookshelf, ignored, then forgotten.

What the partnership seeks, then, is information that determines value (i.e., how and how much its services have made a material difference in the community and if goals are being reached). To do that the partnership wants information that is accessible, is usable, makes a good case, recognizes politics and personalities, and leads to action. When done well, and "well" means practical, it is a most useful investment of time and money. But before the partnership delves into its needs analysis, it needs to be aware of some of the main problems with analysis and data. This is not to discourage a partnership, it is to arm the partnership with information and argument to become comfortable with the tool and the process.

Basically it is tough to measure the public sector, especially public services which are multidimensional (Waldersee, 1999, p. 3). Be aware of the following difficulties lest they distract the partnership from the task at hand, that being what services the partnership should be delivering, and how and where the partnership should be focusing them.

- *Partial assessment.* Outcomes are not well understood, especially in the public sector, and many times are confused with efficiency measures. It is much easier to count attendees than to understand how they have been improved by a service. Numbers can profoundly describe an unimpressive, insignificant project. The misdirected measurement then takes on an aura of proof and believability that leads to bad decisions and wasted resources. Analyze input as long as it is connected to outcome.

- *Aggregation*. When we necessarily reduce truckloads of information to a usable size, important details may be missed or the reduction may mislead. Avoid the temptation to deduce for the whole, a result that applies only to part of the entire matrix. In other words, let good judgment prevail.
- *Manager intuition.* The real problems of analysis and data interpretation predispose managers to make judgment calls without the input of formal investigation. Here, with education and realistic, relevant analyses, senior people can become comfortable with the numbers and what they relate.
- *Context-dependent meaning.* Simply put, it is easier to "see" what needs to be done with measures focused at the lower levels of operation. That is, input and initial output measures, such as resources used and numbers served, are easy to gather and tempting to be used to justify action. Again, this basic analysis needs to be the gateway to insight on effect relative to the partnership's client base (adapted from Waldersee, 1999, pp. 3–6).

Waldersee also aptly comments that numbers do not automatically translate to information. A point well-taken by successful partnership leaders.

The needs assessment, then, seeks to accomplish four things:

- *Respond* to the unique issues and challenges that (children and families) face in the community;
- *Build* on the formal and informal resources of the community;
- Help *avoid duplicate services* and activities; and
- *Plan* in partnership with the community.

Community assessment, especially when it seeks to close a service-to-needs gap, is indeed different from a traditional needs assessment.

- *Involvement*. Residents are involved in design and implementation of the assessment. Their involvement ensures that the right questions are asked.
- *Focus*. Community needs assessment focuses not only on needs but on the concomitant resources to satisfy those needs. Thus, movement is built on community strength.

- *Multifaceted.* Multiple data collection sources and strategies are used to develop an actionable picture of community needs counterpoised to assets and resources.
- *Consensus building and information gathering.* Valid information is only part of desired results. The process allows agreement on what should be done.
- *Systems approach.* The focus on services is defined in terms of community knowledge, will, and skills to help deliver determined services.
- *Practical.* Community needs assessment is a blend of the academic and the realistic. Community has the larger input to the mix of the analysis/decision-making process (adapted from Family Support Centers, 2001, pp. 1–2).

There is nothing worse than for an evaluation to tell somebody what common sense knows. The partnership's analysis does need to avail itself of a range of tools to investigate commonsense characteristics of its environment and clientele. It needs to shed new light on those variables and factors.

Establish the Reassessment Process

How do successful partnerships incorporate research and decision making that lead to meaningful, goal-accomplishing action? Again, it is a process that reflects the needs of both a mature organization about to expand and the community. Following is an effective four-step process to assess its program's service-to-needs gap:

- *Reassess values.* This reaffirmation of commitment to children first reenergizes all stakeholders. Staff and providers, especially, are enthused to be working on a noble cause.
- *Reassess community needs.* Needs are now defined in terms of the larger entity, not largely what the partnership needs to survive and stabilize. This is the first glimpse at the partnership's service gaps and some possibilities for how to close them. This is where the community begins a palpable awareness that change is happening.
- *Reset priorities.* Priorities strike at the core of success. Programming adopted first must produce and, second, must be sustainable. If resources are not ready before the project is undertaken, it is not done.
- *Reset development objectives and benchmarks.* Benchmarking is a widely known and little used natural extension of deciding what a project is to achieve. Benchmarks merely state what is doable, challenging, but doable, and let the partnership know it is making progress. They are another rather simple way to make sure goals are happening. They are

valuable for two reasons: (1) they help conserve limited resources; and (2) they energize participants by offering a visible standard to achieve.

This process provides a snapshot of where the partnership has come and a real sense of the path on which to proceed. This sense of forward movement is vital for the survival of the partnership and improvement of the community. Without value, vision, and direction we have stagnation.

Conduct the Needs Assessment

There are four main steps in the assessment according to the Family Support Centers. The goal is to paint an objective picture of the community to be served according to the available resources and the needs of the target population.

- *Get statistics from secondary sources.* Available data help write a comprehensive profile of the client base. Look for information from the Census Bureau, state and local government, local public agencies, and service agencies. The partnership is looking for a snapshot of conditions to support partnership decisions and baseline numbers that provide a starting (or continuation) point for movement.
- *Gather residents' perspectives.* Doing this adds the necessary qualitative perspective to the community profile. The partnership may want to use client satisfaction questionnaires, focus groups, key stakeholder interviews, or resident surveys. The Chatham County Partnership[3] engaged the considerable talents of the nearby University of North Carolina, Chapel Hill, to help with the aforementioned methodologies. Chatham (2001) produced a professional and impressive collaborative report, *Find the Children*, that is proving most useful; furthermore, it was done for just over $15,000.
- *Conduct resource assessment.* Every community has assets. A statement of what the community can muster to help answer needs is vital. Consider provider, association, and individual capacity surveys.
- *Analyze and prioritize information.* Priority is vital as the partnership operates in austerity even during a robust economy; it is the nature of public service provision. (The Forsyth Early Childhood Partnership has an exceptional assessment program that breaks down data points by initiative; see Exhibit 6.1).

The partnership should try to parcel its needs assessments into smaller more manageable analysis projects that focus on an area of primary concern. For example, Forsyth has focused on the separate areas of family ties, child-care workforce, child-care education, licensure, wages and benefits, parents, business community, and Smart Start projects in successive annual needs analyses. This is quite a creative way to handle an inordinate amount of work and assimilate relevant libraries of information in digestible portions, each contributing to a larger description of the whole. This example of one partnership's take on what could be a daunting undertaking demonstrates the art of combining science, reality, and practicality.

The final step in an efficient needs analysis is that the partnership must distribute the results. Consider internal needs and external customers. Internally, directions suggested by the needs assessment should be itemized and detailed in action format; the strategic plan is the document of choice. The Down East Partnership goes so far as to detail the need, objective, benchmark, measurement, responsible party, and essential activities for every item. There is no mistake about the who, what, when, where, why, and how. This then comprises a positive cycle of evolution. Analysis and introspection lead to direction, then to improvement, which leads to further analysis and betterment. Externally, needs assessments need to be formatted for and distributed to many interested parties. Every item, from the full report, executive summaries, fact sheets, flyers, and brochures, should be distributed in mass mailouts or ready for an envelope when the phone rings. Make sure most of them go on the web and into the ready electronic presentation you have at the ready.

Throughout this overview of the needs reassessment process of a local collaborative, we have stressed practicality. It is a tough part of the local operation due to the dynamic nature of the partnership, the services, the service providers, the community, and those in need. Genevieve Megginson, from the Chatham Partnership, observed, as only the voice of experience can, "The ideal [with needs assessment] is to determine and fill service gaps; the reality is that funds define what gaps will be filled." Still, the most effective partnerships combine this dose of reality with an equal measure of analysis.

DETAIL A LONG-RANGE EXPANSION STRATEGY

Expansion does not happen automatically. Certainly there are forces enough to maintain the status quo if only for the real fact that operating the partnership at the present level seemingly takes all the partnership's time, energy, and resources. Nevertheless, the partnership must devote necessary time to documenting an expansion strategy. The fact that leadership is thinking about moving forward is energizing to the entire organization. Then there is the real possibility, over time, that the partnership will be able to close the gap between services and needs, one need at a time. Leadership has been through the process of planning for change and is quite good at it. The partnership would not be at this phase if its leaders were not skilled and experienced. Thus once again the partnership shold put that hard-won knowledge to work, program by program, slowly and methodically moving forward.

- *Restate vision, mission, and goals.* Vision and mission may not change, though revisiting their original intention is motivating. However, goals certainly will alter to reflect the dynamics of public endeavor and the "morphing" of society. With this process, the partnership should really nail down its greatest need, then target all necessary resources to it. The goal now is to make a measurable improvement in a problem that the partnership may only have been pecking at previously. Leaders should not forget to set new benchmarks too. They have to know if a resource or service fits the mission. This is key decision making that many collaboratives do not make.
- *Identify essential people and resources.* Stakeholders, especially staff, need to have an understanding of intentions and how they individually fit into the plan. Leaders must make sure they really know the impact of any expansion effort on the infrastructure (i.e., the operation and its service providers). This also requires another review of the partnership's most important stakeholder, its client base.
- *Establish a time line.* Outline a time line for the partnership plan according to the most probable sequence of expansion without jeopardizing chances for success. The strategic plan is the place it should be. Be challenging, realistic, and, most of all, flexible.

Again, practicality and experience are the ultimate determinates of when it is time to move ahead. This sense of when a project is right is a knowledge base built on several factors, including the requirement that leadership and staff are trained in and comfortable with resource development. Perhaps their comfort is measured by a move to hire a development officer who may reflect a new way of thinking on the part of the partnership. A development officer represents an indirect benefit and is not a direct service provider. Second, there is the example of other partnerships that have grown successfully. Your partnership should learn from them. Third, leaders should have a sense that the timing is right for their community. And, finally, there is local capacity to support needed resources, especially with hard dollars. In the end, expansion is built on a strong foundation of integrity in the community. If the partnership has established a solid record of successes, kept its promises, and been open about why expectations have not been met, then the integrity of the partnership will continue to strengthen. Successful resource development is the next right step.

INVOLVE KEY SUPPORT VIA CONSENSUS

When the partnership expands, it has to go back to the beginning. Leaders have to revisit all the key stakeholders and shore up relationships in preparation for moving forward. This is a continuous process, but it is particularly acute when new responsibilities and services are considered. Also, often an unsuspecting contact or relationship may take on a new role.

Prepare for Essential Public Relations and Awareness

Essentially, rebuilding support is a matter of having communication tools and staff ready. Update each piece as necessary, from the web site to the partnership's one-page flyers. Leaders have considered their key stakeholders. The must make sure they have suitably formatted information for each, because the corporate chief executive officer has different needs from the parent. Staff should be adequately manned and skilled in handling requests for service and information, and thus project the image of professionalism and competence. For example, the Halifax-Warren Partnership[4] has as its goal for phone referrals to put the requestor in contact with a needed service within two phone calls. In other words, a parent can call in and get a phone number, contact, and request for a return call on progress all on the initial call.

Be aware of and address some peculiar problems of moving the partners ahead. At the beginning of Smart Start in North Carolina, many people mistook the initiative for Head Start, which has a specific purpose and specific target group of at-risk children, which is much different from what our partnership was doing. People were leery of being labeled "underprivileged" if they received services from the partnership, thinking it was Head Start. Businesses did not immediately grasp the economic impact and common sense of quality child care on operation and profitability. And many people just did not see the need for these programs. Parents have often been heard to say, "The program is good, but not for my child." Then there is the real difficulty of reaching those most in need. We have observed, in extreme cases that young parents may both work forty to fifty hours per week. They are most in need of child care and have the most difficulties getting it; yet this type of family is the family your partnership's efforts should reach. It is where your partnership will have the greatest long-term effect.

Every partnership needs a message. That message, if the partnership is addressing the needs of its youngest citizens, is that the well-being of children benefits all. The partnership should have a general campaign that seeks to ensure that as many people as possible know about its efforts and have a good opinion of the organization. Be specific about who does what. Again, if it is school readiness, consider the components:

- *Health.* If a family needs winter heating fuel, ensure they know where and how to get it.
- *Child care.* Obviously, make sure high-quality child care is available for as many as need it. At least prioritize its establishment and be aware of where it is needed.

- *Support and education.* Have a full range of education and training classes available.
- *Other services.* Many North Carolina counties are discovering the real need for translation services, and in more than Spanish.

Remake Essential Collaborations and Partnerships

A local partnership makes scores of contacts. Leaders should pare the list down to those that can help. Think of those essential to any planned project. Remember, to give money, time, or expertise, the givers have to see a benefit to themselves. This may be a sense of accomplishment from participation or via simple, appropriate recognition. It is similar for business. Two examples of how to get business/corporate sponsorship follow:

- *Business family smartness.* The Forsyth Partnership has a survey that is given to local businesses to assess their family smartness. The best are recognized at an awards banquet. Those that do not win are left with a clear understanding of what they need to do to become a winner. In the process, all win.
- *Corporate citizenship.* International Paper began work in the Halifax-Warren area by intending to change the milltown mentality. International Paper became an enthusiastic partnership participant, setting out to become a good corporate citizen by offering office space and supplies, sponsoring corporate volunteering and needed services, providing matches for federal grants, and endorsing a great family-friendly benefits package, including an on-site health facility. Halifax-Warren is enthusiastically involved with International Paper by adopting the philosophy that it does not matter who gets credit for the good works.

Parents can be easily forgotten in the rush to court the influential or the big bank account. Actually, parents are sometimes steamrolled. They may not be as sophisticated as many other board members; the whole process of development leaves them behind. But without parents, children cannot be helped. Step in their shoes for a moment; invite and accommodate their participation. The Smart Start Tool Kit: Family Support and Family Involvement offers the following helpful hints:

- Offer child care on-site or reimbursed as an expense.
- Offer and provide transportation.
- Offer a stipend to replace lost wages of parents who attend your events.
- Meet at convenient and safe locations.

- Survey everyone about convenient times of meetings.
- Provide food at meetings.

The successful partnership is relationship driven. People get involved because they have a reason to get involved, this happens only with the personal touch.

EXPAND SEQUENTIALLY ACCORDING TO WILL AND RESOURCES

> "If you ask enough people for permission, you'll eventually come up against someone who believes his job is to say 'no.' So don't ask."
>
> —Colin Powell, 2001, p. 5

A consistent message from those who are succeeding is that there comes a time when thinking and planning is over! Information is never perfect nor complete. There is never complete consensus. Resources may not be 100 percent. The path also may not be that clear. But progress happens only with prudent forward movement.

Members of the partnership must also be aware of some of the unsuspected pitfalls of expansion and still pursue expanding. Expansion for some may be just an escape from the humdrum routine of managing the same old projects or a distraction from things that are not going well. The supposed expansion might merely be a tradeoff of services, a zero gain proposition. In other words, there is no real expansion, only the trappings of it. There is the temptation to go for an easy grant under the banner of serving the needy without the necessary cautions. Be aware then that the goal at this important juncture is sustainability. The partnership may even channel funds to another service agency because it is more suited to the project. What matters is community betterment. If the partnership can broker a service, a resource, or a grant, it is fulfilling its purpose, its mission. In fact, all the successful partnership executive directors independently noted that only by doing the work of the partnership and services building did they have a functional understanding of how to proceed. Again, the trick is that they do not act imprudently or carelessly, and probably more important, they learn, adapt, and plow on.

GOING FORWARD

We allowed each executive director we interviewed time to pause and to reflect a bit on what the partnership means, where it has come, of what he or she is proud, of what he or she is not proud, and of the road ahead. The universal comment was that a future without partnerships is unimaginable even though that future is most uncertain and crazy with real work and impossible demands. Without a network of needs-based services funneling through a local collaboration, we stand to lose a generation of children to overworked parents, fragmented families, and media-dominated formative years. There would be no forum for collaboration, for differences to be aired and resolved, and for diversity to be explored and shepherded to its potential. There would be one less important avenue for the best leadership, local leadership, to exercise real self-determination for the community. No partnership would be there to break the stereotypes of the inability of counties to collaborate with state and federal governments for the long haul. No partnership means no model for performance-based services leading to real change in the household. As we may imagine, the work to date is just a start.

Just by being part of what is happening, much indeed happens because the partnership is there. We can see it in an office that buzzes with efficiency, in an annual report that relates the facts of meaningful change with meaningful promise. We can see it in happy faces, new and not so new. The individuals in a partnership are universally proud of an entity with high integrity and high ideals that is stable, respected, and dynamic and that really delivers on the promise of services that make a difference, especially for the most needy. Yes, there are regrets, services abandoned, opportunities missed for lack of funding or courage or both, and certainly the daily realization that more can, and must, be done. Partnership stakeholders, especially staff, are aware that this entity is very much alive and is very empowering. They see and feel it when someone is asked to serve. Suddenly, just by association with the partnership new esteem is felt, even by the most accomplished volunteer. Visibility is given to previously invisible people; that is empowerment. And all explore new dimensions as, for example, a senior corporate officer has to learn, perhaps for the first time, how to serve the needs of our youngest citizens. Partnerships do work. There is no going back, nor is there any suggestion that enough has been done.

Now that there are models of successful partnerships, any state, any local community has examples for planning, operating, and expanding a network of partnerships. There are challenges to be sure. The funding base has to be expanded. The concept of the stable, performance-based partnership needs to be expanded. Every community should have a partnership if only for its coalescing effect. We need leadership at all levels of government working, long term, on a national rollout plan for partnership development. Likewise we need leadership, especially at the national level, to raise the visibility of and commitment to early childhood services, instead of the disproportionate effort spent on institutional responses to acute social problems later in life. At the same time that the reach of a local web of services is broadened, that reach also needs to be narrowed and standardized, especially in child care.

The job of raising a child does not end with kindergarten and the public or private school systems. Seeing a child to productive, contented maturity where he or she is ready and able to put back into family and the community needs careful attention, perhaps gentle prodding, all along the way, not only in school. What a shame not to take advantage of the example set by the partnerships in North Carolina's Smart Start initiative—an initiative that is showing us all that it can be done, that we can turn failure into success at the community level.

Notes

1. Forsyth Early Childhood Partnership, Dr. Dean Clifford, Ph.D., Executive Director, 7820 N. Point Blvd., Winston-Salem, NC 27106; tel.: (336) 725-6011; *www.forsythchild.org*.
2. Down East Partnership for Children, Henrietta Zalkind, Executive Director, P.O. Box 1245, 215 Lexington Street, Rocky Mount, NC 27802; tel.: (252) 985-.4300; or via the North Carolina Smart Start Website.
3. Chatham County Partnership for Children, Genevieve Megginsion, Executive Director, 200 Sanford Highway, Ste. #4; Pittsboro, NC 27312; tel.: (919) 542-7449; *chatchld@emji.net; www.chathamkids.org.*
4. Halifax-Warren Smart Start Partnership for Children, Magda Baligh, Executive Director, P.O. Box 402, 24 King Street, Halifax, NC 27839; tel.: (252) 583-1304; or via the North Carolina Smart Start Website.

References

Chatham County Partnership for Children. (2001, April). *Find the Children: A report of the Family Needs Survey and Community Needs Assessment.* Pittsboro, NC: Author.

Family Support Centers. (2001). *A program manager's tool kit: Vol. I—Program planning and evaluation* [On-line]. Available: *www.frca.org.*

Powell, C. (2001). *A leadership primer* [On-line]. Available: *www.freepages.military.rootsweb.com/-rootsrus/powell.html.*

Vancouver Citizen's Committee. (2002). *The citizen's handbook: A guide to building community in Vancouver* [On-line]. Available: *www.vcn.bc.ca/citizens-handbook.*

Waldersee, R. (1999, September). The art of service. V: The science of measurement: Measuring and managing service delivery. *Australian Journal of Public Administration, 58*(3), 1–6.

Exhibit 6.1
Assessment Data

Child Care

- Numbers, categories, locations, and costs of child-care spaces available
- Obstacles preventing access to care
- Educational level of directors, teachers, and other staff
- Educational level of home child-care providers
- Wages and benefits of providers
- Experience/continuity of care
- Licensure/registration/accreditation levels
- Participation in quality improvement programs and results
- Funding streams used by providers
- Variety of program used by parents
- Child-care provider
- Outcomes in children

Family Support

- Information needed by and accessed by parents
- Knowledge regarding child development and parenting skills
- Sources of support and information used by parents
- Family needs (shelter, food, child care, etc.)
- Services used by children with special needs
- Teenage pregnancy
- Birth outcomes
- Family and neighborhood concerns and/or problems
- Satisfaction with services
- Obstacles to service
- Sources of family income
- Family educational levels

Health

- Immunization rates
- Physical and dental screening rates
- Obstacles to services
- Funding for health services

Business and Faith Communities at Large

- Work/life policies and practices in place
- Programs and services offered to children and families
- Interest in offering services
- Needs for technical assistance or other support

Source: Forsyth Early Childhood Partnership

Chapter 7

Providing for the First Need in the Developmental Continuum—Getting Children Ready for School

The previous chapters detailed how to get a local partnership up and running effectively. The partnership's goal is to foster school readiness; that is, what needs to be done to prepare the 0–5-year-old group of children for their entry into a productive school experience. We make that distinction knowing that there are even more specific developmentally appropriate services needed for every age within the 0–5-year-old age range. That is, for example, a 3-year-old has different needs from a 4-year-old, and so on. The point also needs to be made that being ready for schooling also applies to schools. There is much to consider in the appropriate learning/teaching environment when addressing the needs of the preschooler, the kindergartener, and the first-grader. This chapter addresses the larger services needed to help a child be prepared for the first day of formal schooling. There is much to do and in regard to that goal alone.

While the local partnership can and should deliver services according to the need and commensurate resources of the local citizenry, the primary purpose of the local partnership should be to deliver school-readiness services. In fact, the need for school-readiness programs provides the basic motivation to build effective and efficient local service delivery infrastructure. Now, having established an understanding of the process of partnership planning, operation, and expansion, and to be clear about the continuum of developmentally appropriate attention to our children and youth, we will discuss, briefly, what school readiness is, readiness issues, and suggested programming.

We can afford no misunderstanding about the importance of any efforts at every level of government to properly attend to our youngest people. In fact, the importance of this work has been recognized in each generation past, probably none so poignantly as by Maria Montessori nearly 100 years ago, who said:

> The development of the child during the first three years after birth is unequaled in the intensity and importance by any period that precedes or follows in the whole life of the child. . . . If we consider the transformations, adaptations, achievements, and conquest of the environment during the first period of life from zero to three years, it is functionally a longer period than all the following periods put together from three years until death. For this reason these *three years may be considered to be as long as a whole life.* (Lillard, 1972, p. 106; emphasis added)

Recent research bears out this view most emphatically. Thus the real question is, "Why are we still debating the economic and especially common sense of school readiness?" The debate should be long over and much more progress should already have been made.

School readiness has an amoebae-like characteristic. What a community does will be unique to that community; we cannot stress that point enough. We offer an example of how to go about the task with the purpose of getting as many communities as possible working on a developmental continuum of services that begins with getting all children ready for a productive school experience.

Good school readiness, readiness that connects to developmentally appropriate nurturing by family and community, should hinge on one basic question as posed by the Kansas City Partnership for Children: "Is it good for the children?" With that question guiding individual and collective thought, resources, and effort, the local municipality should begin to realize necessary programming in child care and health. In fact, the promises offered by Kansas City's Partnership reflect even better the long-term, continuous task of developing youth from birth to productive young adulthood. Those promises are that there will be caring adults, safe places, a healthy start, marketable skills, and an opportunity to serve (Partnership for Children, *www.pfc.org/promise.shtml*). These promises then consider the dimensions of safety and security, health, early education, the progress of primary education, and progress during teen years. School readiness for children (not to exclude the school being ready to accept children) must be thought of in terms of its connectedness to the age-appropriate needs of youth as they reach and express their potential with the ultimate purpose of returning to the community the measures of strength and human capital the community provided its children as they grew.

SCHOOL READINESS DEFINED

School readiness is defined by developmental conditions manifested as the child enters kindergarten and the capacity of schools to serve their children (School Readiness in North Carolina, *www.ncsmartstart.org/Information/publications.htm*). We will deal with getting children ready for school, which is largely the responsibility of local government, though it be in cooperation/collaboration with the larger network of federal, state, and local interests. There are several dimensions to consider. These dimensions center on the youngsters' ability to think and their awareness of the basics of life and socialization. They are best summarized on the U.S. Department of Education Website (*www.us.ed*).

- *Good health and physical well-being.* Young children need nutritious food, enough sleep, a safe place to play, and regular medical care. Good health for children begins before birth with good prenatal care, nutritionally balanced meals, medical and dental checkups and immunizations, and opportunities to exercise and develop physical coordination.
- *Social and emotional preparation.* Before they come to kindergarten, children must be able to work well in large groups and get along with new adults and other children. They should have at least:

  — *Confidence.* Children must have the feeling of self worth and the personal ability to succeed in a variety of areas of expression.

  — *Independence.* Children must have the ability to work alone.

  — *Motivation.* Children must have a strong desire to learn.

  — *Curiosity.* Children must remain inquisitive.

  — *Persistence.* Children must know how to complete their work or projects.

  — *Cooperation.* Children need to be able to work in diverse groups.

  — *Self-control.* Children must know what is accepted conduct and express appropriate rather than inappropriate behavior, and have the ability to determine and express right from wrong.

  — *Empathy.* Children must be interested in and understand others, especially feelings.
- *Language and general knowledge.* Children must learn to communicate, solve problems, and develop an understanding of the world.

We expect much from our children; they have a right to expect much from adults and parents in particular. Children must believe that no matter what, someone will look out for them; that adults will set a good example, especially in having a positive attitude toward learning and school; that there will be opportunities to learn from repetition; that discipline will be appropriate; that adults recognize that children are capable and will be allowed to do as much as they can alone; and that children will be encouraged to play with other children and be with nonfamilial adults (the foregoing is adapted from *www.ed.gov/pubs/parents/GetReadyForSchoolWhatDoesItMean.html*).

Put another way, to be ready for the first day of kindergarten is to be healthy; to have an involved, nurturing family; and to be able to interact socially with peers and adults in general. Again, we make the distinction between getting the child ready for school and the school being ready to accept the child; both must be considered in the broad topic of school readiness whereas we treat only the readiness of the child in this discussion. The school that is ready to accept the child is concerned with three primary areas of preparedness: The curriculum must be appropriate for the child—not necessarily for the "age group," as it is designed for the individual learner. The school's physical plant must reflect an age-appropriate environment. For example, the classroom for first-graders should be organized in areas for group learning, not just rows of seats. And, importantly, teachers must be ready for their individual learners. A certification in early childhood education for birth through kindergarten is necessarily much different from an elementary school teaching certificate.

It is helpful to review Smart Start (North Carolina Partnership for Children: *www.smartstart-nc.org*) principles for preparing the child for the first day of formal education:

- *Opportunity*. Every child should have the same opportunity to start school ready to succeed, regardless of income or geography.
- *Early involvement.* School readiness begins before birth with good prenatal care, not at school entry.
- *Continuous involvement.* Children's needs must be met throughout their childhood years, thus requiring fewer intervention programs (and social services) later in life.
- *Cooperation*. Local communities must work together to develop comprehensive early educational strategies, using the current infrastructure for children from birth to age 5 that meets their needs (adapted from *www.ncsmartstart.org*).

An effective pre-K program should consider collaboration and appropriate standards, have parental choice and local determination, be accessible to all children, continuously infuse different sources of backing, and be offered continuously throughout the year.

When a comprehensive array of school-readiness programs begins to come together, the more aggressive communities will begin to see definitive local benefits that accrue to the state. Community by community it will become apparent that more children are arriving at school eager; energetic; in the company of an involved, informed family; and ready to learn. They will be ready because more and more, especially the neediest, will be getting preventive health care even if they have to be taken to the service, or vice versa. Obviously, over time, community by community, these real benefits begin to accrue on broader and broader scales simply by focusing on helping children do what is natural, succeed.

LOCAL SCHOOL READINESS PROGRAMMING

Broadly speaking, school readiness programming is executed in three areas:

1. Child care and education;
2. Health care and education; and
3. Family support services.

As always the choice of specific programming is locally determined providing that two overarching purposes are met. First, the child must enter primary schooling already primed for success according to his or her abilities and potential. And any work done to assist the development of the child is seen as only a part of a seamless continuum of attention paid to the youngster until that individual is capable of fulfilling the role of citizen in a democracy. Thus, unless there is a continuum of developmentally appropriate services for the evolving citizen, any break in those services runs the risk of undoing all previous good done. It is common sense; it is equally most rewarding no matter how that reward is defined, whether it be in the monetary sense of hard dollars saved in keeping people independent of social services or the real benefit, though unmeasurable, of someone who understands what it means to be a neighbor and is capable of adding to his or her community in material and intrinsic ways.

Smart Start has a representative array of working ideas by domain (Dombro, 2001, p. 9):

❑ Child care and education

- Subsidies for child care
- Increasing the availability of child-care spaces
- Improving the quality of child care
- Inclusion of children with special needs

- Teacher education and support

❑ Health care and education
- Support for immunizations
- Health and developmental screenings
- Education for parents and child-care providers

❑ Family support and education
- Child-care resource and referral services
- Resource centers
- Family literacy programs
- Transportation

When it comes together, as we have witnessed at many sites, there is evidence of the work both in the numbers and especially in the intangibles that mark progress. When the partnership is working well, other resources and avenues of funding become available and expand. Skeptical foundations, and especially private businesses, can see the business sense of participating. Collaborative efforts multiply resources. The simple expression of this is that volunteers are easier to recruit. A solid service delivery infrastructure provides the basis for a range of services depending on need. One partnership was fully engaged in disaster recovery in addition to working with school readiness. Performance-oriented local partnerships are also well equipped to tackle the complex dynamic of solving neighborhood-level problems. For example, a community advocate has the organization and the pulpit from which to make needed improvements almost household by household.

But now we a need slightly closer examination, on the community level, of the dynamic of offering services in each of these three necessary service areas, the three-legged stool of getting children ready for school. Again, in keeping with the theme of a continuum of developmentally appropriate services, no one program is enough, no specific program is the answer. Designing an array of flexible and long-term answers to unique problems makes progress happen.

CHILD CARE AND EDUCATION

The aforementioned goals for child care are expressed at the local level by improving the quality of child care and making it accessible and affordable. But to be clear, we need a standard for what child care actually is, and for that we use the Smart Start definition. Child care is defined as follows:

- There are three or more unrelated children under 13 years of age.

- Children are receiving care from a nonrelative.
- Children are receiving care on a regular basis, at least once per week.
- That the care is for more than four hours per day but less than twenty-four hours.

Again, the particular mix of programming is highly individual, as determined by local needs and resources. What matters is that the goals of affordability, accessibility, and quality are met.

Child-Care Affordability

Affordable child care is arguably the most difficult aspect of connecting children with quality child care. Neediest young families with child-care-eligible children usually come up against the most barriers to obtaining child care. They need the most persistence and attention to make the connection. Often the affordability issue can only be answered by offering direct monetary aid. Some of the most creative means come via local "scholarships." Child-care and partnership staff found most young parents reluctant to accept outright aid, a problem that was answered by setting up a system of needs-based "scholarships." There is much meaning in a word. Finally, the local child-care advocate can round out services offered perhaps by having child-care resource and referral services with a public information campaign promoting child care.

Child-Care Accessibility

Accessibility is achieved gradually in two ways, by taking the services to the locale and by bringing children to the service. Services are opened on an as-needed basis and as resources permit. Likewise, transportation is provided for children, also on an as-needed basis and as resources permit. The goal is for the local community, via its partnership, to do regular needs assessments that pinpoint child care for the neediest first, then build toward having good child-care services throughout the defined service area.

Child-Care Quality

Child-care quality can be built by three means: program standards of accreditation for a child-care service, credentialing and education for child-care professionals, and compliance history for the type of service. Each state is different. For example, the North Carolina Division of Child Development establishes the following standards outlined in the Stars in Child Care directive (*www.dhhs.state.nc.us/dcd/rateruls.htm*): a child-care facility, depending on whether it is a center, a home, a center for school-age children only, or one that serves preschool and school-age children, has a set of increasingly challenging requirements designated by a star rating from one to five stars. Naturally, centers are not expected to be five-star facilities immediately. But the implication and incentive are to progressively strive for a five-star (quality) rating (extracted from Rated License Highlights, *www.dhhs.state.nc.us/dcd/raterruls.htm*).

A more comprehensive discussion is found on the web site for National Association for Education of Young Children (*www.naeyc.org*). Accreditation criteria alone consider the following:

- Interactions among teachers and children;
- Curriculum;
- Relationships among teachers and families;
- Staff qualifications and professional development;
- Administration;
- Staffing;
- Physical environment;
- Health and safety;
- Nutrition and food service; and
- Evaluation.

Furthermore, child-care quality is markedly enhanced if attention is paid to compensating and educating providers. It helps a great deal if the state can support additional wages and scholarships for active and potential child-care providers. An exemplary program is the Teacher Education and Compensation Helps (T.E.A.C.H.) Program (*www.childcareservices.org/TEACH/T.E.A.C.H%2OPROJECT.htm*). Generally, improving quality takes time—time to improve compensation, programming, and the qualifications of the people in the classrooms. The obvious goal is to increase provider capability and numbers while reducing turnover in conjunction with increasing accessibility and affordability.

HEALTH CARE AND EDUCATION

Health care for children is quite basic. Pregnant women should be encouraged to get early prenatal care and to make sure they get the necessary care when the newborn arrives. This care covers everything from medical and mental health consultation and services, immunizations, and environmental health and safety services. This also includes a campaign to get health insurance coverage for children. When children arrive at the first day of kindergarten their state of health should be that they have had good nutrition, all immunizations, and proper screening. Essentially, the young body, mind, and spirit are ready for the challenges of school.

The local partnership may be the conduit for the following set of health support services, naturally in close cooperation with the appropriate health care professionals and agencies:

- Prenatal health education and coordination;
- Health screenings for preschool children;
- Nutrition education;
- Breastfeeding counseling; and
- Services for children with special needs.

Again, creativity, need, resolve, and resources are in the mix of determining how a municipality prepares its children to be healthy, willing, and able for school. These basic services are relatively easy to deliver, relative, that is, to helping a child who has to face the first day of formal schooling ill prepared and not in the mood to learn, whether it is because the child is hungry, or has a vision problem, or has a preventable childhood disease. There are few things we as a collective, concerned citizenry can do that have such a dramatic, long-term effect as simply nurturing, during the first years of life, the natural curiosity and ability a child has to learn. How well we do this determines the course of each young life.

FAMILY SUPPORT SERVICES

Support for families concerning preparation for primary schooling is generally offered via training, technical assistance, assistance with money issues, outreach, and direct services. Partnerships commonly establish a child resource and referral function which is a catch-all operation for any local school-readiness need with the focus on educating and connecting families with school-readiness-related services, resources, and skills. Furthermore, it is the primary point of local contact for child care.

Skills Building

Obviously there are as many ways to structure this essential service as there are school-readiness professionals handling resource and referral. Indeed, there is a wealth of good programs to augment this operation. One in particular is the Incredible Years training series (Webster-Stratton, 2000). This program offers a series of programs that recognize the interrelatedness of the parent, child, and teacher. Wisely, the program offers developmentally appropriate, progressive training for all three programs to be conducted in the home, community, school, or combination of all three venues. Parents are given, for example, training in the parenting, interpersonal, and academic skills that they will use to teach their youngster. Teachers get a review of classroom management skills. Children have a series in social skill building, problem solving, and classroom behavior. The goals of this and any other family support program, aside from nurturing a smiling, eager young face on the first day of school, should be to reduce conduct problems; promote social, emotional, and academic competence; promote parental competence; strengthen families; promote teacher competence; and strengthen school-home connections (Webster-Stratton, 2000). In fact, these goals are another way to state the point of school readiness for children.

Resource Center and Single Point of Contact

The reality is that there are many resources; research them, pick the most appropriate, and get them working. For example, a local partnership may have, in addition to the foregoing, a program of parenting education, support, and training; a center specifically located and devoted to providing resources; and perhaps a guide to parental resources which summarizes local resources and contacts.

Training, Technical Assistance, and Outreach

Training from the local resource and referral office may include classes specifically for fathers, how to begin a child-care facility, CPR training, substitute child-care provider training, a child discipline workshop, and a workshop on age-appropriate activities for children of new parents. The office can offer a range of technical assistance wherever and whenever needed. It is not uncommon for the resource and referral provider to be called to a child-care center to help solve a problem or help with certification. And there is always outreach. Anyone really in the school-readiness business needs to be ready to spread the word to local organizations and at local events. Articles for the local newspaper and a newsletter are most helpful. Clearly, there is no rule as to what is offered to ensure that children are prepared for school and the next stage in their continuous development.

GIVING CHILDREN THE "FREEDOM TO BECOME"

Our local children have transitioned to elementary school, all is going well, they are on task, on grade level, and, overall, enjoy the school experience. Good school readiness is demonstrated in elevated levels of literacy and numeracy; children who interact well together; capable, involved families; and fewer behavioral problems; happily, this is especially so for at-risk children. But if the community is to realize the potential begun with good school readiness, to realize the real savings in less demand, long term, on welfare assistance, special education, and criminal justice services; less expense for victim services; and the real monetary return on investment, increased taxes from a gainfully employed neighbor, the work must continue into the elementary years and beyond. What we are talking about is the very purpose of education—that is, to facilitate children realizing their potential so that society may enjoy productive, contributing, involved teens and adults.

This process is so much simpler, the result that much more dramatic when the focus is on the youngest of children. Putting these programs in place is a rational thing to do. Furthermore, the main problem is not so much one of organization or one of funding. In fact Maria Montessori, always insightful, commented on the main problem of preparing the young child:

> The main problem is the problem of freedom; its significance and repercussions have to be clearly understood. The adult's idea that freedom consists in minimizing duties and obligations must be rejected. . . . The freedom that is given to the child is not liberation from parents and teachers; it is not freedom from the laws of Nature or of the state or of society, but the utmost freedom for self-development and self-realization compatible with service to society. (Lillard, 1972, p. 119)

The duty of the community is to tactfully, even gently, prepare the way for what occurs naturally in children—wonder, ingenuity, potential, conviction, enterprise, self-reliance, and discipline—properly prepared, they will succeed. When a community embarks on a campaign to prepare its children with a continuum of developmentally appropriate services, it is a journey of developing a body of knowledge which leads to understanding, which comes only from the doing of it. From understanding, people begin to care about this vital pursuit. When people are personally involved and committed, progress is made. In fact, the impossible becomes possible.

References

Dombro, A. M. (2001). *What is Smart Start* [Monograph for the North Carolina Partnership for Children] [On-line]. Available: *www.ncsmartstart.org/Information/publications.htm.*

Lillard, P. P. (1972). *Montessori: A modern approach.* New York: Schocken Books.

Webster-Stratton, C. (2000, June). The Incredible Years training series. *OJJDP Juvenile Justice Bulletin* [On-line]. Available: *www.ncjrs.org/html/ojjdp/2000_6_3/contents.html.*

Part III

Engaging Elementary School Children and Their Parents—Promising and Effective Practices in Parental Involvement

by Meredith B. Weinstein, Ph.D., James R. Brunet, Ph.D., Irvin Vann, Ph.D. (Cand.), and James Klopovic, M.A., M.P.A.

The purpose of Part III is to identify the critical elements in successful school-based initiatives aimed at increasing parental participation.

Over the past several years, a new awareness of the benefit of the role of parental involvement in the education of elementary school children has emerged. Part III is designed to present the research literature that identifies the existing problems with delinquency in youth that can be improved with increased parental involvement at an early age. Parental involvement programs provide benefits to students, parents, families, teachers, schools, and communities. By implementing programs that enhance the home environment, a child's academic and social behavior at school will also improve. According to Cullingford (1999), "A positive and secure home background is found to have a substantial positive relationship with attention at school" (p. 52). Griffin (1996) examined the effects of parental involvement, empowerment, and school traits on academic performance of elementary school students. He concluded that parental involvement is an important element in student academic performance. In the study, parental involvement and empowerment were consistently correlated with student test performance. In another study, Henderson and Berla (1994) found that when parents became involved, grades and test scores went up; attendance rates, attitudes, and graduation rates improved; and and there was an increase in completed homework assignments and enrollment in higher education.

Parental involvement programs take many forms; however, the goal is to increase the positive role parents play in the development of their children. When schools, the community, and families collaborate, children and society as a whole benefit.

Beginning with the earliest stages of program planning and concluding with the later stages of program expansion, Part III provides policymakers and program administrators with practical advice at each phase in a program's life cycle.

Chapter 8 begins a discussion of parental involvement in the lives of elementary school children by focusing on what parents, schools, and communities need to contribute for a successful effort. The importance of parents in the educational, emotional, and social growth of a child is addressed. The chapter concludes with an introduction to program issues which should be considered.

Chapter 9 provides examples from three existing parental involvement programs. By examining successful as well as unsuccessful program designs future programs can learn from the experiences of other programs.

Chapter 10 concludes the discussion of parental involvement with a description of effective program practices. The effective practices identified were shown to be critical elements to program success.

For further resources on parental involvement, see Appendix III-1.

References

Cullingford, C. (1999). *The causes of exclusion: Home, school, and the development of young criminals.* London: Kogan Page.

Griffin, J. (1996). Relation of parental involvement , empowerment, and school traits to student academic performance. *Journal of Education Research, 90*(1), 33–42.

Henderson, A.T., & Berla, N. (1994). *A new generation of evidence: The family is critical to student achievement.* Columbia, MD: National Committee for Citizens in Education.

Appendix III-1

Further Resources

Active Parenting

www.activeparenting.com

Dr. Michael H. Popkin, a former child and family therapist and Coordinator of Child and Family Services for Northside Community Mental Health Centers in Atlanta, Georgia. Center on School, Family, and Community Partnerships, founded Active Parenting Publishers, Inc., in 1980. APP delivers quality education programs for parents, children and teachers to schools, hospitals, social services organizations, churches and the corporate market. APP are the pioneers of the world's first video-based parenting education program.

Children, Youth, and Family Consortium

http://www.cyfc.umn.edu

The Children, Youth, and Family Consortium was established during the Fall of 1991 to bring together the varied competencies of the University of Minnesota and the vital resources of Minnesota's communities to enhance the ability of individuals and organizations to address critical health, education, and social policy concerns in ways that improve the well-being of Minnesota children, youth, and families.

Communities in Schools

http://wwwcisnc.org

Communities in Schools assists communities in connecting community resources with schools. This site provides information on communities in schools of North Carolina.

Family Involvement in Children's Education

http://www.ed.gov/pubs/FamInvolve/title.html

This Idea Book is offered to stimulate thinking and discussion about how schools can help overcome barriers to family involvement in their children's education--regardless of family circumstances or student performance. While this book draws on the successful local approaches studied, we would like to hear about effective programs or practices that have worked in your community.

The Family Involvement Network of Educators (FINE)

http://www.gse.harvard.edu/~hfrp/projects/fine.html

For nearly twenty years, the Harvard Family Research Project has helped philanthropies, policy-makers, and practitioners develop strategies to promote the educational and social success and well-being of children, families, and their communities. As it guides organizations in planning and assists in problem solving, HFRP collects, analyzes, and synthesizes research and information to foster continuous improvement and learning.

Juvenile Justice Bulletin (Families and Schools Together, FAST)

http://www.ncjrs.org/html/ojjdp/9911_2/contents.html

The overall goal of the FAST program, described in this issue of the *Juvenile Justice Bulletin*, is to intervene early to help at-risk youth succeed in the community, at home, and in school and thus avoid problems including adolescent delinquency, violence, addiction, and dropping out of school. The FAST process utilizes the existing strengths of families, schools, and communities in creative partnerships. FAST offers youth structured opportunities for involvement in repeated, relationship-building interactions with the primary care taking parent, other family members, other families, peers, school representatives, and community representatives. The program builds and enhances long-term relationships to provide youth a "social safety net" of protective factors for getting through difficult times.

Juvenile Justice Bulletin (Family Skills Training for Parents and Children)

http://www.ncjrs.org/html/ojjdp/jjbul2000_04_2/contents.html

The Strengthening Families Program (SFP) began in 1983 as a 4-year prevention research project funded by the National Institute on Drug Abuse (NIDA). Because of the project's promising results, SFP has been replicated, revised, and adapted for diverse population groups throughout the Nation. The program was designed as a drug abuse prevention program for high-risk, drug-abusing parents to help them improve their parenting skills and help their children avoid drug use.

National Association of Partners in Education

http://www.partnersineducation.org/

Partners in Education has direct links to local school districts and community leaders throughout the country. Through thousands of grassroots member programs, Partners in Education connects children and classroom teachers with corporate, education, volunteer, government, and civic leaders. These community partners play significant roles in changing the content and delivery of education services to children and their families.

National Association of Elementary School Principals

www.naesp.org

The mission of the National Association of Elementary School Principals is to lead in the advocacy and support for elementary and middle level principals and other education leaders in their commitment to all children. NAESP strongly urges principals to take an active role in providing parents with skills that develop intellectual and reasoning abilities as well as personal and social development of their children from birth through the formal schooling process. Suggested concepts for parenting programs in the school are not limited to, but include: nutrition and health; prenatal care; educational activity suggestions for neighborhood day care providers; developmentally appropriate activities to foster school readiness; developing positive self-esteem; home activities that support learning at school; materials describing available family services and educational programs, e.g., public health department, community service organizations, adult education, literacy education; and information regarding school goals and objectives relating to behavioral and specific academic expectations.

National Coalition for Parent Involvement in Education (NCPIE)

http://www.ncpie.org

NCPIE advocates the involvement of parents and families in their children's education, and fosters relationships between home, school, and community to enhance the education of all our nation's young people. NCPIE seeks to:

- Serve as a visible representative for strong parent and family involvement initiatives at the national level.
- Conduct activities that involve the coalition's member organizations and their affiliates and constituencies in efforts to increase family involvement.

- Provide resources and legislative information that can help member organizations promote parent and family involvement.

National Network of Partnership Schools

http://scov.csos.jhu.edu/p2000/

The National Network of Partnership Schools was established by researchers at Johns Hopkins University, The National Network of Partnership Schools brings together schools, districts, and states that are committed to developing and maintaining comprehensive programs of school-family-community partnerships.

The Parent Institute

http://www.par-inst.com/

The mission of The Parent Institute is to encourage parent involvement in the education of their children. The Parent Institute publishes a variety of materials including newsletters, booklets, brochures, and videos. The Parent Institute is a division of NIS, Inc., an independent, private corporation founded in 1989 by educators with extensive experience working with public and private schools in the U.S. and Canada.

National Parent Teacher Association

www.pta.org

National PTA is the largest volunteer child advocacy organization in the United States. The PTA is a not-for-profit association of parents, educators, students, and other citizens active in their schools and communities. One of the PTA's stated purposes is to bring into closer relation the home and the school, that parents and teachers may cooperate intelligently in the education of children and youth.

National PTA's National Standards for Parent/Family Involvement Programs

http://www.pta.org/programs/invstand.htm

The National Standards for Parent/Family Involvement Programs are guidelines for leaders of institutions with programs serving parents and families. Developed in 1997, the standards are designed to help direct leaders as they move from discussion to action in developing dynamic parent involvement programs that are meaningful, well planned and long lasting. The program standards are also a tool to evaluate the effectiveness of long-term school reform efforts to involve families in their child's education.

Parenting Resources (U.S. Department of Justice)

http://www.parentingresources.ncjrs.org/

Parenting Resources for the 21st Century links parents and other adults responsible for the care of a child with information on issues covering the full spectrum of parenting. This site, federally sponsored through the Coordinating Council on Juvenile Justice and Delinquency Prevention, strives to help families meet the formidable challenges of raising a child today by addressing topics that include school violence, child development, home schooling, organized sports, child abuse, and the juvenile justice system.

Partnership for Family Involvement in Education (U.S. Department of Justice)

http://pfie.ed.gov

Staff at the U.S. Department of Education established the Partnership for Family Involvement in Education in September 1994. Because family participation in children's learning is often influenced by work schedules and time constraints, it is crucial that businesses, community and religious organizations, and especially families and schools support parent and employee involvement in education. To encourage such support, the Department of Education administers the Partnership and offers resources, ideas, funding, and conferences relevant to family involvement in education.

Strengthening America's Families (Office of Juvenile Justice and Delinquency Prevention)

http://www.strengtheningfamilies.org/

The Office of Juvenile Justice and Delinquency Prevention (OJJDP) in collaboration with the Substance Abuse and Mental Health Service's Center for Substance Abuse Prevention (CSAP) provides the results of the 1999 and 1997 search for "best practice" family strengthening programs. The website provides links to summaries of the programs divided into categories based upon the degree, quality and outcomes of research associated with them. There is a program matrix that may be helpful in determining "at a glance" which programs may best meet a community needs.

Chapter 8

Parental Involvement—A Key Dimension In Enhancing Childhood Development

Parental involvement involves collaborative interaction between family, school, and the community. Parental involvement programs can take on many forms to achieve positive results. The key element of all programs that seek to involve parents is to "engage" parents in the educational, social, and emotional development of their child; it is important to make parents partners in these areas of their children's development. Henderson and Berla (1995) indicated, "the best results are gained when parents are involved in both learning and decision making" (p. 16). Also, there has been debate as to the definition of a parent, resulting from the differing composition of families in the United States. There is no longer a "typical" family structure. Some researchers believe that instead of parental involvement, programs should be designed for family involvement to encompass all family forms. Epstein and Connors (1995) emphasized the importance and potential influence of all family members, not only parents, and all family structures, not only those that include the birth parents. In addition, they recognize the need for students to join the partnership. For our purposes, parental and family involvement are considered interchangeable.

PARENTAL INVOLVEMENT DEFINED

Over the past decade, a great deal of attention has been paid to parental involvement in the education of elementary school children. Definitions of parental involvement vary. However, parental involvement centers on the idea that parents must become engaged in the life of their children in order for the children to develop appropriate social and academic skills. Parental involvement definitions also recognize the collaborative relationship between family, school, and community. Parental involvement has traditionally involved three aspects: preparing children to enter school (teaching the alphabet and reading to the child), attending school events (parent teacher conferences and PTA), and performing any requests made by teachers (assistance with homework or other projects). However, current theory contends that parents must do more to truly be involved in the education of their child. The National Parent Teacher Association (2000) defines parent involvement as the "participation of parents in every facet of children's education and development from birth to adulthood, recognizing that parents are the primary influence in children's lives" (p. 8).

Importance of Community Collaboration in Parental Involvement

In addition to involving families in the upbringing of children it is essential to collaborate with the community to prevent delinquency. This is best stated in the African proverb, "It takes the whole village to raise a child." This saying is as true in U.S. society today as in the rural villages of Africa. A partnership must be forged between the family, school, and community to produce positive educational and social effects on the child while being mutually beneficial to all other parties involved (Lueder, 1998). The collaborative relationship is complex and should be built on trust, mutual regard, caring, and shared beliefs. There must be a shared belief that all are "equal" partners in education, both academic and social. It is important to recognize that the social development of today's youth is important to all of society in that as children grow older, they will become either productive members of society or a burden.

Role of the Federal Government in Promoting Parental Involvement

The federal government has recognized the importance of parental involvement in two recent pieces of legislation. The Goals 2000: Educate America Act signed in 1994 (Pub. L. 103-227, 108 Stat. 125) established a national goal on parent participation, "Every school will promote partnerships that will increase parental involvement and participation in promoting social, emotional, and academic growth of children" (U.S. Department of Education, 1994, p. 11). Schools were asked to help parents strengthen home learning activities and involve them in school decision making. In addition, the Improving America's Schools Act of 1994 (Pub. L. 103-382, 108 Stat. 3518) reauthorized aid to low-income and low-achieving students (Title I). Title I requires parents to be consulted in the development and review of local school improvement plans. Moreover, one percent of Title 1 funding must be set aside for parental involvement programs in districts that receive $500,000 or more (Booth & Dunn, 1996). Numerous federal agencies, including the Department of Education and the Office of Juvenile Justice have identified parental involvement programs as essential.

Parental Involvement as a Form of Delinquency Prevention

Parental involvement in the education of elementary school children has been identified as a way to prevent future antisocial behavior, dropping out of high school, and delinquency. The nature of youth delinquency has become increasingly violent, shifting from what is considered simple delinquent behavior (i.e., truancy or shoplifting) to that which is criminal (i.e., murder, rape, and assault). Many states are dealing with the change in youth crime by treating youth as adults and sentencing them as such. However, an alternative to punishment is prevention of delinquency. Current research suggests that effective prevention of delinquency should begin at the early stages in a child's life, during elementary school or sooner (Kazdin, 1985). Thus far, efforts at prevention have yielded little long-term success as a result of the intervention's being brief and focused on single dimensions of the problem (e.g., parenting) (Kazdin, 1985; Lytton, 1990). Parental involvement has been identified as an element that can be combined with other services such as after-school programs, mentoring, tutoring, mental health, and social services to assist in the prevention of delinquency.

IMPORTANCE OF THE PARENT AND FAMILY TO SUCCESSFUL PROGRAMS

Parents play a significant role in the education of their children. "It has long been acknowledged that the genesis of delinquency lies in the home" (Cullingford, 1999, p. 153). Parents are the first nurturers, socializers, and educators of children. As stated by Boyer (1991), "Home is the first classroom. Parents are the first and most essential teachers" (p. 33). The social abilities of young children are established before they can express themselves. As such, the earliest relationships are of the greatest importance (Cullingford, 1999).

Research has shown that children who do not form attachments to others during their first two years are often unable to form bonds later in life. Based on this finding, it is essential to target families in the early stages of children's lives and assist families in forming positive relationships with their children. In addition, programs should assist families in helping their children develop socially and academically. For children, the development of bonds with others depends on the family environments in which they were raised. The particular family management practices and family communication styles have an impact on youths' behaviors. Family factors that enhance social development include the development of bonds (Sokol-Katz et al., 1997), attendance and encouragement with educational and social activities (Felner, 1982; Smith et al., 1995), and spending quality time with the children (Benson, 1993). Children who are raised in a family with a warm and uncritical parenting style are more likely to demonstrate prosocial behavior. Parents who communicate clear expectations of behaviors (Hawkins & Catalano, 1992), clear values, expectations for educational standards and goals (Felner et al., 1982), and proactive ways to manage stress and conflict (Werner, 1990) are more likely to encourage positive emotional development in their child.

Behavior Patterns of Elementary-Age At-Risk Youth

Delinquency, violence, drug abuse, and other problem behaviors in youth are a significant problem in the United States. Over the past decade, violent crimes committed by adults have decreased while violent crimes committed by youths have dramatically increased. According to Middleton and Cartledge (1995), "Aggressive, disruptive behaviors of children and youth are increasingly a major concern of our schools and the larger society" (p. 192). Hughes and Cavell (1995) reported a significant increase in aggressive behaviors among school-age youth. Teachers describe aggressive students as argumentative—individuals who frequently take things, fight, and tease other students. Parker and Asher (1987) indicate that these aggressive students prevent an orderly classroom environment, have academic difficulties, and are future school dropouts. Kenneth Kamminger (1988) identified at-risk youth as those showing persistent patterns of underachievement and maladjustment. These children are typically unmotivated and too distracted to be successful in school. Kamminger found that patterns of underachievement identified in third grade were significantly correlated with dropping out of school.

Early Interventions: Need for Parental Involvement in Elementary Education

One possible method to combat the problem of juvenile crime is the implementation of early intervention programs. Parent and community involvement is emerging as the vital "missing link" to reaching educational goals in many communities. On the other hand, knowing how to involve parents remains a big mystery for many professional educators and community leaders (Batey, 1996).

Several researchers have found that improving parenting practices and the family environment is the most effective and longest-lasting solution to delinquency. Cullingford (1999) indicates the root problem of crime "lies in the experience of home and school. Crime is a manifestation of something having gone wrong earlier. It is the last outcome of feelings of exclusion and dysfunction" (p. 1). Social deprivation is a factor in delinquency though it does not by itself explain delinquency. Peer influence is also important to future delinquency; however, its extent and nature depend largely on the early relationships developed in the home. "Friends might come and go and are formed for pleasure rather than learning, but parents dominate. They teach, however inadvertently. They present attitudes and interests and are the first example to young children both of the importance of the point of view and how individual and idiosyncratic they can be" (p. 16).

For some families parental involvement comes naturally. Some parents volunteer at their children's schools, are members of the PTA, attend sporting or musical events, and talk with their children's teachers on a regular basis. Moreover, these families also tend to promote the importance of education in the home by assisting their children with homework and supporting their children in the learning process. However, some families lack the skills to participate in the educational and social development of their children. According to Lueder (1998), "The major parental involvement issue facing this country is that many parents are not engaged in the education of their children at home. It is this group of 'missing families' that should be the focus of involvement programs" (p. 4). Comer (1987–1988) defines human capital as one's skills and capabilities. Typically human capital encompasses the resources parents possess, including educational, economic, and social status. Social capital, on the other hand, includes the relationships and interactions that take place among people. Typically at-risk families are deficient in both human and social capital. Parents can restore social capital by becoming involved in their children's school. When schools incorporate activities that support educational achievement they increase the human capital of the parents. To assist these at-risk families, Liontos (1992) suggests that schools can help offer training and services to promote the basic obligation of at-risk families to their children's safety and health. Liontos recognizes that a gap exists for at-risk children between home and school. For these children, different cultures tend to exist between home and school; the values, expectations, and environments are significantly different.

MODELS OF FAMILY INVOLVEMENT: PAST, PRESENT, AND FUTURE

Parental involvement has been identified in current research and policy literature as a resource for school and social success (Henderson & Berla, 1994). In a 1996 report, the U.S. Department of Education indicated that when schools and families work together to support learning, children are inclined to succeed both in school and throughout life.

The traditional model of family involvement has been single dimensional whereby family resources flow to the school in the form of money, time, and expertise. Limitations to this approach result in many families not being involved or receiving the support they need (Lueder, 1998). In contrast, Davies (1991) identifies the recent shift in the paradigm of parental involvement from a parent focus to a comprehensive family focus. This paradigm shift involves several dimensions:

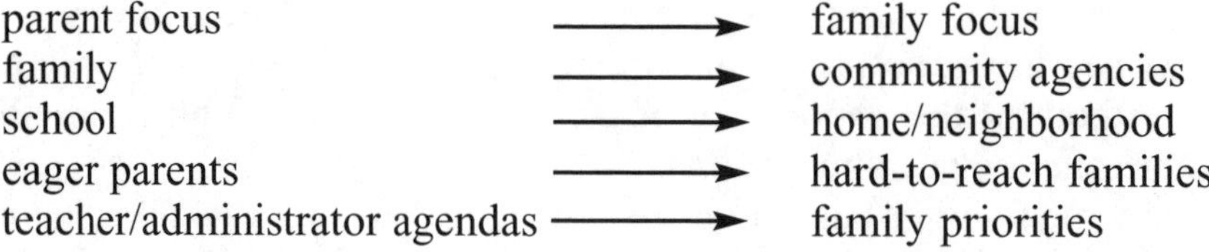

This model suggests that community agencies are becoming involved in assisting families through nontraditional means such as providing workshops or creating family resource centers in the schools. Moreover, there has been a shift in the view that the school is solely responsible for education to one that recognizes that education must also be emphasized in the home and in one's neighborhood. In addition, schools are attempting to target hard-to-reach populations rather than focusing activities on those few parents who typically volunteer to participate whenever needed. It has been recognized that hard-to-reach families are those whose children are most at risk for future failure, and whose families are most in need of assistance. Finally, input from families is solicited as to what they would like to have included in family programs as opposed to what teachers or administrators think interests the families.

Role of the School in Facilitating Family Involvement

Current research has focused on the role schools play in the facilitation of parental involvement and in the academic achievement of the child. It is critical that relationships develop between teachers, parents, schools, and communities (Booth & Dunn, 1996). When developing parental involvement programs school districts need to establish policies by gaining the input of parents either through surveys or parent advisory councils. Schools must initiate policies to encourage parental involvement. Moreover, it is essential for schools to train teachers in methods of engaging families (Fuller & Olsen, 1998).

Essential Role of the Parent in Parental Involvement Programs

The role of the parent is an essential consideration in program design. That role should be emphasized and considered equal to or greater than that of the school. The National PTA (2000) identified four key roles of parents that are consistently identified in the research literature:

- *Teachers/nurturers.* Parents are involved with the physical, moral, intellectual, emotional, and social development of their child.
- *Communicators/advisors.* Parents serve as communicators between the home and the school, therefore, it is important to have effective two-way communication. In addition, parents need open communication with their children in order to serve as advisors.
- *Supporters/learners.* Parents can assist their children by obtaining skills and knowledge to enhance their children's educational and social development.
- *Collaborators/decision makers.* Parents can help solve problems, make decisions, and develop policies.

In *Beyond the Bake Sale,* Henderson, Marburger, and Ooms (1996) describe parent roles as being more complex than traditionally believed. If parents are to truly be involved in the development of their child, they must serve numerous roles to support their child. These roles include partners performing basic obligations for educational and social development, collaborators and problem solvers reinforcing the school's effort and helping to solve problems the school may encounter, audience members supporting their child and others by attending and appreciating such school functions as athletic events and musical productions, supporters volunteering in the school when needed, and, as advisors/decision makers, providing input on school policy. Berger (2000) presented another perspective on the role of parents which includes eight levels of parental involvement:

- *Parent as an active partner and educational leader at home and at school.* Parents must be highly committed to the educational and social success of their child.
- *Parent as a decision maker.* Parents should serve on school boards, management, or advisory councils to contribute to the policy making process.
- *Parent as an advocate to help schools achieve excellent educational offerings.* Parents should volunteer to participate in fundraisers to raise money for the school and write letters to newspapers or policy makers to advocate for their school.
- *Parent actively involved with the school as a volunteer or paid employee.* Parents can become involved with the school either on a paid or voluntary basis.
- *Parent as a liaison between school and home to support homework and*

be aware of school activities. Parents should be aware of what is required of their child and confirm that any assignments are completed and that their child participates in school activities.

- *Parent as learner.* Parents can participate in parent education classes to improve their ability to help their child. Additionally, parents can share information to help with common problems or situations.
- *Parent, though not active, supporting the educational goals of the school and encouraging the child to study.* Parents may not have the time to actively participate in school activities but can encourage their child's achievement.
- *Parent as recipient of education and support from the school.* Parents can utilize school and community resources to improve their personal situation.

Essential Design Elements of Programs to Involve Families

When designing a parental involvement program, one must question why some parents are involved and others are not. Family status variables (e.g., income, education, ethnicity, and marital status) are often related to parental involvement and children's school success. However, it has also been established that family status variables do not explain fully parents' decisions to become involved in their children's education (Hoover-Dempsey & Sandler, 1997). Hoover-Dempsey and Sandler developed a model to explain the decision to become or not to become involved in their children's education. They believe there are three fundamental issues related to involvement: (1) the parents' construction of their role in their children's lives; (2) the parents' sense of efficacy for helping their children succeed; and (3) invitations, demands, and opportunities for parental involvement. When these three issues are considered in the development of parental involvement programs, the likelihood of success increases.

In discussing the design of parental involvement programs, Cullingford (1999) stresses the importance of recognizing that parents' attitudes toward school are influenced by their own experience when in school. "Parents who come from economically deprived backgrounds are found to have the greatest sense of awe at, and alienation from, schools" (Cullingford, 1999, p. 52). Due to the potential feelings of alienation, schools must reach out to the parents of at-risk youth to make them want to become involved in the educational process. Comer (1994) indicates that parental involvement is influenced by cultural dissonance between the parents and school or negative prior experiences with school. Schools tend to punish what they understand as bad behavior and to hold low expectations for underdeveloped children. This results in a "culture of failure" in school. As a result, the relationship between the school and home is built on distrust, anger, and alienation. Parents and staff are thus unable to support the level of development needed for school success.

Epstein (1995, 1987) categorized six types of involvement to enhance a school-family-community collaboration:

- *Basic obligations of families.* Parents have a basic obligation to provide for the economic and social needs of their family. Parental involvement programs can help parents develop skills and an understanding of child development to help them create a supportive home environment. Schools can help families develop positive skills through workshops, parent education, training, and information giving.
- *Basic obligations of schools.* The schools must communicate with families regarding the child's progress and school programs. Communication must be two way. The school can communicate with families through notices, telephone calls, visits, report cards, conferences, and activities.
- *Involvement at school.* Parents should be involved at their child's school by volunteering for temporary or permanent activities. The school must provide recruitment, training, and flexibility in volunteer opportunities.
- *Involvement in learning activities at home.* Parents need to recognize that learning does not take place only in the school. Schools should provide parents with activities that can be used to enhance learning at home.
- *Involvement in decision-making, governance, and advocacy.* Parents can become involved in the PTA/PTO, advisory councils or site management teams. For parents to participate in decision making, the school must teach parents decision-making skills.
- *Collaborating with community organizations.* Schools should integrate community services to strengthen school and home conditions. Parents are thus able to use community resources to assist in the development of their child.

Many authors have identified what they view as the most important elements of parental involvement programs. The U.S. Department of Education (1997) recognizes that there is no "one size fits all" approach to partnerships. Programs must build on what works and incorporate flexibility and diversity to enhance program success. Moreover, programs must recognize that change takes time. Morrison (1994) found that a mix of formal and informal activities works best. Parents become engaged through participation in social and recreational activities, which, in turn, results in parents being more likely to work on school-related activities. Liontos (1992) identified ten elements of successful programs:

- *Committed dedicated leadership.* Successful programs have leaders who possess energy, patience, and persistence.

- *An innovative, flexible approach.* Successful programs realize that they must use innovative approaches to reach out to parents who may need assistance but must also be flexible to address changing needs of families.
- *Strong, personal outreach.* Successful programs must reach out to families using multiple personal means such as telephone contacts and home visits.
- *Warm, nonjudgmental communication.* Successful programs include two-way communication which is nonthreatening in nature.
- *Nonthreatening activities.* Successful programs promote activities that are enjoyable for the participants.
- *Active support by administrators and staff.* Successful programs have ongoing active support from administration.
- *Attention to environment, format, and scheduling.* Successful programs consider environmental factors that may influence a family's participation in a program as well as the need to be flexible to accommodate parents' work schedules.
- *Meaningful activities.* Successful programs incorporate activities that are beneficial to the families.
- *Provide for the essentials.* Successful programs provide for the essential needs of families such as child care, transportation, and meals.
- *High visibility.* Successful programs market themselves to families through positive publicity from the school as well as current and past participants.

Kumpfer (1999) contends that an early intervention in a nonthreatening environment can help prevent antisocial behavior by improving family relations and communications. Programs should be long term, enduring, and comprehensive interventions that promote parent-child bonding and alter family dynamics. The focus of parental involvement programs should be on the family at sufficient intensity levels determined by the needs of the families involved. Liontos (1992) recognized that teachers and administrators must change their mind-set if parental involvement programs are going to be successful. Schools must recognize that all families have strengths, parents can learn new techniques, parents have important perspectives about their children, most parents really care about their children, cultural differences are both valid and valuable, and many family forms exist and are legitimate. Henderson et al. (1996), stress that all aspects of the school's climate must be "open, helpful, and friendly" and communication with parents should be "frequent, clear, and two-way." The school should treat parents as "collaborators in the educational process," sharing in the decision-making process. The school administration should "actively express and promote the philosophy of partnership with all families" and recognize its responsibility "to forge a partnership with all families in the school."

Elizabeth Sandell (1998) examined effective parental involvement programs and found six qualities shared by successful programs.

- *Responsibility*. Staff and sponsors take responsibility for providing comprehensive, flexible, and responsive programs.
- *Creative marketing.* Programs are marketed creatively and intentionally to their community. Service providers persevere in their outreach efforts.
- *Theoretical foundations.* Programs have strong theoretical foundations which organize their activities toward long-term prevention and empowerment.
- *Trust and respect.* Participants and staff trust and respect each other. Sponsors create accepting environments and build relationships with families.
- *Community context.* Staff members deal with the child in the context of the family, neighborhood, and community. Several generations are involved with responding to the concerns of different individuals and populations.
- *Highly qualified staff.* Highly competent, energetic, committed, and responsible individuals are involved on the staff and as volunteers. Workers are allowed to make flexible, individualized decisions (pp. 177–178).

When determining program design, the opinions of parents should be solicited and incorporated. Lindle (1989) identified characteristics of parental involvement programs which parents believed were necessary for the success of a program; parents prefer frequent, informal relationships with teachers who take the time to see the parent's perspective.

EXAMINATION OF EXISTING PROGRAMS: SITE DESCRIPTIONS

In addition to an examination of the research literature regarding parental involvement in elementary school programs, an examination of existing programs that involve parents is essential to illustrate the "lessons learned" from existing parental involvement programs. (See Appendix III-1 on page PIII-3.)

Eight parental involvement programs, at varying stages of development, were selected to examine the implementation process of programs designed to engage elementary school children and their parents. Of the eight programs studied, the three most developed programs were studied extensively (see

Exhibit 8.1). The first program is a pilot program implemented locally in North Carolina. Victory-in-Partnership (VIP) is currently implemented district wide in Winston-Salem/Forsyth County schools. VIP encourages parents to become more involved in their child's education through parenting sessions and weekly progress reports. Two nationally recognized exemplary programs were also examined. These programs were developed based on extensive research and evaluation of the effectiveness of program elements. The first program, Families and Schools Together (FAST), is a two-year, school-based, elementary-level program aimed at building bonds within families. The program begins with eight weeks of family group activities designed to improve communication and build bonds within the family unit. Upon completion of FAST, families enter Fast Works, which reinforces skills learned during the eight-week program. FAST has been replicated in over 450 schools in the United States and in five countries. The second exemplary program, Fast Track, is a multisite research program designed to prevent serious and chronic antisocial behavior identified as high risk in kindergarten. Fast Track incorporates in-class curricula, parent training, home visits, social skill training groups, child tutoring, and child friendship enhancement. Fast Track is a longitudinal research study implemented in four locations in the United States. (Chapter 9 details some of the existing programs that highlight parental involvement.)

THE CHALLENGE OF INVOLVEMENT

Engaging parents in the educational process may seem an easy task given the natural inclination of all parents to wish the best for their children, but then try to make it happen. Go to an open house or an orientation or even a field hockey game after school. You'll see the same relatively few faces—relative, that is, to the numbers of parents who should be there. Even at a school open house, when parents have their first opportunity to meet the teachers who shape their children, where the parents are supposed to take their child's seat, notice how many places are empty or attended only by one parent (usually the mother). Again, we see the same faces. But what can be done to engage the at-risk parents of at-risk children, the parents who really should not have any excuse not to attend? The school community has the obligation, albeit an impossible task, to engage these parents.

Schools have to battle time restraints imposed by the dual incomers, or the single parent, or parents just too tired at the end of the day for another meeting or event. There is too much or too little—too much on the schedule or too little energy to get engaged even for the annual open house. Or, the next sitcom episode takes precedence. Society seems to be set up to undermine efforts to make a connection between schools, parents, and their children—a connection that needs to be made early and often. Soon, especially after the elementary years, it becomes impossible to make connections that translate into a really successful primary educational experience. Yet parents bemoan these missed opportunities after the fact.

Engaging parents on any socioeconomic plane is difficult these days, but it is worth it. Any time spent, especially during the elementary years, on a concerted, single-minded effort to help parents connect with their children, and children connect with their parents is most productive. A program to do so needs to be designed for all families of a particular school, and it is especially rewarding to target the neediest of families. Go at it with an attitude of possibility and gains will be made. It is neither simple nor easy, but it is worthwhile. We have noted in this chapter only a few examples of the many successful efforts that demonstrate that it can be done.

References

Batey, C. S. (1996). *Parents are lifesavers: A handbook for parent involvement in schools.* Thousand Oaks, CA: Corwin Press.

Benson, P. (1993). *The troubled journey: A portrait of 6th–12th grade youth.* Minneapolis, MN: The Search Institute.

Berger, E. H. (2000). *Parents as partners in education: Families and schools working together* (5th ed.). Upper Saddle River, NJ: Merrill.

Booth, A., & Dunn, J. F. (1996). *Family school links: How do they affect educational outcomes?* Mahwah, NJ: Erlbaum.

Boyer, E. L. (1991). *Ready to learn: A mandate for the nation.* Princeton, NJ: Carnegie Foundation for the Advancement of Teaching.

Comer, J. P. (1987–1988). School power: A model for improving black student achievement. *The Urban League Review, 11*(1–2), 187–200.

Comer, J. P. (1994). *Introduction and problem analysis. School development program research monograph.* New Haven, CT: Yale Child Study Center.

Cullingford, C. (1999). *The causes of exclusion: Home, school, and the development of young criminals.* London: Kogan Page.

Davies, D. (1991). Schools reaching out: Family, school and community partnerships for student success. *Phi Delta Kappan, 72*(5), 376–382.

Epstein, J. L. (1987). What principals should know about parental involvement. *Principal, 66*(3), 6–9.

Epstein, J. L. (1995). School/family/community partnerships: Caring for the children we share. *Phi Delta Kappan, 76*(9), 701–712.

Epstein, J. L., & Dauber, S. L. (1991). School programs and teacher practices of parental involvement in inner-city elementary and middle schools. *The Elementary School Journal, 91*, 289–305.

Felner, R. D., Ginter, M. A., & Primavera, A. (1982). Primary prevention during school transitional: Social support and environmental structure. *American Journal of Community Psychology, 10*, 227–240.

Fuller, M. L., & Olsen, G. (1998). *Home-school relations: Working successfully with parents and families.* Needham Heights, MA: Allyn & Bacon.

Griffin, J. (1996). Relation of parental involvement, empowerment, and school traits to student academic performance. *Journal of Education Research, 90*(1), 33–42.

Hawkins, J. D., Catalano, R. F., & Miller, J.Y. (1992). Risk and protective factors for alcohol and other problems in adolescence and early adulthood: Implications for substance abuse prevention. *Psychological Bulletin, 112*(1), 64–104.

Henderson, A. T., & Berla, N. (1994). *A new generation of evidence: The family is critical to student achievement.* Columbia, MD: National Committee for Citizens in Education.

Henderson, A. T., & Berla, N. (1995). *A new generation of evidence: The family is critical to student achievement.* Washington DC: Center for Law and Education.

Henderson, A. T., Marburger, C. L., & Ooms, T. (1996). Beyond the bake sale: An educators guide to working with parents. Columbia, MD: The National Committee for Citizens in Education.

Hoover-Dempsey, K. V., & Sandler, H. M. (1997). Why do parents become involved in their children's education? *Review of Education Researc*h, *67*(1), 3–42.

Hughes, J. N., & Cavell, T. A. (1995). Cognitive-affective approaches: Enhancing competence in aggressive children. In G. Cartledge & J. E. Milburn (Eds), *Teaching social skills to children and youth* (3rd ed., pp. 199–236). Needham Heights, MA: Allyn & Bacon.

Kamminger, K. (1988). Early intervention with children at risk. Marquette County.

Kazdin, A. E. (1985). *Treatment of antisocial behavior in children and adolescents.* Homewood, IL: Dorsey.

Kumpfer, K. L. (1999). *Strengthening America's families: Exemplary parenting and family strategies for delinquency prevention.* Washington, DC: U.S. Department of Justice, Office of Justice Programs, Office of Juvenile Justice and Delinquency Prevention.

Lindle, J. C. (1989). What do parents want from principals and teachers? *Educational Leadership*, *47*(2), 12–14.

Liontos, L. B. (1992). *At-risk families and schools: Becoming partners.* Eugene, OR: ERIC Clearinghouse.

Lueder, D. C. (1998). *Creating partnerships with parents.* Lancaster, PA: Technomic.

Lytton, H. (1990). Child and parent effects in boys' conduct disorder: A re-interpretation. *Developmental Psychology*, *26*, 683–697.

Middleton, M. B., & Cartledge, G. (1995). Effects of social skills instruction and parental involvement on the aggressive behaviors of African American males. *Behavior Modification*, *19*(2),192–211.

Morrison, M. T. (1994). *Increasing parental involvement by motivating parents of fourth and fifth grade students to become more meaningfully involved in children's education.* Miami, FL: Nova University Press.

National PTA. (2000). *Building Successful Partnerships: A guide for developing parent and family involvement programs.* Bloomington, IN: National Educational Service.

Parker, J. G., & Asher, S. R. (1987). Peer relationships and later personal adjustment: Are low-accepted children at risk? *Psychological Bulletin*, *102*, 357–389.

Sandell, E. J. (1998). Family involvement models in early childhood education. In M. L. Fuller & G. Olsen (Eds.), *Home school relations* (pp. 177–183). Boston: Allyn & Bacon.

Smith C., Lizotte, A. J., Thornberry, T. P., & Krohn, M. D. (1995). Resilient youth: Identifying factors that prevent high-risk youth from engaging in delinquency and drug use. In J. Hagan (Ed.), *Delinquency and disrepute in the life course* (pp. 217–247). Greenwich, CT: JAI Press.

Sokol-Katz, J., Dunham, R., & Zimmerman, R. (1997). Family structure versus parental attachment in controlling adolescent deviant behavior: A social control model. *Adolescence*, *32*(125), 119–215.

U.S. Department of Education. (1996). *Policy guidance for Title I, Part A: Improving basic programs operated by local educational agencies*. Washington DC: Author.

Werner, E. E. (1990). Protective factors and individual resilience. In S. J. Meisels & J. P. Shonkoff (Eds.), *Handbook of early intervention* (pp. 97–116). New York: Cambridge University Press.

Exhibit 8.1
Resources

Fast Track Project

http://www.fasttrackproject.org/

Fast Track is a comprehensive, multisite intervention designed to prevent serious and chronic antisocial behavior in a sample of children selected as high-risk at school entry because of their conduct problems in kindergarten and home. The intervention is guided by a developmental theory positing the interaction of multiple influences on the development of antisocial behavior.

Families and Schools Together (FAST)

http://www.wcer.wisc.edu/fast

Families and Schools Together (FAST) is a prevention program developed by Dr. Lynn McDonald in 1988, in Madison, Wisconsin. FAST is collaborative, starts early, works with families in groups, and puts research into practice. FAST starts by creating culturally representative teams based on collaboration between parents and professionals from the local school and two community-based agencies. The team is then trained to do outreach to stressed, isolated, and often low-income families to invite them to attend a multi-family group meeting. 80 percent of the families who attend one FAST session, continue to attend, and then graduate from the 8–10 weekly sessions. The sessions focus on building relationships within the family (with the parent being in charge of her/his children), across families (with parents from the same school getting to know other parents of their child's classmates), and with school and community personnel.

Victory-in-Partnership (VIP)

http://wsfcs.k12.nc.us/parents/vipprog.html

The Victory-in-Partnership program is a collaboration between schools, parents and the community in Winston-Salem/ Forsyth County, North Carolina. There are three models, based on needs of parents and students at the pre-kindergarten, elementary/middle school, and high school levels.

Chapter 9

Cases in Point—Benefits of Parental Involvement

This chapter is designed to illustrate the "lessons learned" from existing parental involvement programs, including an examination of the design, program components, evaluation methods used, and a description of extensive implementation for the programs most thoroughly developed. It is essential to examine these programs in addition to the research literature, which supports parental involvement in elementary school programs.

VICTORY-IN-PARTNERSHIP

Program Design

The mission of Victory-in-Partnership (VIP) (see Exhibit 8.1 on page 8-15) is "to create a more pronounced partnership between the school, parent and community for the purpose of building stronger support for student success." VIP was piloted in Winston-Salem elementary schools in July 1999 as a collaborative effort between Wachovia Corporation, the Greater Winston-Salem Chamber of Commerce, and the Winston-Salem/Forsyth County Schools. The program was expanded to all elementary schools in the 2001–2002 school year. VIP is funded through in-kind contributions, school district funding, Title I funds, and donations from private foundations.

The main components of the VIP elementary school program include weekly progress reports, parental involvement sessions, Saturday academy for parents, and on-site VIP coordinators. Parental involvement is enhanced through the use of weekly progress reports designed to provide parents with information on their child's performance, attendance, and behavior. Parental involvement sessions are held before and after school to assist parents with skills necessary to help their child academically and socially. Another component is the Saturday Academy for parents, which includes consumer mathematics, GED, computer skills, Spanish, reading, and English as a second language (ESL). Each school has a resident VIP coordinator who serves as a liaison between teachers and parents. An outcome evaluation of the VIP has not been conducted; however, two surveys were distributed in May 2001 to parents and teachers to ascertain their reaction to the VIP program.

Parent Survey

During the 2000–2001 school year, parents were surveyed to ascertain their opinions regarding the VIP program. The survey asked parents to evaluate key features of the VIP program, including weekly progress reports and parenting sessions. The on-site VIP school coordinators and classroom teachers administered the surveys. The first element of the VIP program is the weekly distribution of progress reports.

- Almost all parents/guardians (95 percent) said that they "usually" or "always" receive progress reports.
- Parents at one school (a school in the first year of program implementation) reported elevated levels of nonreceipt compared to other schools. About 8 percent of parents at this school indicated that they "never" or "seldom" receive progress reports and an additional 17.3 percent stated that they "sometimes" received the progress report. In short, 25 percent of parents at this particular school did not consistently receive the reports.
- No other school reported more than 2.4 percent of parents indicating that they never or seldom received progress reports.
- Approximately 96 percent of parents noted that the weekly progress reports were clear and understandable.
- Most respondents (92.7 percent) indicated that the reports "usually" or "always" helped them and their children.
- Interestingly, 8.8 percent of parents at the elementary school who reported high levels of nonreceipt said that the reports "never" or "seldom" helped their families. This result may be related to the inconsistent receipt of reports by parents.
- Parents reported overwhelmingly that they "usually" or "always" responded to the weekly reports in a timely manner (94.4 percent).

- In sum, a large majority of parents received the progress reports on a consistent basis, judged them to be clear and understandable, viewed the reports as helpful, and responded to the reports in a timely manner.

The second element of VIP is participation in parenting sessions and meetings. Parents split evenly in terms of their participation in parenting sessions and other monthly meetings.

- About half reported that they regularly attended parenting sessions (usually/always). The other half infrequently or never participated (never/seldom/sometimes).
- There appeared to be wide variation in participation rates among the schools. On the high end, two-thirds of parents at two schools stated that they regularly attended parenting sessions. Conversely, four schools had over 40 percent of parents say that they "never" or "seldom" participated in parenting sessions.
- A majority of parents (68 percent) reported that the parenting sessions were "usually" or "always" helpful to the family.
- In sum, about half the parents regularly participated in VIP meetings while a solid majority found the sessions helpful.

One goal of VIP is to improve academic performance, attendance, and behavior for the students participating in the program.

- Most parents stated that their child's performance, attendance, and behavior "always" improved. However, there was some minor variation among schools on these student outcome measures.
- Parents at one school recorded the highest scores for student outcomes. For each of the outcomes, over 90 percent of the respondents from one school, which was in its third year of operation, said that their child "usually" or "always" improved.

Teacher Survey

Elementary school faculty who participated in the VIP program during the 2000–2001 school year were asked to evaluate the program by completing a written questionnaire. The purpose of the survey was (1) to gauge teacher satisfaction with specific program components (e.g., weekly reports, technology, and VIP coordinator) and (2) to see if teachers viewed the program as a valuable resource for improving parental involvement and various student outcomes.

Teachers had mixed feelings about core program elements such as progress reports, technology, and on-site VIP coordinators. The teachers objected to the time commitment required for VIP paperwork. Several teachers acknowledged that it took upwards of six additional hours to complete the weekly progress reports. A majority (59 percent) agreed that the weekly progress report form was well organized. Over three-quarters reported that technology was a major problem in preparing the reports. However, more than half noted that the technology had improved during the year. An overwhelming number of teachers (90 percent) found their VIP coordinator to be helpful and understanding. As a whole, teachers did not see parents as holding up their end of the partnership. A slight majority did not find parental feedback after progress reports constructive. Almost 80 percent of teachers did not think that parents were fulfilling program requirements.

Teacher responses were collapsed into two categories: those who agreed that the VIP program had been a success and those who disagreed with the same statement. Teachers at four schools reported extremely high negative responses for this question. In fact, every respondent at one school felt that the program had not been a success. A second group of four schools had 57–65 percent of teachers not finding the program successful. Teachers at three other schools generally split 50/50 on this question. Small majorities at three schools agreed that the program had been a success. Teachers at two schools recorded extremely positive scores (82 percent and 90 percent, respectively) on the issue.

Overall, the teachers participating in the survey, understandably, were fairly negative about program outcomes due to the increased paperwork and job duties. On a positive note, two-thirds of teachers disclosed that the weekly reports improved communication with parents. However, a similar percentage did not agree that the reports helped to improve student grades and attendance. Almost 70 percent of teachers did not think that VIP had increased parental involvement for students having academic problems. Only 43 percent of teachers agreed that the VIP program had been a success. In short, teachers were generally pessimistic about the effectiveness of the program. That is, the program did not appear to improve student outcomes or parental involvement. Time-consuming paperwork and computer hardware breakdowns were commonly cited problems with the program. On the positive side, the teachers seemed pleased with their VIP coordinators and saw improvements in the technology over the course of the school year. This reluctance of teachers to be enthused about the program is understandable considering the increased paperwork and needs to be seen in light of the strong endorsement by parents.

FAST TRACK PROJECT

Program Design

The Fast Track project was developed as a comprehensive, multisite intervention to prevent antisocial behavior in students identified as high risk in kindergarten. The Fast Track project was designed to develop, implement, and evaluate a comprehensive intervention to prevent conduct problems. Fast Track is especially noteworthy in that it is a longitudinal examination of prevention activities over time, which were designed based on developmental theory and research. The Fast Track project followed three cohorts of high-risk students at four sites selected based on crime and poverty statistics (Durham, North Carolina; central Pennsylvania; Seattle and Highline, Washington; and Nashville, Tennessee) to determine ways to prevent future antisocial behavior. The study includes approximately 440 intervention and 440 control children. The Fast Track project is funded by the National Institute of Mental Health, the National Institute on Drug Abuse, the U.S. Department of Education, and the Center for Substance Abuse Prevention (Conduct Problems Prevention Research Group, 1999, 2000).

Fast Track uses a two-phased approach, one designed for elementary school students and the other for adolescents. Fast Track used a home-school partnership intervention to improve academic achievement, peer relations, classroom atmosphere, parenting and socialization, and child coping and problem-solving skills. To achieve such goals, Fast Track stresses increased adult supervision and monitoring, achievement and bonding to school, involvement with nondeviant peer groups, and healthy identity development and coping skills.

In each of the four geographic areas selected for the program, schools were randomly selected to either be intervention or control sites. A total of fifty-four elementary schools were selected to participate in the program. Teachers evaluated the behavior of all kindergarten students; the parents of the most aggressive 40 percent in each school were then contacted. Parents were asked questions related to the child's behavior at home. The highest scoring 10 percent based on teacher and parent evaluations were identified as high risk and invited to participate in the program. The program consisted of a universal teacher-led classroom curricula for all students, parent training groups, home visits, child social skills training groups, child tutoring in reading, and child friendship enhancement (Conduct Problems Prevention Research Group, 1999, 2000). Program staffing included a family coordinator to conduct home visits, parent groups, and parent-child sharing time; an educational coordinator to conduct friendship groups and supervise teachers and tutors; a classroom teacher to teach curriculum; and a tutor to conduct the reading tutoring and peer pairing.

The teacher-led curricula was taught two to three times per week from grades 1 through 5. The curriculum was designed to strengthen emotional understanding, increase self-control, increase social problem-solving skills, and improve peer relations. The curriculum was universal in that all students in the selected schools received the intervention regardless of risk identification.

The intervention for at-risk students included two-hour family group meetings, in which the parents were paid $15 per meeting and provided transportation and child care. Family group meetings were held weekly for twenty-two weeks in first grade, biweekly for fourteen weeks in second grade, and monthly for eight sessions in grades 3–5. The sessions included parent training groups, social skills training for children, tutoring, and a parent-child sharing session. The parent training groups were designed to promote positive family-school relations, to encourage parent self-control, to teach parenting skills, and to set reasonable expectations that parents should have for their child. The parent groups were developed with the needs of the parents in mind; often the parents determined their needs. Parents visited the school for positive purposes to reduce apprehension and feel more at ease with the school environment. The child-training group (friendship group) increased emotional understanding, self-control, and social problem solving. Activities were designed to improve cooperation, negotiation, and conflict management. The reading-tutoring component promoted basic reading skills through supportive adult-child relationships.

Home visits occurred once a week for one year, allowing program staff to build positive relationships with the family and assisting the parents' development of problem-solving and time management skills. The goal of the home visits was to improve parent empowerment by teaching parents how to become self-sufficient and have the skills necessary to deal with family problems at home.

Finally, child peer enhancement time-paired students with peers to strengthen self-efficacy. High-risk children were paired with peers, with whom they had weekly thirty-minute play sessions. The sessions were designed to build friendship skills and create friendships with other students.

Impact Evaluations

One evaluation of the Fast Track program was conducted when all three cohorts had completed at least third grade (i.e., first cohort was completing fifth grade, second cohort was completing fourth grade, and the third cohort was completing third grade). Using the classroom as the unit of analysis, the evaluation of the classroom-based program found that the control classrooms displayed more aggressive, disruptive, and disobedient children. In addition, children in the intervention classrooms reported fewer classmates demonstrating aggressive behavior and reported fewer classmates they disliked as compared to the control groups. The Spache Diagnostic Reading Scale was used to measure reading ability. Findings showed that the intervention children had significantly higher scores than did the control group. The evaluation of the child social and coping skills groups found that the intervention group had more accurate emotion recognition scores, more positive responses to hypothetical emotional experiences, more competent responses to hypothetical social problem solving, and fewer aggressive responses to hypothetical provocations than did the control children. Findings related to parenting behavior and values showed no difference between the intervention and control parents on measures of values and consistency and punitiveness of discipline.

Intervention parents did report higher use of loss of privileges as a form of discipline, rather than use of physical punishments, than did control parents. Teachers reported that parents of intervention children were more involved in school activities than the parents of control children. In addition, teachers reported that intervention parents demonstrated a higher value placed on education than did the control group parents (Conduct Problems Prevention Research Group, 1999, 2000).

A second assessment of Fast Track examined each program element using multiple instruments. Assessments were made through home visits, teacher reports, peer ratings, and school observation data. All instruments were shown to be valid and reliable in prior studies. On the dimension of child social cognition, the intervention groups improved their scores to a greater extent than did the control group in the areas of emotional recognition and emotion coping/social problem solving and decreased their score in aggressive retaliation. The intervention group displayed higher scores on the Spache Word Attack instrument and received higher language arts grades. On the dimensions of child peer relations and social competence, the intervention group spent significantly more time taking part in positive peer interaction and received higher peer social preference scores. In regard to the parenting behavior dimension, the parents in the intervention groups reported lower levels of using physical punishment on their children. In addition, teachers reported that there was a higher level of parental involvement in school for the parents in the intervention group. Parents in the intervention group reported increased satisfaction in parenting as well as satisfaction with the Fast Track program in general. Evaluation of the dimension of child aggressive-disruptive behavior, showed significantly less aggressive behavior in the intervention group (Conduct Problems Prevention Research Group, 1999).

FAMILIES AND SCHOOLS TOGETHER

Program Design

Families and Schools Together (FAST) was developed in 1987 to help at-risk youth develop relationships through a multifamily group approach to improve family communications, as well as to prevent juvenile delinquency and drug abuse. Since its development, FAST has been implemented in more than 450 schools. FAST implementation requires a collaborative team consisting of the school, parents, substance abuse agency, and one other community agency. The FAST team is trained to conduct weekly meetings. FAST has been recognized as an effective parental involvement program by numerous national organizations, including the U.S. Department of Health and Human Services, the U.S. Department of Education, the U.S. Office of Substance Abuse Prevention, the U.S. Department of Justice, the United Way of America, Harvard University and Ford Foundation, and the Family Resource Coalition.

The primary goal of FAST is to provide early intervention to help at-risk youth succeed in the home, community, and school. FAST categorizes parental involvement in four areas; involvement with their children, involvement with other parents, involvement with the school, and involvement with the community. Specific goals of FAST are to accomplish the following:

- Enhance family functioning;
- Promote a child's success in school;
- Prevent substance abuse by the child and family; and
- Reduce the stress that parents and children experience from daily life situations.

The FAST program builds on existing family strengths to encourage relationship building within the family and between the family and the school and community. FAST enhances family functioning by strengthening parent-child relationships and empowering parents to serve as prevention agents for delinquent behavior and to become active partners in the education of their child. FAST assists youth in building long-term relationships which serve as protective factors against future delinquency. FAST achieves its goals by building bonds, trust, and support networks for families.

FAST begins with home visits, followed by eight weekly school-based evening activities for families, and two years of monthly multifamily FAST-WORKS meetings. The individual school determines eligibility for FAST participation. In each FAST session, ten to fifteen families meet for two and a half hours and participate in a family meal, family activities, parent support groups, peer support groups, and parent-child communication. The FAST meetings begin with an opening tradition, the FAST hello and FAST song lasting approximately twenty-five minutes. Next, parents spend forty-five minutes with their family participating in activities followed by one hour of peer support time. Families then meet together for fifteen minutes of one-on-one parent-child communication. The meeting concludes with a closing tradition. The elements of the FAST program are designed to position parents to take charge of their families. Parents lead their family in each of the following activities:

- *Family flag.* One element of the FAST program is the creation of a family flag. The family flag is set on the family table each week during the FAST program. The family creates the flag by having each member add one element to its design. The development of a family flag is based on a systems theory approach to strengthen the family unit by drawing a boundary around the family (McDonald, 2000; McDonald & Moberg, 2000).
- *Family dinner.* A second element of the FAST program is the family dinner. Each week one family is chosen to prepare a dinner for the group. The FAST program provides money for the family to purchase supplies

to cook the meal. Eating together as a family has been found to strengthen the family unit. The children serve their family as a means of teaching children respect for their parents. The family that prepares the meal is selected using a fixed lottery. The winning family receives both a gift basket and the benefit of "winning" (McDonald, 2000; McDonald & Moberg, 2000).

- *Music.* A third element of the FAST program is the inclusion of music. Families share songs that they are encouraged to bring to the FAST meetings and sing the FAST song together each week. This promotes a positive mood in the participants (McDonald, 2000).
- *Scribbles.* A fourth component of FAST is family scribbles. Scribbles is a drawing and talking game used to improve communication within the family (McDonald, 2000; McDonald & Moberg, 2000).
- *Charades.* Family feelings charades is a fifth component of FAST. This activity assists in providing opportunities for families to express their feelings through play acting within the family with the goal of family members guessing and talking about feelings (McDonald, 2000; McDonald & Moberg, 2000).
- *Parent time.* The sixth component of FAST is parent time whereby parents meet as a group to discuss issues relevant to parenting. Parents discuss both difficulties and successes in raising their children. Research has shown that informal peer relationships between parents helps provide necessary social support (McDonald, 2000). While parents are meeting, the children also participate in kids' play that includes organized age-appropriate activities.
- *Special play.* The seventh component of FAST is special play. Parents and children spend one-on-one time together whereby the parent follows the lead of the child and is forbidden to teach, direct, or judge the child.

FAST can be implemented by repositioning existing personnel or hiring new staff. Depending on current staffing, the cost of FAST operation varies. The estimated expenditure to implement FAST for one pilot cycle is $24,000, which includes training and evaluation. The personnel needed for FAST include a lead facilitator (180 hours per cycle), mental health partner (50 hours per cycle), school partner (90 hours per cycle), substance abuse partner (50 hours per cycle), parent partner (100 hours per cycle), community organizer (50 hours per cycle), and two child-care providers (50 hours per cycle).

Impact Evaluations

FAST requires all sites to continuously evaluate program effectiveness. One element of the implementation of FAST is the requirement that representatives from the FAST National office evaluate programs. Each new FAST program receives evaluation feedback and program monitoring to ensure quality assurance. Each new program is assigned a certified FAST team trainer who conducts three site visits to observe implementation and provide necessary technical assistance. (McDonald & Moberg, 2000).

FAST uses a number of validated instruments to determine program effectiveness. The program uses the Revised Behavior Problem Checklist (RBPC) to screen child behavior in schools, which has been found to correlate with school success and future substance abuse problems. The Parenting Stress Inventory, Social Insularity Subscale measures parents' perceptions of social support and family social isolation. The Social Skills Rating System assesses social skills of the child at home and school. The Parent Survey on School Environment/Parent Involvement Scale rates family involvement in the schools. The Family Involvement Scale and the Family Adaptability and Cohesion Evaluation Scales (FACES II) measure family cohesion, expressiveness, and conflict. The Families and Schools Together Program Evaluation allows parents to describe the impact of FAST on their life. The Site Information and Participation Survey reports the demographic make-up of the school. The Parenting Stress Index measures the stress level of participants.

Evaluations are required for each FAST site. Data from fifty-three schools in thirteen states have shown significant improvements in child behavior (McDonald & Frey, 1999). In addition, FAST has performed a comprehensive evaluation of the effectiveness of program elements (see McDonald & Sayger, 1998; McDonald & Frey, 1999).

An evaluation of FAST found that two to four years after participation in FAST, 91 percent of families reported increased involvement in community activities, 75 percent of parents were still very involved in the schools, 86 percent were still friends with other parents they met in FAST, 55 percent obtained employment, 44 percent of parents pursued further education, and 26 percent self-referred to family counseling (McDonald & Frey, 1999).

Abt Associates conducted a five-year study on FAST as part of a congressional inquiry in New Orleans. Families were randomly assigned to FAST or a control group. The study found statistically significant improvements in the behavior and social skills of the FAST group (McDonald & Moberg, 2000).

An experimental study of FAST was conducted in Milwaukee. Families were randomly placed into FAST or a low-level control intervention. Families in the FAST group showed significant improvements in measures of social support. In addition, the FAST group had significantly lower behavioral problems following program participation (McDonald & Moberg, 2000).

An evaluation of the statewide implementation of FAST in Wisconsin was conducted. The RBPC was completed by parents and teachers. Parents reported significant improvements in their child in conduct disorder, socialized aggression, attention span problems, anxiety/withdrawal, and psychotic behavior. Teachers reported significant improvements in FAST participants in conduct disorders, attention span problems, anxiety/withdrawal, and motor excess (McDonald & Frey, 1999).

LEARNING FROM THE EXPERIENCES OF THOSE WHO ARE SUCCESSFULLY ENGAGING FAMILIES

Wherever we went during our research we saw schools engaged with parents; it is just that there are various levels of engagement. The three programs discussed in this chapter are some of the more successful ones. The essential element or theme of these successes is that program leadership and staff have a very positive attitude in the face of real frustration or what could be defeat. The program director at Victory in Partnership almost defied parents to give her excuses why they "couldn't." If a parent said she didn't have transportation to a school event, the director arranged for it. If another parent said he could not possibly to help his child with homework because he didn't understand it, she arranged for Saturday tutoring for the parent. If school staff told her there was no time for after hours and Saturday duty to engage parents she told the local bank president she needed volunteers; and they came. If she heard that parents couldn't get off work or couldn't find a baby sitter, she changed schedules and got volunteer baby sitters until parents ran out of excuses and became engaged. Wherever there was success there was this kind of attitude.

Does this "can do" attitude precede success, or does a little success breed this attitude? It is some of both. What is more important is that there is example. There is no cookie cutter to produce successful parental involvement. Anyone who suggests that there is does not understand the dynamic. Each success is a unique success. Victory in Partnership is the brainchild of one woman, a lifetime educator who grew frustrated at the missed opportunity of less than acceptable education that could be remedied by patching up the collective interest in the education of all her children, especially the children floating through school on the fringes. Fast Track is a sophisticated scientific experiment meant to study the effect of the best techniques of education for the at risk. Lessons learned add to the wealth of knowledge on how to get education done with a demanding population in a demanding environment. Families and Schools Together demonstrates that a good idea can be replicated. It further demonstrates the workable combination of prescribed format and local determination. In combination, programs like these provide scores of good ideas and a framework, a process that suggests how to proceed. Success in engaging families of elementary aged children then lies only in taking the first step with the resolve not to look back.

References

Conduct Problems Prevention Research Group. (1999). Initial impact of the Fast Track prevention trial for conduct problems: I. The high risk sample. *Journal of Consulting and Clinical Psychology*, *67*(5), 631–647.

Conduct Problems Prevention Research Group. (2000). Merging universal and indicated prevention programs: The Fast Track model. *Addictive Behaviors*, *25*(6), 913–927.

McDonald, L. (2000). *Research article: Pre-certification seminar homework.* Madison, WI: FAST National Training and Evaluation Center.

McDonald, L., & Frey, H. E. (1999). *Families and schools tTogether: Building relationships.* Washington, DC: U.S. Department of Justice, Office of Justice Programs, Office of Juvenile Justice and Delinquency Prevention.

McDonald, L., & Moberg, P. (2000). Families and schools together: FAST strategies for increasing involvement of all parents in schools and preventing drug abuse. In W. B. Hansen, S. M. Giles, & M. D. Fearnow-Kenney (Eds.), *Improving prevention effectiveness* (pp. 235–250). Winston-Salem, NC: Tanglewood Research.

McDonald, L., & Sayger, T. V. (1998). Impact of a family and school based prevention program on protective factors for high risk youth. *Drugs and Society*, *12*(1/2), 61–85.

Chapter 10

Effective Program Practices for Involving Parents of Elementary School Students

This chapter describes the promising practices we found to be effective based on a review of the research literature and an examination of the design and operation of eight existing programs. We are defining effective practices as those activities which programs have used and found to be successful in achieving the goal of engaging elementary school parents. It is important to recognize that simply because a program element was or was not successful in one location, it will or will not be successful elsewhere. Programs must recognize the characteristics of the population being served and make adjustments to program elements accordingly. The purpose of proving effective practices is to assist programs to "look in the right direction" in their effort to engage elementary school parents and their children. It is possible to identify a number of key programmatic features that come to define the most successful parent involvement initiatives.

PHASE 1: EFFECTIVE PRACTICES IN PROGRAM PLANNING

Build a Collaborative Group of Local Leaders and Expertise

A collaborative group of school administrators, mental health professionals, social service agencies, nonprofit service providers, and parent representatives should come together to discuss the needs of the local community. The National Parent-Teacher Association (2000) recommends the creation of an action team. The action team should include school administrators, teachers, parents, and community members. This team should guide program development and focus on the individual needs of the community. It has been demonstrated that links between the school, community, and family are an effective method of engaging parents in the educational and social development of their children. Davies (1989) indicates that neither the schools nor low-income families can solve these problems alone. Schools and families both need each other and other community resources and support. The creation of links between the schools, community, and families may be a difficult challenge. Chapman (1991) indicates, "The development of these links will take a great deal of effort, because both the schools and the social service agencies are accustomed to operating autonomously" (p. 356). Liontos (1992) stresses the importance of collaboration as the schools cannot solely provide support services. Many families have multiple needs that are best addressed through multiple service providers. In an effort to build successful community partnerships, Kibel and Stein-Seroussi (1997) identify five essential elements; build joint efforts with others striving for the same goal, acknowledge importance of all groups involved, identify common beliefs and values, bond and network, and accept mutual responsibility.

Collaborating with the community will provide numerous benefits for schools and families, including strengthening schools, strengthening families, and increasing learning. Collaborative efforts will help schools and community agencies distribute information on cultural, recreational, academic, health, social, and other resources available to families. Moreover, partnerships with local businesses, service groups, community service agencies, and community volunteers can all provide necessary services to assist families in becoming engaged in the life of their child (National Parent-Teacher Association, 2000). The U.S. Department of Education (1997) also recommends the utilization of external supports for partnerships through collaboration with businesses, health care, service agencies, and universities. Also, projects need to take advantage of the training, assistance, and funding offered by these sources.

The importance of a collaborative team was seen in some of the programs we studied. The FAST (Families and Schools Together) program requires new sites to build collaboration prior to training and implementation. At a minimum, a collaborative team must be formed with a parent representative, a school representative, a substance abuse community agency representative, and a mental health community agency representative. This organization ensures representation from both consumers (parents) and providers (both from the schools and the local community). FAST allows the collaborative group to be expanded to a maximum of ten members; however, 25 percent of the team must consist of parent representation. The insistence on 25 percent of the team being composed of parent representatives ensures that the needs of the families will be addressed. The collaborative team works together as a cohesive group to plan, implement, and operate the FAST program. The team goes through FAST training to learn the necessary skills and information to run the FAST sessions.

The VIP (Victory-in-Partnership) program tapped nontraditional partners in the local business community to help start the program. The local Chamber of Commerce, Wachovia Bank, and Subway provided early financial and volunteer support to the fledgling program. VIP relied on these community partners in the planning and operation phases of the program. In the planning phase, community partners assisted program designers in developing essential program components as well as providing financial support.

Examine Current Practice and Develop an Improvement Plan

The action team should examine current school and community practices prior to developing a plan to improve parental involvement. The National Parent-Teacher Association (2000) recognized that prior to program development, the collaborative team should look at current school policies. The team should examine elements of current polices which encourage parental involvement and those which serve as a barrier to parental involvement. Based on an analysis of existing policies, the collaborative team can develop a plan to engage families. During the planning phase, the leadership team should determine the governance structure for the program by defining the duties of leadership and administrative support. In addition, it is important to conduct a needs assessment by analyzing relevant data on the target population.

VIP examined current policies in the schools relevant to families. The school recognized that additional efforts were needed to engage families. By conducting a needs assessment, VIP planners examined the makeup of the elementary schools in Winston-Salem/Forsyth County to determine the schools in greatest need of a program to engage families. Based on this needs assessment, individual schools were identified. Moreover, the needs assessment identified the elements of the program seen as essential. VIP identified problems that prevented parents from fully participating in programs, including a lack of transportation to the program site, an inability to secure child care, and difficulties in meeting during the traditional 9-to-5 workday. VIP structured its program based on the deficiencies in current school policy while considering the potential barriers to parental involvement.

Achieve Consensus on a Vision, Mission, and Goals for the Project

Prior to program design, it is critical that leaders achieve a consensus on a vision, mission, and goals for the project. The first step is to define the vision of the action team. The importance of a vision is borrowed from the business field where Peters and Waterman (1982) note that it is commonplace to consider the long-term vision for the organization. The vision should be in written format and include the strategic aims of the organization. The vision should be revised as needed to maintain flexibility and adjust to the changing needs of the families and community. Following the development of the vision, the action team should create a mission statement. Stephen Covey (1989) discusses the importance of the mission in *The Seven Habits of Highly Effective People.* According to Covey, every organization needs a clear, direct mission and must establish goals by a committee or decision-making team. The mission is a clear, concise statement of the purpose of the program. The next step is to develop a set of measurable goals the program seeks to achieve. These goals will be the foundation of the program elements as well as future program decision making. Research literature stresses the importance of goal setting to prevent confusion and misdirected program elements. The program goals must reflect the needs of the parents, school, and community. Finally, a formal parental involvement policy should be written. The policy should guide decision making at the school level emphasizing the importance of parental involvement and the school's level of dedication to both the academic and social development of children and their families (National Parent-Teachers Association, 2000).

The VIP program defined its mission early in the planning process. The development of the mission helped to guide the planning process. The mission of VIP is "to create a more pronounced partnership between the school, parent and community for the purpose of building a stronger support for student success."

As previously stated, parental involvement programs should develop a set of program goals. The FAST program identifies four program goals, which include "enhancing family functioning, prevent the target child from experiencing school failure, prevent substance abuse by the child and family, and reduce the stress that parents and children experience from daily life situations."

Gain Commitment From School Leadership

The school's administrator must have a firm commitment to the program and convey the importance of the program to staff. The National Parent-Teachers Association (2000) stressed the importance of a firm commitment from school administration for a successful parental involvement program. Administrators are seen as the key to providing friendly access to school buildings. "To make parent involvement work, administrators need to provide direction and leadership and model a welcoming attitude toward parents and families" (p. 27). Fuller and Olsen (1998) also view the role of the school administration as critical in the success of a parental involvement program. The principal sets the climate for parental interaction by motivating teachers to include parents by coordinating, managing, supporting, funding, and recognizing parent achievement. Administrators must encourage activities to bring parents into the schools. Batey (1996) recognizes that it is the principal's job to create a positive climate between teachers and parent groups. The principal must create a climate such that parents will know they are welcome. The principal should explain the school's goals and how parents can help to achieve those goals. The National Parent-Teachers Association (2000) identifies several roles of the school principal to facilitate parent/family involvement, including the following: provide feedback, assist in and encourage collaborative decision making, identify common goals, promote professional development in teachers, and encourage districtwide parental involvement policies. Henderson, Marburger, and Ooms (1996) indicate that the school should recognize its responsibility to form partnerships with families and the principal and administrators should promote the partnership approach.

In sum, the research literature has identified numerous strategies school administration can use, which include the following:

- Extending an invitation to parents and families;
- Helping parents feel welcome by removing fear and intimidation;
- Making the school more inviting by using welcome signs;
- Ensuring safety for parents and children;
- Recruiting parents and community members;
- Sharing decision making;
- Providing professional development for teachers;
- Providing materials, space, equipment, and staff;

- Blending diverse interests; and
- Communicating with parents.

The program sites we visited also stressed the importance of dedication from the school administration. The FAST program stressed the importance of the principal in the success of the program. In each school that implements FAST, it is the responsibility of the principal to establish guidelines for who is eligible to participate in the program. The principal determines the criteria for who is invited to participate in the program. For instance, the school principal can determine that an entire grade level is eligible to participate, or only a classroom, or even only first-grade girls. It is the principal's responsibility to understand the needs of the students and to select the group of participants who would benefit most from being invited to participate in FAST.

The VIP program also stresses the importance of dedicated leadership. The superintendent fully supported expansion of VIP to all schools. Thus, in the 2001–2002 school year the VIP program was expanded. VIP is implemented in each school with the support of the school principal. The school principals and assistant principals are fully supportive of the effort to incorporate VIP into their schools. Moreover, the school district has created positions of VIP coordinator in each school to oversee the daily operations of VIP in the school.

Remove Barriers to Program Participation

When considering program elements, possible barriers to program participation should be identified and steps should be taken to eliminate potential barriers. Researchers have found that the families most in need of interventions and assistance have multiple barriers that prevent participation. Barriers have been characterized by Lueder (1998) as those related to psychological factors such as apprehension, fear, and alienation; those related to physical factors such as time, distance, and child care; and factors resulting from the lack of skills or knowledge. Liontos (1992) discusses the psychological barriers for parents that result from feelings of inadequacy, failure, and poor self-worth. Some parents feel insecure about involvement in their children's education due in part to low expectations of themselves and in turn their children. Some parents hold negative attitudes or had bad experiences with schools themselves. Thus they often have high levels of suspicion or anger that schools are not treating them equally. The National Parent-Teachers Association (2000) identified the following psychological and physical barriers to parental involvement: not enough time, not feeling valued, feeling unwelcome, not knowing how to contribute, not understanding the school system, need of resources, lack of child care, language barriers, disabilities, and lack of transportation.

In addition to barriers that prevent families from becoming involved, there are also barriers for schools and teachers (Liontos, 1992). These barriers include the following:

- Level of commitment of parental involvement;
- Confusion about the role of teachers (i.e., how to maintain role and include parents);
- Concern about turf and territory;
- Doubts about their abilities to work with at-risk parents;
- Belief that at-risk parents do not care and will not keep commitments;
- Low teacher expectations for at-risk children;
- Communication from schools focuses on the negative;
- Failure to focus on strengths all families have;
- Lack of time and funding; and
- Lack of adequate training.

In the implementation phase of the FAST program, potential barriers for families are identified. To encourage participation, FAST provides transportation, child care, a family meal, and an opportunity for parents to spend time with other adults. Of the families that attend the first FAST meeting, 80 percent will complete the eight-week program. One of the reasons attributed to this high completion rate is the removal of barriers. Transportation and child care are logistical problems that can prevent families from participating. By providing such services, the program eliminates physical limitations. In addition, FAST is held in the evenings to encourage maximum participation. The family meal and socialization encourage participation by making the experience enjoyable for the family and a means to reduce stress levels. Another aspect of the FAST program designed to eliminate barriers is the requirement that those operating FAST represent the racial and ethnic background of the participants. In some locations FAST is even provided in Spanish to encourage participation from the Spanish-speaking community.

VIP also examined potential barriers to participation. VIP eliminated transportation and child care as potential barriers. The VIP program provides free bus passes to parents to encourage participation as well as providing child care during meetings. VIP also recognizes the importance of overcoming language barriers. When conducting the evaluation of VIP, a Spanish version of the survey instrument was distributed to ensure that Spanish-speaking parents could voice their opinions on the program.

Provide for Teacher Training

Teachers should receive training related to child development and methods of working with parents and community members. According to the U.S. Department of Education (1997), training and staff development are essential investments for a successful parental involvement program. Teachers need to have a greater understanding of child development, parental involvement, and the needs of at-risk families. Moreover, teachers need the skills to work to help families in ways other than academic. Rich (1987) believes that there is a new role for teachers to coordinate what is learned in class with what is learned elsewhere: Teachers must work with adults on that which they are not trained to do.

The Council of Chief State School Officers (1989) recommend in-service training to help teachers develop better relationships with families. This training first needs to address the teachers' attitudes toward and motivation for working with at-risk families. Then teachers learn knowledge and research regarding parental involvement. Finally, teachers can develop skills necessary to work with families. Cahvkin and Williams (1988) also identify three components for teacher training: an understanding of the framework of being a teacher, understanding of the effective models of parental involvement, and knowledge of the research on parental involvement.

The FAST program involves intensive training for the team running the program. FAST training is conducted from FAST-certified trainers from the FAST national office. FAST training involves several dimensions, including foundations of child development theory, skills to engage families, and program design features. The structure of FAST team training involves three phases. Phase I is a planning process whereby a two-day orientation to the program is held. During Phase I, the group works to become a "team." Phase II of team training involves three on-site visits by a certified FAST trainer during the program cycle. Phase III involves debriefing the team and a graduate of the FAST families. Upon completion of training, the FAST team becomes certified to operate a program.

Fast Track also included a teacher-training component. Teachers who participated in the program taught a specially designed curriculum to an intervention group. The teachers were trained in the methods of delivering the special curriculum.

When training is not provided, negative effects are often seen. The VIP program did not adequately train the teachers on the fundamental skills necessary to work with families or on use of the technology required to submit information. Thus, many teachers reported negative opinions related to the overall success of the program.

Plan for the Future

In addition to planning for the immediate needs of the program, planning for the future of the program is also important during the development phase. Program planners should also determine how they intend to evaluate the success of the program. Measures of success and benchmarks should be identified early in the planning process. In addition, program planners should consider how they propose to achieve continued collaboration with community groups. Finally, program planners must consider how they plan to maintain financial support for their program. Without continued financial support, it would be impossible for the program to be successful.

The VIP program did consider the future of the program in the planning process. VIP designers worked to maintain strong collaborative efforts with community organizations and businesses. Moreover, VIP worked with the school district to integrate the program into the school's funding structure. VIP was able to achieve permanent funding by encouraging the school district to include VIP in the annual budget.

FAST also plans for the future of the program. The FAST National Office evaluates every FAST site. This evaluation process ensures that the program is having a positive impact and program elements are correctly in place. Moreover, FAST works with a number of local, state, and national organizations to secure continued funding. For instance, many of the FAST programs are partly funded by school districts, Communities in Schools (CIS), and federal grants (see Appendix III-1).

PHASE 2: EFFECTIVE PRACTICES IN PROGRAM OPERATION

Provide a Welcoming Atmosphere

All aspects of the school's climate should be open, helpful, and friendly. The U.S. Department of Education (1997) recognized the need to restructure schools to support family involvement. To support family involvement, schools must promote a welcoming environment by bridging school-family differences (i.e., language, cultural, and low levels of parental education). The research literature has provided numerous examples of ways schools can promote a welcoming atmosphere: teachers and principals can greet parents outside the school when parents drop the child off for school, to foster a nonthreatening means of communication; schools can post signs indicating that parents are welcome; staff working in the front office must be friendly and welcoming to parents because they are often the first point of contact when the parent enters the school; and the principal and teachers should encourage parents to "drop in" to observe their child in class and to encourage parents to take part in school-related activities.

FAST works with families to help them feel welcome in their child's school. FAST operates in the school outside regular school hours. Parents are "invited" to participate in FAST, and that helps them feel less isolated and more inclined to participate in the program. One parent indicated that even though she lives only a block from the school she never felt welcome; however, FAST helped form a bond between her family and the school. Another FAST participant indicated the importance of the program director coming up to her at the first meeting, which made her feel more welcome. She indicated that if the director had not approached her and welcomed her she probably would not have returned to the program. The FAST program takes some pride in its family retention rate. Over 80 percent of parents graduate from the program if they make it to the first session. FAST staff cite the positive and welcoming environment created during the first meeting as a reason behind the high repeat participation.

The Fast Track project encouraged parents to feel welcome in their child's school. Representatives from the program would go with parents to visit the school under positive circumstances. A representative from Fast Track would go with the parent into the child's school to help the parent feel more comfortable with the school's teachers and administrators. This encouraged parents to feel more at ease with the school environment.

VIP also encourages parent visits. At one of the VIP sites the VIP coordinator went to the homes of parents who were unable to find transportation to the school and brought the parents into the school to meet with the teacher. In another instance, the VIP coordinator facilitated a meeting between a teacher and an alcoholic parent by sitting with the parent until she was sober enough to go to the school to meet with the teacher.

Encourage a Healthy Home Environment

Parental involvement programs should work with families to meet both physical and emotional needs of the family as a whole. Schools can help establish home environments that foster preparation for school, effective discipline, and positive conditions for learning and behavior. In addition, schools can help prepare families to provide for basic physical needs. Successful programs integrate learning activities into each family's daily routine. Successful programs also teach families how to create a home environment that encourages development and learning (Liontos, 1992). Families need to work on communication skills and spending time with one another on a regular, ongoing basis. Through the use of collaborations with community agencies, schools can work with families to meet basic physical needs such as housing, food, and clothing, as well as assisting families in providing for the emotional and developmental needs of their children.

One aspect of the FAST program is the gift basket the family receives the night the family wins the lottery and is asked to prepare the next week's dinner. Each basket contains games as well as other items the family may need. The gift baskets help with providing for some of the basic physical needs of the family. In addition, FAST works with community agencies to assist family members in locating additional services they may need. In relation to the home environment, FAST assigns "homework" to the family each week. The homework assignments include fifteen minutes of one-on-one special playtime between the parent and child to enhance communication within the family. By requiring each family to communicate on a daily basis, it becomes a routine part of their day.

Fast Track also worked to promote a healthy home environment. One element of the Fast Track project was weekly home visits during the first year. These visits encouraged positive relationships with the family in addition to teaching parents problem-solving and coping skills. The parent groups also encouraged a healthy home environment by helping parents develop self-control and parenting skills.

Develop Learning Opportunities For Parents

Schools can promote parents as learners by offering workshops in areas such as child development and parenting skills. Because parents are their children's first and most influential teachers, they need the skills necessary to help their children learn. Many parents lack the necessary skills. The school can help by providing workshops or classes to teach parents how to help their children. The National Parent-Teacher Association (2000) stresses the importance of parents participating in student learning. Parental involvement programs should help parents identify what is required from children, identify how parents can foster learning, provide interactive homework, and set student goals with parents. The U.S. Department of Education (1997) recommends that parental involvement programs provide information and training to parents and school staff especially in the area of information and skills to promote two-way communication.

Several home conditions can enhance the development of children. Parental involvement programs can teach families the skills that can assist in learning. The National Parent-Teacher Association (2000) identified five conditions that aid learning. Positive family work habits promote a sense of discipline and work ethic in children. Academic guidance and support from parents are important for children to achieve scholastically. Parents should participate in activities with their children to stimulate exploration and discussion. Language development is initially taught in the home. Thus it is vital that parents provide an environment that fosters development. Finally, academic ambitions and expectations are initiated in the home. Parents who stress the importance of education and expect their children to succeed have a positive influence on the academic achievement of children.

VIP offers a series of educational opportunities for parents. The Saturday Academy was created in reaction to parent requests for courses in applied mathematics, computers, the GED, and English as a Second Language. By enhancing their own education, parents are better equipped to help their children with homework. Parents are also invited at the start of each term to a session at which teachers explain the concepts that will be taught in the upcoming months. Parents are instructed on how to reinforce school lessons at home to help their children achieve.

Fast Track extends the learning process into the home environment. During home visits, Fast Track staff instruct parents in home management skills. Fast

Track staff work with the family in the home to teach skills necessary for the family to work together as a unit.

Solicit Parent Volunteers

Schools should use volunteer opportunities to involve parents in their child's school. There are a multitude of volunteer opportunities for a parent in the school. Fuller and Olsen (1998) identify numerous ways parents can serve as volunteers, such as assisting in the classroom, serving as tutors, sharing skills, assisting in fundraisers, and organizing or attending social events. When parents volunteer they provide support and assistance in the school while developing a personal relationship with school staff and administrators. Schools should encourage volunteer participation from parents and the community.

In promoting voluntary opportunities, schools should contact all parents throughout the year. There may be circumstances in which a parent may not be able to volunteer due to scheduling conflicts. Schools should not interpret a parent's being unable to volunteer as a lack of interest. All parents should be contacted when volunteer opportunities arise. Schools should design differing volunteer activities to promote all parents' participation. Schools must recognize that parents have different strengths and abilities. Through varied activities, all parents would be able to participate. In addition, volunteer activities should be meaningful. Volunteering should be an enjoyable experience for parents that encourage their involvement in the education of their children. If parents are participating in activities they see as having little value, they are less likely to participate in the future.

Parents participated in voluntary roles in many of the programs we examined. For instance, in the FAST program, parents who successfully complete the program can become parent partners and work with future FAST groups. FastWorks also encourages voluntary activities. Many of the activities in which FAST families participate once they enter FastWorks are designed to help the school or community at large.

Involve Parents in Decision Making

Schools should encourage parents to become active participants in the policy- making process for their school. The National Parent-Teacher Association (2000) indicates the importance of parental involvement in school decision making and advocacy. Parents should be treated as full partners in decisions that affect children and families. Moreover, when they are organized, parents can be a powerful voice as advocates for their children (National Parent-Teacher Association, 2000). Fuller and Olsen (1998) indicate that it is the responsibility of schools to involve parents in goal setting and to inform parents of leadership opportunities. Schools need to look beyond the traditional definitions of parental involvement (PTA, signing report cards) to a view of parents as full partners. The National Parent-Teacher Association (2000) stresses the need for schools to ensure that parents are aware of current information on policies, to encourage parents as partners in setting goals, and to respect parent concerns. Fuller and Olsen (1998) identify ways in which parents can become involved in the governance of their school. including parent councils, parent-teacher groups, planning teams, budget review, and school boards.

A hallmark of the FAST program is its emphasis on parental decision making. Parents are seen as the primary authority in the child's life. The primary role for the school and community is to support the parent's decisions regarding the child. Parents actually take the lead in running many FAST activities. Many of the activities within the FAST program are designed to teach parents how to be leaders both within their family and within the community. Parents are encouraged to serve as decision makers on school boards and committees.

Promote Two-Way Communication With Families

Parental involvement programs should encourage two-way communication between the school and home as well as between parent and child. The research literature has stressed the importance of frequent two-way communication between the school and the home. The U.S. Department of Education (1997) found that communication is the foundation of effective partnerships. Communications with parents should be "frequent, clear, and two-way" (Henderson et al., 1996). Batey (1996) contends that clear communication is necessary to keep things running effectively. Parents and schools need to know what is going on, and what others are thinking. According to Liontos (1992), "the lack of information flowing between home and school may lie at the root of the dissonance between teachers and parents"; it is typically the "initial contacts that can make or break relationships" (p. 35). Schools should assure that initial contacts with parents are positive and encouraging.

There are numerous ways in which a school can foster communications. Liontos (1992) identifies memos, conferences, and home visits as effective means of communication. However, Liontos believes that face-to-face contacts are most effective especially in the way of home visits. Decker and Decker (1988) also recognize the importance of home visits to assist the school in gaining insight into the parent-child relationship. Decker and Decker identify several benefits of home visits, including:

- Providing information about the student which the teacher may otherwise not know;
- Observing situations that account for problem;
- Providing information and support for parents;

- Learning about the home environment; and
- Providing a more relaxed form of communication.

The VIP program is based on open communications between the parent and school and parent and child. The weekly reports used by VIP are meant to facilitate communication between parents and teachers. One teacher described VIP as "constant communication with parents of children on a weekly basis so that they know what's going on." Moreover, another teacher indicated that increased communication enhances accountability. The enhanced communication encourages teachers to be prepared to discuss how the child is doing due to the ongoing documentation; the parent is not surprised when grades are given. Through weekly contact, teachers and parents can work together to solve problems before the problems become too serious. Each week the parent receives a report which outlines aspects of his or her child's behavior and academic achievement in the prior week. In a survey of parents, a large majority reported that they found the reports helpful. Some parents noted that they actually sit down with their child and go over the reports every week. The reports have the ancillary result of increasing communication between parent and child.

FAST helps families improve communications. Many of the FAST activities are developed to help families communicate. The feelings game, scribbles, and the one-on-one special play time all promote effective communication within the family (see Chapter 9). Parents are taught to talk with their children about their feelings as well as discussing topics that are relevant to their children. One FAST parent indicated to her child, "I am your best friend when you have no one else"; she attributes her actions to participating in FAST. "FAST taught me how be my child's best friend, how to talk things out."

Empower Parents to Lead Their Family

Schools should assist in empowering parents. Empowerment is especially important when designing involvement programs because many parents feel a sense of exclusion and powerlessness that they often pass on to their children. When parents get involved they gain a greater sense of adequacy and self-worth that can have a ripple effect on families. For example, parents may decide to go back to school themselves, which would emphasize the importance of education to their children and lead to community involvement and participation in the political process (Liontos, 1992). According to research conducted by Lewis and Henderson (1997), lower-income parents become involved in their children's school when the school adopts a policy such that the family feels valued, encouraged, and supported. Davies (1989) believes schools can increase empowerment by providing opportunities for parent participation in decision-making matters. Parental participation will result in building skills for empowerment.

Empowering parents is a key element of the FAST program. FAST works with parents to give them the support they need to take charge of their lives and their family. Each activity is designed to help parents take control over their family and the education their child receives. Parents are taught skills to facilitate family discussions and activities.

VIP is also founded on the belief that parents must be empowered to take charge of their families. VIP has worked to improve parental involvement by simplifying the language used and eliminating jargon to help parents understand what is being discussed. Parents are also empowered by being trained to work within the school system to help their children get the most from their education.

Actively Recruit Families

Parental involvement programs should develop systematic and inclusive recruitment procedures. Parental involvement programs can be universal (i.e., any family may participate) or targeted (i.e., aimed at at-risk families). Parental involvement programs should determine the purpose of the program and direct recruitment procedures toward that end. Liontos (1992) identifies ways which parental involvement programs can improve their recruitment process:

- *Assign a recruiter who understands the culture and background of parents.* The recruiter must be interested in and dedicated to the mission of the program.
- *Survey your community.* Determine how many different groups of families would be interested, the specific interests and needs of families, barriers to participation, and other organizations to which the families belong.
- *Vary techniques.* Recruitment should use multiple techniques such as views from former participants, brochures or letters, visits by staff, door-to-door techniques in the community, posters in community locations, and radio.
- *Arrange home visits.* Successful recruitment needs personal contact that can be achieved through home visits.
- *Follow up visits or invitations.* Recruitment should be ongoing and encouraging.
- *Post teachers and principals outside the school.* School staff can greet parents outside of the school to make them feel welcome.
- *Ask parents what they would be interested in doing.* Successful programs are tailored to the agenda of families and should include aspects which the parents are good at. If the program is interesting to families they are more inclined to attend.

- *Don't hold the first activity at school.* Activities outside the school help make apprehensive families feel more at ease.
- *Make first event fun and capture the parents' attention.* By holding an interesting activity, families are more likely to continue to participate in the program.

The school principal determines participant eligibility for the FAST program. The principal extends an invitation to the entire school, grades, or classes. Everyone is contacted and invited to attend. FAST stresses the importance of its universal provision. The program is founded on the belief that every family could use assistance and should be provided the opportunity to participate if the members so desire. Specific families are not individually targeted for program participation. Some sites, which selected families through referrals, found that there was a lack of trust between the families and staff due to the referral process.

VIP avoids the problem of whom to recruit as all families participate in the program. A teacher indicated that universal participation was positive and noted that one would not want to use the program only for children with discipline problems, explaining that "you set up a hierarchy of children who get bad notes. What's wrong with telling a child consistently, on a weekly basis, you are doing a great job."

Measure Performance

Programs should develop systems to monitor their effectiveness. Research has shown that programs that develop systems to monitor themselves encourage flexibility in the program. Through constant program monitoring, changes can be made as needed when program elements are found to lack efficacy. Moreover, parental involvement programs should measure program performance. Fuller and Olsen (1998) indicate the importance of evaluating parental involvement programs on a regular basis. Elements that should be included in an evaluation are consideration of the amount, quality, and outcomes of parental involvement. The level of parental involvement can be measured by collecting information regarding the number of visitors, volunteers, decision makers, advocates, opportunities, and participants. The U.S. Department of Education (1997) also recognizes the importance of programs to regularly assess the effects of the partnership using multiple indicators. Programs should develop measures examining participation levels and satisfaction levels for families, school staff, and community members. In addition, programs should develop measures of quality of school-family interactions and improvements in the student educational progress.

Because Fast Track was developed as an empirical research study aimed at determining successful parental involvement elements, measurement of performance was a key program component. Fast Track established a data center to collect data relevant to the program. Fast Track used numerous validated measures to determine program success. Fast Track recognized the importance of testing the effectiveness of each intervention used in the program.

FAST is also founded on empirical research-based strategies to engage families. FAST stresses the importance of continuous evaluation and feedback. Evaluation is necessary for the program to evolve and keep staff on track. FAST National Training and Evaluation Center offers an evaluation of the FAST program using a pre- and posttest design. The evaluation uses seven measures to assess the program's impact on behavior, family functioning, social isolation, and parental involvement. FAST uses a number of evaluation instruments as previously discussed, including the Revised Behavior Problem Checklist, Parenting Stress Inventory, Social Insularity Subscale, Social Skills Rating System, Parent Survey on School Involvement, Family Environment Scale, Families and Schools Together Program Evaluation, and the Site Information Survey and Participant Survey.

PHASE 3: CLOSING THE GAP: EXPANSION AND REPLICATION

Program expansion and replication are important issues to be addressed. Prior to expansion, programs must examine findings from performance measurements. Programs must be sure they address any problems within the program prior to expansion. Moreover, programs must demonstrate that the program is indeed successful at meeting the desired goals. Finally, programs must consider the availability of sustained funding for program expansion and continuation. Without locating a long-term funding source, programs should not consider expanding services or replicating the program in new locations.

Expansion

In three short years, the VIP program has expanded from one pilot site to all forty elementary schools in the Winston-Salem/Forsyth County school system. Teachers had mixed feelings about this expansion. One teacher indicated that it was a positive step because all students have equal access to the program. However, other teachers stressed the importance of eliminating any "bugs" from the program prior to expansion. Teachers encountered problems with technology and changing formats of the program.

Replication

Replication should also be contingent on need within the community. Program administrators must resurvey the needs of the community prior to determining that the program should be replicated. The FAST program has had great success with regard to program replication. FAST has been replicated in over 600 sites in five countries. One key feature of FAST replication is the continued oversight by the FAST National Office. FAST conducts impact evaluations at each site to maintain program integrity. Moreover, FAST monitors program sites to watch for program drift, whereby programs shift from the empirically tested elements of the FAST program. Due to the empirical basis of FAST it has proven to be successful in a multitude of locations with significantly different target populations.

PLAN TO ACT

Several important aspects of planning are not apparent in the overall process or the individual action step. Yes, the element of preparing to act is essential. But more than that, a disparate group of people begin the process of coagulating into a force with direction. This is one of the most significant aspects of planning, actually the reason for planning. People become a group with a purpose. The best result of this is that each person is motivated to lead in his or her way whether it is to be the champion of the entire effort or to be involved in the life of one child at a moment that makes all the difference.

Another important, slightly hidden aspect of planning is that the point is to lead to action. Many times this is forgotten; planning becomes the occupation. Planning without action is just bureaucracy looking good; it is just the appearance of getting work done. Taking appropriate action—that is, deciding what is best to do when confronted by the reality of engaging people—is enhanced by a plan. But nothing takes the place of the day when most agree it is time to make ideas happen. No plan ever anticipated the totality of what the day brings. The time to begin is never really right; there is always more to be done; there are never enough resources; there are many arguments for continuing the planning; and there are always those who "know" it can't be done. Ignore them. Though it may be obvious, we observed over and over again, from those who are succeeding, that action with speed, not the foolhardy kind, must happen. Thus there is an element of courage that is necessary to the planning process because it must inevitably and soon lead to the commitment of money, resources, and the most important commodity, time.

Furthermore, the better plan is the one that is least ironclad; a good plan is constantly being rewritten as it plays out in daily operations, which is another reason that planning has to end: It is imperfect and must be tested by making the idea it supports a reality. It then becomes what it should be, a learning tool instead of any one of the common dictates that propose the way to do things such as a "roadmap," a "best practice," a "blueprint," or any other impossible suggestion from a far-away observer. The better plan is the product of the people who must eventually sweat under it. Furthermore, the plan will be in continuous use as the project develops from start-up to expansion; it has to evolve. Learn from those who have learned by doing, then do it.

References

Batey, C. S. (1996). *Parents are lifesavers: A handbook for parent involvement in schools.* Thousand Oaks, CA: Corwin Press.

Cahvkin, N. F., & Williams, D. L. (1988). Critical issues for teacher training for parental involvement. *Educational Horizons*, *66*(2), 87–89.

Chapman, W. (1991). The Illinois experience. *Phi Delta Kappan*, *72*(5), 355–358.

Council of Chief State School Officers. (1989). *Family support: Education and involvement.* Washington, DC: Author.

Covey, S. R. (1989). *The seven habits of highly effective people.* New York: Simon & Schuster.

Davies, D. (1989, March 27–31). *Poor parents, teachers, and the schools.* Paper presented at the annual meeting of the American Educational Research Association, San Francisco.

Decker, L. E., & Decker, V. A. (1988). *Home/school/community involvement.* Arlington, VA: American Association of School Administrators.

Fuller, M. L., & Olsen, G. (1998). *Home-school relations: Working successfully with parents and families.* Needham Heights, MA: Allyn & Bacon.

Henderson, A. T., Marburger, C. L., & Ooms, T. (1996). *Beyond the bake sale: An educators guide to working with parents.* Columbia, MD: The National Committee for Citizens in Education.

Kibel, B., & Stein-Seroussi, A. (1997). *Effective community mobilization: Lessons from experience.* Rockville, MD: U.S. Department of Health and Human Services, Center for Substance Abuse Prevention.

Lewis, A. C., & Henderson, A. T. (1997). *Urgent message for parents.* Washington, DC: Center for Law and Education.

Liontos, L. B. (1992). *At-risk families and schools: Becoming partners.* Eugene, OR: ERIC Clearinghouse.

Lueder, D. C. (1998). *Creating partnerships with parents*. Lancaster, PA: Technomic.

National Parent-Teacher Association. (2000). *Building successful partnerships: A guide for developing parent and family involvement programs.* Bloomington, IN: National Educational Service.

Peters, T. J., & Waterman, R. H. (1982). *In search of excellence: Lessons from America's best Run companies.* New York: Warner Books.

Rich, D. (1987, May 15). Testimony of D. Dorothy Rich, The Home and School Institute. *Congressional Record*, *133*(79).

U.S. Department of Education. (1997). Family involvement in children's education. Washington, DC: Author.

Part IV

The Local Alternative School—Strategies and Effective Practices for Making It Work

by Douglas L. Yearwood, M.S. and James Klopovic, M.A., M.P.A.

Alternative learning programs are a primary part of community infrastructure that address the needs of at-risk children. Every municipality has youth who thrive in regular public schools as well as those who need a different focus and environment. Evidence shows, though, that both can succeed when schooled properly according to individual needs. After visiting numbers of alternative learning experiments, two things are evident: Some succeed against real odds and some can stand improvement. We set out to discover and illuminate the process of what determines success in an alternative school environment.

It is our intent not to duplicate or cloud the relevant body of written work on alternative schooling, although we do use it to set the stage for the process of "doing" alternative schooling. Rather, we intend to add to what is commonly found in the research about alternative schools by offering something as practical as possible. This is not the way to construct alternative learning services; it is a way. It is a point of departure. This work is different in that we have looked for and found those little things happening every day at well-working schools. These effective practices that we have observed actually define the differences between success and failure.

Is it the entire process, element after minute element? No. But it is the complete process of planning, building, and expanding the idea of alternative schools. Each suggestion is illuminated and sanctioned by school administrators, principals, teachers, students, and parents who confirm what works by doing it. These effective practices must be interpreted anew by those seeking to build a program from nothing or to enhance an existing one. The plan on which you embark will be much more detailed and unique to your circumstances, but you should follow a logical sequence. In the end, action must be taken. We recall speaking to a principal who, after an afternoon spent talking about planning, summed things up by saying, "In the end, there is nothing like doing it." We propose to put a little order to your activity, but nothing succeeds like action. Plan, then get going!

Chapter 11 discusses alternative school programs, addressing necessary issues such as definitions and typologies that have been used to categorize these programs. Chapter 12 outlines basic characteristics of alternative learning programs. Chapter 13 provides a discussion of field-proven effective practices to document what alternative school attributes work well and those conditions that define the proven practice. Benefits, and conversely criticisms, of these programs, are addressed in order to assess the efficacy of alternative school programming. Several model programs are highlighted.

Chapter 14 provides a detailed explanation for planning and operating as well as expanding your school. The focus of Chapter 14 is the practitioner. School administrators and educators should find this chapter useful as they consider and realize their alternative school program.

Chapter 11

The Broad Range of Alternative-School Types

DEFINING ALTERNATIVE-SCHOOL PROGRAMS

Many definitions, or explanations, of alternative schools actually confuse the understanding of the concept. These definitions have been derived from numerous factors, including the nature of the educational curricula, the location of the alternative school itself, and the purpose or goals of the alternative school. Other definitions use student attributes as the basis for describing what alternative school programs are and what they seek to accomplish. In this chapter we develop a framework for analyses by providing definitions for both alternative schools and alternative learning programs.

As Lange (1998) suggests, defining exactly what is, and what is not, an alternative school has been controversial since the early 1970s and continues to remain so thirty years later. The lack of a standardized or consistent definition of alternative educational programming presents numerous issues for educators and school administrators. This deficiency poses serious concerns and obstacles which affect such issues as defining the goals and purposes of an alternative school; funding and staffing considerations; justification for funding and resources; student and teacher selection criteria; and evaluating program process, impact, and outcome. Indeed, as Boss (1998) notes, the prevalence of numerous and divergent definitions poses a serious challenge for ascertaining the effectiveness and efficacy of alternative schools and the impact that these programs have on their respective students. The following definitions demonstrate this dilemma.

Gold and Mann (1984) employed a broad definition that skirted the issue of just what constitutes an alternative school. They simply included all programs and educational instructional methods that somehow differed from the standard curriculum offered to the largest majority of a community's school students as "alternative." Reflecting on the divergent and often vague definitions for alternative schools, Raywid (1999) asserts that "alternative schools are designed for many purposes and function as empty glasses to be filled with any sort of liquid and are even sometimes used for something other than a glass" (p. 47).

Other scholars offer more concrete and specific definitions when discussing alternative educational programs. "Alternative schools are public schools which are set up by states or school districts to serve populations of students who are not succeeding in the traditional public school environment" (Boss, 1998, p. 4). Coeyman (2000, p. 2) expands on this definition and notes that "alternative schools work outside of the conventional mode, catering particularly to students who haven't succeeded in traditional academic settings and recruit from the extreme ends of the academic spectrum appealing to kids who struggle in ordinary school and to those who are highly academically gifted." We prefer the following definition as a guide and foundation for discussion. Alternative learning programs or schools are "services for students at-risk of truancy, academic failure, behavior problems and/or dropping out of school and more adequately meet the needs of individual students" (Hawes, Brewer, Cobb, & Neenan, 2000, p. iii).

ALTERNATIVE-SCHOOL TYPOLOGIES

There have been numerous attempts to more clearly define alternative programming methodologies and schools which consider the multitude of services offered by these educational programs. Raywid (1990), a leading authority and scholar in the area of alternative schools, offers a three-tiered typology formulated by the overall goal or purpose of the alternative school.

Typing by Purpose

Type I, or *educational,* alternative schools typically operate on a multiyear curricula with the students attending full time. These alternative schools enroll a wider variety of students that span the entire academic and conditional spectrum. They include at least:

- Gifted, or advanced placement students;
- Students with development or special education needs;
- Students with behavioral problems, which includes students who are violent;
- Students with substance abuse problems;
- Students with other special issues, such as truancy or pregnancy; or
- Students with a disruptive home life.

The scope and understanding of the range of students is most important because each classification of student requires different services, sometimes an entirely separate school. Student enrollment and teacher selection typically occur on a voluntary basis. Examples of Type I alternative schools include schools that offer vocational-based instruction, experiential learning schools, home schools, and magnet or charter schools.

Type II, or *disciplinarian*, alternative schools typically offer short-term enrollment periods with the students being mandated to attend by authorities from the juvenile justice system and/or the public school system. The focus of these programs is segregating disruptive students from mainstream classrooms and correcting unruly and undesirable behaviors. Examples include in-house suspension rooms, programs in juvenile correctional facilities, and other "last chance" schools.

Type III, or *therapeutic*, alternative schools also offer short-term enrollment periods and serve students with social and emotional problems which impede academic performance. Emphasis is placed on individual and group counseling, life skills training, and other therapeutic modalities such as anger management, token economies, and Glasser's (1986) control therapy. As Raywid (1990) comments, these typologies serve to partially differentiate alternative schools with each not being mutually exclusive (i.e., one school may possess attributes of one, two, or all three types).

Typing by Intended Outcome

Raywid (1999) proposes a more recent typology that divides alternative schools into three types based on the magnitude of their intended outcomes or impact. Some alternative schools seek a conservative outcome with the primary purpose of changing behavior. Commonly, these programs seek to alleviate or at least modify academic, social, and behavioral deficiencies among their students. Other programs seek a moderate degree of impact just by changing the school through innovative and creative educational curricula. Students serve as "test subjects" with the goal of using their improved performance as a springboard for expanding the curriculum to the entire student body. Finally, some alternative school programs have a more liberal goal of changing, or altering, the entire school system or district. Once improved performances have been documented for the "test subjects" and their school peers, these types of programs focus on replicating their successes and expanding the educational methods from one school to the next until the entire district has adopted the new policies, goals, and operational and administrative features of the pilot alternative experiment.

Typing by Relationship to Traditional Schools

Brewer, Blackwelder, Aragon, Langmeyer, and Cobb (1998) subdivide alternative educational programs into two distinct categories, alternative schools and alternative learning programs, based on three factors. Alternative schools are located in separate facilities away from any traditional public school buildings. They also have autonomous funding streams and independent transportation services for their students. Conversely, alternative learning programs coexist with a mainstream public school by being housed in the regular school or in a modular unit on school grounds. These programs receive funding from the public school system and use the same school buses that serve mainstream students.

Koethe (1999) delineates a similar typology that categorizes alternative schools by their relationship with the traditional public school system. Some alternative schools are outside or independent of the public school system. Koethe (1999) includes home schooling and experiential schools within this category. Other alternative schools are inside or dependent on the public school system. Schools of this type include in-house suspension programs and other programs serving children who are at an increased risk of dropping out of school or who display behavioral or other social problems that must be addressed by public school teachers and administrators.

Hefner-Packer (1991) lists eight different types of alternative educational programs used for serving at-risk students.

- *Alternative classrooms.* Alternative classrooms within a regular public school facility.
- *Schools within schools.* Schools within schools are alternative schools that coexist within regular public school buildings but have separate operational, managerial, and administrative features.
- *Remote alternative schools.* These are separate alternative schools located off public school grounds.
- *Continuation schools.* Here students spend half their day either in the regular public school classrooms or at work. Then they attend an alternative program until the end of the school day and/or into extended evening hours.
- *Magnet schools.* Magnet schools focus on specific academic courses.
- *Schools without walls.* These schools are experiential or hands-on schools in which at-risk students work and/or participate in extensive field trips but do not learn through the traditional method of sitting in a classroom.
- *Residential schools.* Examples of residential schools are juvenile detention facilities or group homes.
- *Alternative learning centers.* These schools may be housed in places such as motels, museums, YMCAs, and other nontraditional educational settings.

What is important is that the community fully profile and define its population of need. Then, based on resources, offer the best, affordable learning environment for each category of student. At the very least, a range of learning/teaching programming can be offered even if several separate schools cannot be opened and operated.

HISTORICAL OVERVIEW

Applying a broad definition of alternative schools within an historical perspective documents the presence of home schooling, a type of alternative education, as early as the colonial and industrial revolution periods in American history. As Gregg (1999) comments, these early alternative schools focused strictly on education and academic instruction at the exclusion of disciplinarian or punitive approaches which later emerged. Garrison (1987) notes the historically significant role of alternative education by suggesting that American education today is the collective product of countless past alternative schools.

Alternative schools experienced their first "boom" period during the decades of the 1920s and 1930s as a result of the Progressive Educational Reform Movement. Led by John Dewey, the movement sought to revitalize the educational field and create a warm and nurturing classroom environment in which the needs of the child became the primary focus. Montessori and Waldorf schools became fashionable among the wealthier and American elite who sought to enroll their children in these new progressive educational environments. Despite their popularity during this period, alternative schools, and the entire alternative educational philosophy, fell into disfavor during the mid 1940s and 1950s. The advent of World War II and the subsequent involvement of American troops, coupled with the emergence of teachers' unions, crippled alternative schools during this period in American history (Coeyman, 2000).

The alternative educational philosophy reemerged during the 1960s with A. S. Neill's seminal book, *Summerhill*, serving as a significant catalyst or manifesto for the concept of alternative schools. Neill successfully taught "problem" children by tapping into their natural intellectual curiosity and empowered them by allowing students to have input into their own educational plans and curricula. Much of Neill's work and philosophy can be found in today's alternative schools and their internal operational procedures (Lamb, 1995).

As Raywid (1999) argues, these programs persisted and were highly adapted during the 1960s, yet they never completely received legitimacy with public school teachers and administrators. Programming reflected the turmoil and paralleled the larger societal problems of the period with inner-city alternative schools being reserved for intractable, incorrigible youth experiencing academic difficulties. Consequently, many of these programs were nothing more than quasi juvenile detention facilities for poor inner-city minority males which did little more than create "make work" for these students in order to keep them from dropping out of school and delaying their possible downfall to public dependence or into criminogenic street life. Conversely, suburban alternative schools focused on academic remediation and offered more innovative and creative curricula and instructional methods. There is the argument that many parents used these exclusive suburban alternative schools as a means of subverting the integration of public schools.

Hadderman (2000) notes that alternative schools of the 1970s and 1980s demonstrated a renewed commitment to children at risk with "hands-on" or experiential learning through field trips and "real world" work experience. Realizing that many students were at a disadvantage in the traditional public school that only offered lectures and note taking from the chalkboard, alternative school teachers began to shake free from standardized instructional methods. These teachers acquired a greater appreciation and understanding of the value of matching teaching styles to the individualized special needs of the students. Students had real input into the design of their own educational plans and coursework with self-paced and individualized instruction the norm in alternative schools. Courses were developed to help students cope with and overcome many behavioral, social, and emotional deficiencies or obstacles that impede academic performance.

CURRENT VIEW ON ALTERNATIVE SCHOOLING

Today alternative schools not only flourish but have gained a greater degree of legitimacy within America's public school systems. Educators appreciate the necessity for alternative learning programs and praise these programs for their ability to educate nontraditional students and offer them a second chance to obtain the education that many of their predecessors were denied. Alternative schools will continue to grow in the future and serve an increasing number of children who demonstrate such at-risk behaviors as delinquency, truancy, poor academic performance, and other undesirable social and behavioral problems.

Much of this growth can be attributed to an increase in school violence and school-related tragedies as witnessed in the San Diego, Columbine, and Paducah massacres. Hadderman (2000) argues that the adoption of zero-tolerance policies for violence and weapons possession within the nation's public school systems will force the creation of more alternative schools as federal and state legislatures mandate the removal of violent students yet still seek alternatives to expulsion and juvenile detention facilities. Indeed, Congress passed zero-tolerance legislation in 1994 and at the time of Hadderman's (2000) research, twenty-two states had passed legislation to establish alternative learning programs.

Katsiyannis and Williams (1998) surveyed administrators from public school systems within all fifty states and the District of Columbia and found that twenty states not only had alternative schools enabling legislation but also had standard definitions and minimum standard guidelines for curricula, instructional methods, and evaluation plans for assessing these alternative schools. Coeyman (2000) found 10,000 public and private alternative schools in the United States.

Jones (1999) reported that in the 1996–1997 academic calendar year, there were 2,874 alternative public schools across the nation enrolling 410,000 students. The most recent data from the National Center for Education Statistics (U.S. Department of Education, 1999) reveals a total of 3,605 alternative public schools that serve 511,882 students, or 1.1 percent of the nation's public school students. Observed trends show these numbers continue to increase dramatically. More than ever education needs to understand what makes a well-working alternative school and how to establish it.

ALTERNATIVE SCHOOLS ARE HERE TO STAY

The future of alternative educational services for at-risk youth is positive and promising. The sheer growth in the number of alternative schools and their documented successes imply that they will continue to serve as viable and needed educational programs within the community; but not without real work, commitment, and perseverance. We found that every successful school we visited provided an invigorating, energizing experience. The people there, from the students on up, know and show that something important is under way. Even visitors are compelled to pitch in and help. The message of all the suggestions organized in the process of making a network of alternative learning programs is that it is really workable. Your path will be different and your rewards are incalculable. If there is a challenge here, it is to get started today!

References

Boss, S. (1998). Learning from the margins. *Northwest Education Magazine*, *3*, 3–11.

Brewer, D., Blackwelder, S., Aragon, A. T., Langmeyer, D., & Cobb, C. (1998). *Alternative learning programs evaluation: 1997–98.* Raleigh, NC: North Carolina Department of Public Instruction.

Coeyman, M. (2000). More no. 2 pencils at alternative schools. *Christian Science Monitor*, *92*, 13.

Garrison, R. (1987). *Alternative schools for disruptive youth. NSSC Resource Paper.* Malibu, CA: National School Safety Center.

Glasser, W. (1986). *Control theory in the classroom.* New York: HarperCollins.

Gold, M., & Mann, D. (1984). *Expelled to a friendlier place: A study of effective alternative schools.* Ann Arbor: University of Michigan Press.

Gregg, S. (1999). Creating effective alternatives for disruptive students. *EBSCO Clearing House*, *73*, 107–114.

Hadderman, M. (2000). *Trends and issues: School choice: Alternative schools.* Eugene, OR: Clearinghouse on Educational Management, College of Education, University of Oregon.

Hawes, J., Dillard, L., Brewer, D., Cobb, C., & Neenan, P. (2000). *Case studies of best practices: Alternative schools and programs: 1998–99.* Raleigh, NC: North Carolina Department of Public Instruction.

Hefner-Packer, R. (1991). *Alternative education programs: A prescription for success* [Monographs in Education]. Athens: University of Georgia Press.

Jones, C. (1999). The rise of alternative schools. Office of External Relations: Chalkboard. School of Education. Indiana University at Bloomington [On-line]. Available: www. indiana.edu/~education/chalkboard/fall99/alternative.htm.

Katsiyannis, A., & Williams, B. (1998). A national survey of state initiatives on alternative education. *Remedial and Special Education*, *19*, 276–284.

Koethe, C. (1999). *One size doesn't fit all [Tech-Nos Quarterly]*. Bloomington: IN: The Agency for Instructional Technology.

Lamb, A. (1995). *Summerhill School: A new view of childhood.* New York: St. Martin's Griffin.

Lange, C. M. (1998). Characteristics of alternative schools and programs serving at-risk students. *The High School Journal*, *81*, 183–198.

Raywid, M. (1990). Alternative education: The definition problem. *Changing Schools*, *31*.

Raywid, M. (1999). History and issues of alternative schools. *Education Digest*, *64*, 47–51.

U.S. Department of Education. (1999). *Digest of education statistics.* Washington, DC: National Center for Education Statistics.

Chapter 12

Characteristics and Benefits of Alternative Schools

SCHOOL LOCATION AND ENVIRONMENT

Turpin and Hinton (2000) studied fifty-eight alternative schools in Kentucky and found that 81 percent of these schools were housed in separate facilities outside traditional public school grounds. Alternative schools can be found in a variety of facilities and settings in addition to being housed within an existing school or having their own separate building. These programs have been housed in old farmhouses, hotels, museums, and even shopping centers. Unfortunately, many alternative schools have less than adequate physical facilities and resources and are often placed in facilities that have been, or should be, condemned. Surveying alternative school administrators in North Carolina, Brewer, Blackwelder, Aragon, Langmeyer, and Cobb (1998) report that 25 percent of those surveyed commented that their facilities were inadequate due to overcrowding or physical deterioration, with many not being in compliance with Americans with Disabilities Act (ADA) requirements to provide adequate access to handicapped students. Despite the variety of physical locations and the divergent conditions of their facilities, all alternative schools share a common learning environment.

The environment or atmosphere within an alternative school concentrates on the students' needs, improving their academic abilities, and helping them to understand other issues that impede progress in regular school. A positive, warm, friendly, and caring environment is the rule. Given the fact that many potential alternative-school students display violent and other undesirable behaviors in their respective traditional public school classrooms, one assumes that this behavior would persist in the alternative setting. Surprisingly, maintaining order is not the primary priority within alternative schools. Alternative-school students are treated as adults and are expected to police themselves. Consequently, they demonstrate remarkable prosocial behavioral changes. Enthusiasm, respect, responsibility, creativity, maturity, progress, success, and a sense of belonging are all good descriptors or buzz words that are commonly seen and heard within the alternative school environment.

ADMINISTRATION AND ORGANIZATIONAL STRUCTURE

As Paglin and Fager (1997) remark, funding sources and the administration of alternative schools vary considerably across the nation. Many alternative schools receive funding from the local or state public school district either through direct funding, per-student tuition paid to another entity such as a community-based organization, or an educational district or on a contractual basis. Foundation, federal, state, and local grants have also been used as either the sole source of funding or supplemental funding. In-kind or cash donations from local businesses and other community organizations are also potential funding sources for alternative schools. Volunteers also fill a large peripheral manpower gap. Alternative schools or programs are administered by school districts, cooperatives affiliated with the school district, education service districts, local nonprofit organizations, and private contractors or firms.

Alternative schools also vary in the extent to which they maintain ties to or relationships with the alternative-school students' regular public schools. Many alternative schools have no contact with these feeder schools while other alternative programs maintain extensive and ongoing relationships with the regular public schools. Often a full-time alternative-school staff person serves as a liaison to the feeder schools and provides feedback about the students' academic progress and behavioral development. The liaison is really indispensable, serving, for example, to screen students before entry for proper placement and to assist in devising an individual learning plan. The liaison then follows that student's transition to and performance in the regular school. This function alone changes the philosophy of the alternative program from one of "warehousing" to one of academic and personal progress.

The extent of staff involvement with alternative school students ranges from situations in which only the student's teacher monitors academic progress to other examples that use a team or case management approach. Alternative schools that use this approach involve not only the student's teacher but also the school principal, parents, other school staff such as clerical and food service personnel, and representatives from the student's regular public school. This case management approach is more holistic and closely monitors not only academic progress but other behaviors both inside and outside the classroom. Many alternative schools use these same teams, with student representatives also, to establish school policies and procedures, to handle disciplinary infractions, to recruit teachers, and to select which students will be admitted to the school program.

Community involvement with alternative school programs varies. Some schools remain completely autonomous from the local community; others actively embrace the community and its members. In addition to providing funds, local businesses may employ alternative school students, offer career days or job shadowing opportunities, and have their members serve as volunteers and teachers.

EDUCATIONAL CURRICULA AND INSTRUCTIONAL METHODS

Commenting on the diversity of alternative school curricula and the wealth of instructional or teaching methods, Coeyman (2000) notes that these run the gamut from straight classroom lectures to the use of the Socratic method to programs in which the students own and operate a business. Because many alternative-school enrollees are not amenable to traditional learning through lectures plus have other academic, social, and behavioral issues that they must face, most alternative schools use other nontraditional curricula and teaching methods.

In addition to reading, math, and English, other courses, which are more relevant to the students' real-world experiences, are offered. Courses on life and parenting skills, substance abuse, anger management, and vocational skills classes are common across the nation's alternative schools. Individual and group counseling sessions are also common. Students are often required to work through internships, apprenticeships, and job-shadowing programs. Field trips and guest speakers are routinely employed in an effort to bridge the gap between the alternative school classroom and the students' external surroundings.

Students often design their own educational plans and learn through self-paced work with course credits being awarded once they demonstrate subject proficiency. Students repeat assignments until competency is demonstrated. Many alternative schools shun homework assignments; they allow all work to be done in the classroom. Computer-based training (CBT) has proven to be a major instrumental tool within the alternative setting as it supports the individualized self-paced mode of learning. Students get rewards for completing assignments more often than punishment for noncompletion as they are often subjected to in their regular public school classes. Some alternative schools allow students to leave early on Friday afternoons or hold pizza parties and other special events for those students who complete all weekly assignments. Other schools use point systems where students receive points or credits for completing assignments, demonstrating prosocial behavior, and adequately coping with issues and other problems. Students can then cash in their points for rewards and privileges.

Alternative schools shun student comparisons and favor a noncompetitive learning environment, with the traditional public school grading system being rejected or nonexistent (Hadderman, 2000). Many educators feel that this is a common mistake when managing alternative schools. Competitions and comparisons are an inevitable fact of life that students will face when returning to the home school or searching for a job. Alternative educators should construct programs that include healthy and appropriate opportunities for productive competition. This teaches alternative-school students an important life skill—how to cope with winning and losing.

Student assessment methods vary from having them complete projects, or portfolios, to being evaluated on attendance and progress on their individual education plans. The issue of requiring alternative school students to successfully pass standardized tests at the end of their courses and end-of-year competency tests remains a topic of much heated debate among the nation's public school educators and administrators with these requirements varying considerably from state to state.

TEACHER ATTRIBUTES

Teaching alternative school students poses greater and more formidable challenges for those educators who find themselves within an alternative-school classroom. In addition to dealing with students who have academic difficulties, these teachers must also be prepared to handle disruptive and violent students, students who are pregnant or have children, and students who have low self-esteem and poor impulse control and who have rejected, and been rejected by, the public school system. These teachers must have dedication and discipline, demonstrate compassion, never give up on their students, and always be positive and "cool" in class. Despite rigorous and demanding job responsibilities, our own research indicates that alternative-school teachers are dedicated and truly believe in their work. Most important, they possess an undivided and often inspiring commitment to their students.

Lange (1998) surveyed a stratified sample of Minnesota's alternative-school teachers and found that 66 percent of them were employed by the alternative school on a full-time basis and 64 percent volunteered to teach within these programs. The majority of these teachers had been employed by the alternative school for five years or less, with 8 percent having more than a decade of alternative school teaching experience. Despite poor conditions in the classroom and less than adequate supplies and resources, 89 percent reported having greater control and freedom, whereas 73 percent reported greater job satisfaction than teaching experiences in their regular schools.

STUDENT ATTRIBUTES AND PROGRAMMING

Alternative-school students mirror the diversity found in regular school student bodies. Some alternative schools offer advanced curricula for the academically gifted, others have students with special education needs, some have students with violent tendencies, some have students who are under court supervision, and many alternative-school children are simply "at risk."

Defining At-Risk Children

The categorization of at-risk children is broad and varies by school district, with different alternative schools defining which at-risk students they enroll in their educational programs. As a general rule, at-risk children are those who are involved in or demonstrate a higher probability of future involvement in behaviors that impede their academic performance. Social and behavioral indicators of at-risk status include low-income households, single-parent households, pregnancy, drug abuse, attention deficit disorders, learning disabilities, and delinquency (University of Missouri, 2000). These children often grow up in crimogenic environments and commit acts of delinquency with many developing substance abuse and alcohol dependencies. Children with children, or who are pregnant, are also defined as at risk for academic failure. Obviously, children who have already demonstrated truant behavior, have been suspended or expelled from a public school, lag behind in their academic studies, or have repeated one or more grade levels are also considered to be at an increased risk of not completing their education.

Analyzing data from the National Center for Education Statistics, Cantelon and LeBoeuf (1997) report that nearly 5 percent of the nation's public school students do not graduate from high school. Failing grades, habitual suspensions, conflicts with teachers, family problems, and job-related issues were cited as the most common reasons for dropping out of school. Commenting on the breadth of this definition, Knutson (2001) notes that as many as 25 percent of America's public school students fit the definition of at-risk children.

Hawes, Dillard, Brewer, Cobb, and Neenan (2000) provide a succinct characterization of these at-risk children and their commonalties in relation to their academic performance and classroom behaviors. These children demonstrate "a gnawing sense of inadequacy and failure within the regular classroom; a sense of futility, ineptitude, and purposelessness, frequently exacerbated by constant negative feedback from parents, teachers and peers" (p. xvi). Often this feeling produces violent and defensive reactions within the children who seek to control their environments through aggressive behavior or other forms of "acting out." "*In a nutshell these are students that no one expects to amount to much or even make it to graduation*" (Hayes, 1997, p. 1, emphasis added).

Conversations with, and self-reported surveys of, alternative-school students document and validate their problematic behaviors and their at-risk status. Castleberry and Enger (1998) surveyed 173 alternative-school students in Arkansas and specifically inquired into the reasons that the youngsters were in these schools. Students confessed to having bad attitudes about education and their normal public schools. Frequent absenteeism, extracurricular distractions, personal problems, and poor teaching methods were also revealed by students to explain why they were currently in an alternative school.

Data from the Youth Risk Behavior Surveillance System (YRBS) indicate that alternative-school students engage in more at-risk or high-risk behaviors than do their traditional public school counterparts. A greater percentage of alternative-school students reported engaging in unprotected sexual intercourse, having multiple sexual partners, and using alcohol or drugs prior to sexual activity (U.S. Centers for Disease Control and Prevention, 1998).

Selection and Enrollment Process

The selection or enrollment criteria of these students into alternative schools is also diversified and ranges from mandatory enrollment by public school or juvenile court authorities to voluntary enrollment by students in consultation with parents, teachers, and school administrators. Many alternative schools use student contracts in which students agree to maintain high attendance levels, complete academic subjects, and refrain from fighting and other inappropriate behaviors. These contracts are periodically reviewed by students, their teachers, and principals to assess student progress and to rectify and remove deficiencies or obstacles that might impede student achievement. Lange (1998) found that 68 percent of the Minnesota alternative schools in her sample allowed students to draft their own learning plans and goals. (See Lange, 1998, for an exhaustive list of enrollment criteria used in Minnesota's alternative school programs.)

North Carolina's alternative schools use a school services management team that evaluates prospective alternative-school enrollees to assess their academic aptitudes and behavioral records (North Carolina Department of Public Instruction, 2000). This team consists of the student's public school principal, parent(s), school counselor, a representative from the alternative school, and a representative from the central school district. If an alternative school placement is made the team, in conjunction with the student, develops a personal ized education plan (PEP). The PEP outlines academic and behavioral goals, timelines for completion, and an evaluation plan for monitoring the student's progress. At a minimum, the PEP includes what the school will do, what the student will do, and what the parent(s) will do. It may also include what the community will do, current levels of academic functioning, and a parental contact log. A working PEP that continually responds to the needs of the student is essential for success. The team should review the student's PEP at least annually.

The length of a student's alternative school enrollment can vary from as short as a few weeks or one school semester to several years. Some alternative schools operate strictly on the premise that students will return to their respective regular schools once they have demonstrated academic "recovery" or completed agreed-on student contracts. Other alternative schools allow the student to complete all requirements for their high school diploma on site and then return to the traditional public school to participate in graduation ceremonies. Still other alternative programs operate a full high school curriculum with graduation ceremonies separately for their students who have earned a diploma or GED equivalency certificate.

Brewer et al. (1998) report that 41 percent, of the alternative schools studied for their mandated statewide evaluation of alternative learning programs, had enrollment periods of one year or more. They note that enrollment periods were usually longer for alternative schools serving high school age youth versus those schools that offer services to middle or junior high school age children.

BENEFITS OF ALTERNATIVE SCHOOLS

The importance of understanding and proving the benefits and evidence of a program cannot be overstated. A succinct, professional presentation of a program's contribution, factual, perhaps dramatic in proof, is compelling. It is more than compelling—justifying an alternative schooling program is the life blood of the program, as it must successfully compete with other municipal needs for limited funds and resources. Until an evaluation program is under way it seems daunting. Picking a few of the indicators suggested in this section or developing a few new ones, then ensuring that the numbers and stories that support the measure are collected every day is a good beginning. Make sure telling the story is routine. It seems that evaluation is the first critical task of services building abandoned, yet, it is genuinely invigorating to see accomplishment build one child at a time, by the numbers. That growth and success will, likewise, be enjoyed by the people controlling the flow and direction of money!

Academic Improvements

Attendance Increases. Research on the efficacy and impact of alternative schools documents substantial and significant improvements in the academic performance of those students enrolled in alternative learning programs. Because many alternative school students report that they do not want to return to their home schools, it is not surprising that attendance rates at the alternative schools is higher among those children. In addition, truant behavior is less problematic than when these children were in their regular schools. Lawrence Lytynsky, and D'Lugoff (1982) found increased attendance rates among alternative school students enrolled in a Maryland alternative school. Cox (1999) employed an experimental design within an alternative school and found a similar finding with attendance substantially improving among the treatment group. King, Silvey, Holiday, and Johnston (1998), employing a case study method, reported an increase in the average daily attendance rate for alternative-school students, climbing from 65 percent to 80 percent by the end of the school year.

Suspensions and Expulsions Decrease. Many alternative-school students are enrolled in the program because they have been suspended or expelled from the traditional public school. Research suggests that suspensions and expulsions from alternative schools are significantly less frequent than the rate at which students are suspended or expelled from traditional schools. Brewer et al. (1998) studied more than fifty alternative schools in North Carolina with a total of 14,821 students and found that less than 2 percent were expelled from an alternative learning program. Hadderman (2000) reports reduced disruptive incidents and suspensions in a Passaic, New Jersey, alternative school.

Graduation Rates Increase. Transitioning alternative-school children back into their respective home schools is a crucial phase for these children as they return to the same environment in which they had prior difficulties and academic and behavioral problems. Hayes (1997) studied an alternative school in Virginia and commented that long-term follow-up on the transitioning of students back into home schools appeared to be successful with 50 percent of the alternative-school students making the transition and going on to graduate. Lawrence et al. (1982) found a 50 percent successful transition rate as well.

Grades Improve. Improvements in academic performance, as measured by student grades, standardized tests, and aptitude tests, were shown in numerous studies of alternative schools. Sowell (2000) notes that reading scores among students at an inner-city Brooklyn alternative school were the second highest in the state. He concludes that alternative schools produce higher test scores than do the traditional public schools. Turpin and Hinton (2000) surveyed staff of fifty-eight alternative schools in Kentucky and reported that 91 percent of respondents noted significant improvements in student grades. Lawrence et al. (1982) found substantial improvements in reading and math test scores among their alternative school study's population. Cox, Davidson, and Bynum (1995) conducted a meta-analysis of prior studies on the effects of alternative schools and concluded that the literature suggests that alternative-school education has a small positive effect on academic performance. Dugger and Dugger (1998) found significant improvements in reading, English, and math scores of alternative-school students, while King et al. (1998) noted that a third of the alternative-school students in their sample obtained districtwide honor roll status. Brewer et al. (1998) report that by the twelfth grade, 72 percent of alternative-school students passed nearly all of their courses and 88 percent successfully passed the state competency examination.

Rates of Further Education, Training, and Employment Increase. Longitudinal studies of alternative-school students indicate positive successes in both graduating from high school and attending college or holding steady employment. Fix (2000) studied an alternative school in South Carolina and discovered a 76 percent graduation rate. Cantelon and LeBoeuf (1997), commenting on a study of communities that had some schools with alternative learning programs, found a low 7 percent dropout rate with a high proportion of the students remaining in school until graduation. Paglin and Fager (1997) highlight numerous successful alternative schools in the northwestern United States and report graduation rates as high as 80–90 percent. High employment rates were also reported for alternative-school graduates, with one school sending 50 percent of their graduates on to a four-year college or technical school. Brewer et al. (1998), commenting on the status of their alternative-school students at the end of the school year, noted that 70 percent of high school students graduated or went to college.

Behavioral Improvements

Research findings on how alternative-school education affects current and future disruptive or delinquent behavior are mixed, with most noting significant short-term effects that dissipate over time. Hadderman (2000) found reduced disruptive behavior among alternative-school students in New Jersey and reports that 50 percent of alternative-school students in a Missouri alternative school demonstrated improved behavioral measures and had fewer disciplinary infractions once they returned to their respective home schools. Boss (1998) likewise found reduced disciplinary problems among the alternative-school students in her study. Lawrence et al. (1982) reported significant reductions in delinquency as measured by declining juvenile court appearances. Mann and Gold (1981) suggested that the alternative-school environment is more effective at starting the maturation process, which in turn helps to lower delinquency rates. However, Cox et al. (1995) noted that the literature discussing the ability of alternative schools to reduce delinquency does not offer support that alternative-school education affects delinquent behavior. Clearly these schools have a positive effect on behavior; all that is needed for confirmation is a quick walk through an alternative school on a school day. More research is needed, not so much to confirm the effect of alternative schools on behavior as to describe the methods used to introduce better behavior, to assist the evolution of the alternative-school experiment.

Cognitive/Affective Improvements

Attitude Becomes More Positive. Research on the impact of alternative schools, on the cognitive and affective attitudes of these youngsters clearly documents significant improvements in these domains. Nichols and Utesch (1998) studied the impact and effects of a midwestern alternative school on student motivation, goal orientation, and self-esteem. Pre- and posttesting on a sixty-six-item Likert scale indicated significant increases in extrinsic motivation and self-esteem among those students who completed the alternative school program. Peer self-esteem and home self-esteem were also significantly improved among these students.

Self-Esteem Improves. Other researchers have also reported the significant progress that alternative school programs have for raising student self-esteem (Cox, 1999; Cox et al., 1995). Castleberry and Enger (1998) discuss the numerous positive effects that these schools exert and impart to their students, while Johnston and Wetherill (1998) add that these programs improve the social skills of their attendees. The development of extrinsic motivation and the sense of belonging and community that pervades the alternative school classroom have a direct and profound impact on not only shaping children's academic performance but also teaching children new cognitive skills and coping methods (De La Rosa, 1998; Dugger & Dugger, 1998).

Additional Benefits

Evidence of Cost-Benefit and Cost-Effectiveness. Fix (2000) comments on the cost-benefit and cost-effectiveness of alternative schools and notes that every $1,750 invested in alternative-school students produces a cost saving of $18,300 which would have been spent on juvenile incarcerations or welfare programs. Each student that is "saved" from repeating a grade saves $5,623 and each hour that is conducive to learning (i.e., free of disruptive behavior) saves $23,429 per class (American Teacher, 1997). Thus alternative schools appear to be better investments than the alternative of juvenile court and correctional system involvement, substance abuse programs, and unemployment and welfare assistance. General facts such as these, combined with locally generated evidence of effectiveness and a few personal success stories, make a solid argument for program justification, continued operation and improvement, and expansion.

Citizenship and Character Development. The participation of alternative-school students in community programs also reintegrates them back into the community as productive and responsible citizens. The sense of belonging and giving back profoundly shapes the students and their lives. Community involvement also imparts an important message to community organizations and their members as they no longer view alternative-school students as delinquents, misfits, outcasts, and throwaway children (Hawes et al., 2000).

RESPONDING TO CRITICISMS OF ALTERNATIVE SCHOOLS

Alternative Schools are Dumping Grounds

Alternative-school educators must constantly address and resist the stereotype that their schools are "dumping grounds" for bad and problematic children. Often members of the public school system and the community view these programs as "bad" schools for "bad" kids. Johnston and Wetherill (1998) note that in many areas alternative schools are defined or described as mere euphemisms for places to house and detain the most incorrigible, maladaptive, and seditious students. Stereotypes of this nature can become obstacles to recruiting and retaining the best teachers, resource allocation, and the distribution of public school dollars. Often these programs are criticized on the grounds that they are throwing good money at bad students (Hawes et al., 2000). In fact, this criticism can be true if policy does not address this fiscal criticism at the outset of the formation of the alternative learning program.

Alternative Schools "Label" Students

Alternative-school programs have also been criticized for labeling and segregating "problem" children. Some argue in their favor as a convenient way to remove unruly and unappreciative students, thus creating orderly and safe public schools, but this attitude realizes the self-fulfilling nature of "dumping" difficult youngsters. Others focus loudly on the negative effects of being sent to a "school for bad kids." Fears of labeling children often raise concerns that these are the very children who do not need to be labeled or categorized as being special or different. It is argued that such children have enough personal issues and concerns to deal with and should not run the added risk of seeing themselves in a more negative light than many people already see them. Alternative-school programs have also been misjudged as segregating poor inner-city minority males in little more than temporary shelters from unemployment and possible future incarceration. Still other critics argue that alternative-school children are being rewarded for not adapting to the normal curricula and rigors of the traditional public school by being allowed to study what they want, go on field trips, and, in some cases, avoid homework assignments.

Policy and philosophy circumvent the difficulty of labeling. School policy needs to be clear that entry into the alternative situation is based on criteria. Staying in an alternative school is based on performance, and reentry to regular school and graduation based on standards is expected. It helps to have a philosophy of respect for, appreciation of, and expectation of high standards from the entrant.

ALTERNATIVE SCHOOLS EMPOWER AT-RISK YOUTH

The research literature on alternative educational programs clearly documents their efficacy and utility for offering a second chance to youth who are at a greater risk of academic failure and/or a heightened probability of engaging in delinquency and other antisocial behaviors. Worse yet, failed children disappoint the community and especially themselves when they fail as citizens and neighbors. These educational programs offer promise for keeping at-risk children in the classroom and off the streets, thus enabling and empowering these youngsters to become productive adults who give back to the community versus preying on it or burdening it.

References

American Teacher. (1997). Order in the classroom: Why alternative placements are crucial to giving all our students the chance to learn. *American Teacher*, *81*, 8.

Boss, S. (1998). Learning from the margins. *Northwest Education Magazine*, *3*, 3–11.

Brewer, D., Blackwelder, S., Aragon, A. T., Langmeyer, D., & Cobb, C. (1998). *Alternative learning programs evaluation: 1997–98.* Raleigh, NC: North Carolina Department of Public Instruction.

Cantelon, S., & LeBoeuf, D. (1997). *Keeping young people in school: Community programs that work.* Washington, DC: Office of Juvenile Justice and Delinquency Prevention.

Castleberry, S., & Enger, J. M. (1998). Alternative school students' concepts of success. *NASSP Bulletin*, *82*, 105–111.

Coeyman, M. (2000). More no.2 pencils at alternative schools. *Christian Science Monitor*, *92*, 13.

Cox, S. M. (1999). An assessment of an alternative education program for at-risk delinquent youth. *Journal of Research in Crime and Delinquency*, *36*, 323-336.

Cox, S. M., Davidson, W. S., & Bynum, T. S. (1995). A meta-analytic assessment of delinquency-related outcomes of alternative education programs. *Crime and Delinquency*, *41*, 219–234.

De La Rosa, D.A. (1998). Why alternative education works. *The High School Journal*, *81*, 268–272.

Dugger, J. M., & Dugger, C. W. (1998). An evaluation of a successful alternative high school. *The High School Journal*, *81*, 218–228.

Fix, S. (2000). *Alternative schools offer second chance for education* [On-line]. Available: *www.charleston.net/news/education/altern0430.htm.*

Hadderman, M. (2000). *Trends and issues: School choice: Alternative schools.* Eugene, OR: Clearinghouse on Educational Management, College of Education, University of Oregon.

Hawes, J., Dillard, L., Brewer, D., Cobb, C., & Neenan, P. (2000). *Case studies of best practices: Alternative schools and programs: 1998–99.* Raleigh, NC: North Carolina Department of Public Instruction.

Hayes, L. (1997). Alternative schools boast of their role in education. *Counseling Today* [On-line]. Available: www.counseling.org/ctonline/archives/ct1197/alt.htm.

Johnston, B. J., & Wetherill, K. S. (1998). HSJ special issue introduction alternative schooling. *High School Journal, 81,* 177–182.

King, L., Silvey, M., Holliday, R., & Johnston, B. (1998). Reinventing the alternative school: From juvenile detention to academic alternative. *The High School Journal, 81,* 229–243.

Knutson, G. (2001). *Alternative high schools: Models for the future?* [On-line]. Available: *http://horizon.unc.edu/projects/HSJ/Knutson.asp.*

Lange, C. M. (1998). Characteristics of alternative schools and programs serving at-risk students. *The High School Journal, 81,* 183–198.

Lawrence, C., Litynsky, M., & D'Lugoff, B. (1982). Day school intervention for truant and delinquent youth. In D. J. Safer (Ed.), *School programs for disruptive adolescents* (pp. 177–192). Baltimore: University Park Press.

Mann, D. W., & Gold, M. (1981). Alternative schools for disruptive secondary students—Testing a theory of school processes, students' responses and outcome behaviors. Washington, DC: U.S. Department of Health, Education and Welfare, National Institute of Education.

Nichols, J. D., & Utesch, W. E. (1998). An alternative learning program: Effects on student motivation and self-esteem. *The Journal of Educational Research, 91,* 272–278.

North Carolina Department of Public Instruction. (2000). *Clarification of guidelines for alternative learning programs and schools.* Raleigh, NC: Division of School Improvement.

Paglin, C., & Fager, J. (1997). *Alternative schools: Approaches for students at risk.* Portland, OR: Northwest Regional Educational Laboratory.

Sowell, T. (2000). Success of alternative schools ignored. *The Austin Review* [On-line]. Available: *www. austinreview.com/articles/92.html.*

Turpin, R., & Hinton, D. (2000). *Academic success of at-risk students in an alternative school setting: An examination of students' academic success out of the mainstream school environment* (ERIC Document No. RC022409). Campbellsville, KY: Campbellsville University Press.

U.S. Centers for Disease Control and Prevention. (1998). *Youth risk behavior surveillance—National alternative high school youth risk behavior survey.* Atlanta, GA: Author.

University of Missouri. (2000). *Alternative schools* [On-line]. Available: *http://web. missouri.edu/~C674813/alt.htm.*

Chapter 13

Real-World Practices for Alternative Schools

GENERAL EFFECTIVE PRACTICES

School Location and Environment

Locate School in Separate Facility. Research on alternative schools indicates that these programs operate most effectively and efficiently when they are housed in separate facilities as opposed to being located within traditional public schools or public school classrooms. Duke and Griesdorn (1999) conducted an extensive field study of thirty-two alternative schools in Virginia and recommended that the alternative school be apart from, yet in close proximity to, the feeder public school. This is also advantageous because many local school board policies prohibit suspended/expelled students from being on school property during this suspension/expulsion period; thus they could possibly be excluded from attending alternative-school programs that are maintained on any public school properties. These schools should also have access to social service providers and be easily accessed through public transportation (Dugger & Dugger, 1998). We also advocate for the existence of assembly halls, indoor and outdoor recreation facilities, ample facilities for vocational training (e.g., automotive mechanics or brick masonry), and a fully equipped media center in order to maintain an exceptional alternative school. Ideally, numerous alternative schools will exist within a school district, with these schools providing services that match the specific needs of the students. It is preferable for a school district to maintain and operate a continuum of alternative-school services as not all at-risk students have the same academic and social problems (Duke & Griesdorn, 1999; Hawes, Dillard, Brewer, Cobb, & Neenan, 2000). Paglin and Fager (1997) suggest that the most successful alternative schools maintain a unique identity separate from other traditional public schools.

Maintain Low Teacher to Student Ratios. Low teacher-to-student ratios should be strictly adhered to and maintained with no more than 75 to 150 students being enrolled in the entire school and ideally only 12 to 15 students per class (Kellmayer, 1998). We found that many alternative school candidates simply could not function in the "larger" world of the regular school. Classes are larger; there is more reason to "act up"; the pace sometimes ignores individual needs. Simply having a smaller environment, smaller classes, and a little more attention makes the difference between a graduation cap and gown and dropping out or worse.

Maintain Safe, Positive, and Nurturing Environment. The school environment or climate should be warm and conducive to the learning process and not reflect a punitive or disciplinarian atmosphere (Gregg, 1999). Dugger and Dugger (1998) suggest that the school program be highly structured and yet extremely flexible. Black (1997) studied alternative schools in seven states and found that the most successful schools have a family or home-like atmosphere, full of care, compassion, and individualized attention. Hawes et al. (2000) describe the ideal alternative school environment as being permeated with a sense of belonging, serious but fun, relaxed, full of trust and respect, with the children being treated more as adults and not being targeted or labeled as "problem kids." The most promising alternative schools have designed and maintain school safety plans and crisis contingency plans in the event that a serious and significant threat occurs at the school or on school grounds. These plans should be developed through a team approach including students, parents, school administrators, and members of the community. Safety drills or mock disaster sessions are also recommended (North Carolina Department of Public Instruction, 2000). Successful alternative schools also have clearly delineated, reasonable, and enforceable rules—rules that teach values and instill responsibility in the students.

Administration and Organizational Structure

Maintain Autonomy With Tactful Oversight. Successful alternative-school programs are given a high degree of autonomy by central school districts, with the alternative-school staff having independent control over school administration and operational policies and procedures. Nonetheless, these alternative schools constantly maintain contact with the central school districts in order to provide feedback on student progress, inform others about school activities, and handle financial matters (Hawes et al., 2000; Lange, 1998). As Kellmayer (1998) suggests, the central school district should provide full support for its alternative schools, including providing financial, personnel, logistical, and technological assistance at equivalent levels to its traditional public schools.

Encourage Vigorous Community Involvement. Model alternative schools maintain strong ties to the community and its citizens and businesses. These programs keep the community informed and involved, use community volunteers, solicit financial contributions, and involve their students in community projects such as litter removal and delivering food to senior citizens. It is suggested that alternative schools have a teacher serve as a community public relations officer and maintain constant contact with community members and organizations (Virginia Commonwealth University, 2001).

Manage by Teams. The most promising alternative schools use team management concepts involving shared decision making among parents, staff, and students (Lange, 1998). These teams should develop clear and consistent goals, objectives, mission statements, and operating policies and procedures for the alternative school and its students. Research indicates that alternative schools that have a clear purpose and mission statement stand a better chance of succeeding (Black, 1997). Examples of excellent goals and objectives include the following:

- *Comprehensive primary education requires alternative solutions.* A school system must consider alternatives for students unable to successfully participate in a regular school.
- *Prevent and engage the dropout.* Students must be encouraged to stay in school; dropouts must be given an opportunity and encouraged to return to school and complete their education.
- *Prepare for citizenship.* The goal of learning, especially alternative solutions, is preparing students to become productive citizens and lifelong learners who have a strong sense of ethical and moral obligations to oneself, others, and the community (Hawes et al., 2000, p. xvii).

Establish and Require Challenging Expectations and Standards. These model alternative schools also set clear expectations and standards for the students, adopt and enforce class attendance policies, and establish policies that discourage avoidant behaviors (May & Copeland, 1998; Paglin & Fager, 1997). It has been demonstrated over and over again that if, in a tough but nurturing environment, exemplary performance is expected, that is what is given. This works especially well for the at-risk child.

Maintain an Active Circular Flow of Information. Successful alternative-school administrators maintain and encourage open communications with the feeder public schools in order to help their students experience a smooth transition back into the regular public school environment or transition to community, work, or further education. Many have full-time staff who serve as transition counselors and act as student liaison representatives in this capacity. Successful alternative-school administrators have strong leadership abilities and charismatically communicate and sell the school's mission and goals on a daily basis to anyone who will listen.

EDUCATIONAL CURRICULA AND INSTRUCTIONAL METHODS

Successful alternative schools and their administrators and teachers understand several vital facts about the at-risk students who are enrolled in their programs. One of the most obvious is the fact that these students learn at different rates, have differing abilities and deficiencies, and are not amenable to the traditional and mechanical method of public school instruction. Quoting an alternative-school administrator, Hawes et al. (2000) capture this basic understanding of alternative school students: "If it looked like, smelled, or tasted like education the kids did not want it; we had to disguise [education] and make it fun" (p. 59). Echoing that observation, Brewer et al. (1998) state, "one thing is certain—alternative school students do not need more of the same thing they have had before; they need different and effective approaches" (p. 95). Consequently, the best and most productive alternative schools use a variety of nontraditional curricula and incorporate an eclectic mix of instructional methods. This leads to situations in which the students become engaged in the learning process and consequently choose to do their assignments.

The best alternative schools focus first and foremost on improving the students' academic abilities in the basics of reading, writing, and arithmetic and try to improve their comprehension of these core subjects. As Hawes et al. (2000) comment, academic accomplishments produce increased self-esteem and instill discipline and responsibility in at-risk children. Strive for skills and characteristics that empower the kids to master life and not just academics. Life skills and parenting classes, computer classes, and group and individual counseling are all commonly found in successful alternative education programs. Daily physical education components should be included. It is here that the alternative-school students practice the coping skills that they have learned in the classroom and in counseling. These schools develop curricula that are directly related to the students' lives and interests and allow staff and students to jointly develop individual student learning plans and educational goals (Lange, 1998)—the more experiential or hands-on the better, with classes being student-centered and related to the students' concerns and interests (Kellmayer, 1998). Courses and instructional methods should be engaging and fun and hold the interests of the alternative-school students (Gregg, 1999). Dugger and Dugger (1998) advocate real-world learning experiences by requiring the students to attend school half a day and work the other. Hawes et al. (2000) provide excellent examples of real-world instruction, including teaching geometry through the shooting of basketball free throws and learning ecology by planting a school garden. In essence, the learning needs to come alive for these students.

Research on the planning of alternative-school curricula and instructional methods illuminates numerous other effective practices, including the following:

- Devise thematic and product-related curricula.
- Recognize and reward achievements and personal growth.
- Include a physical education component.
- Use technology extensively.
- Use community volunteers and mentors.
- Provide extensive one-on-one attention.
- Request waivers from mandated state public school curricula to enhance school flexibility.
- Match instructional methods to each student's best, or most, productive, learning style.
- Avoid a "watered down" curriculum at all costs.

Obviously, academic proficiency and improving student abilities are tantamount for alternative schools; however, it takes a special breed of teacher to work in these alternative-school environments. As Raywid (1999) astutely points out, in many cases it is the teacher-student relationship, as contrasted with the actual curriculum, which emerges as the most salient and significant factor when explaining what makes a successful alternative school.

Teachers and Staff

Recruit, Hire, and Retain the Best Staff and Faculty Possible. Paglin and Fager (1997) note that the best alternative school administrators remain aloof from the hiring process for teachers and staff. They prefer to leave this authority in the hands of capable staff and students. Exemplary administrators seek out training and professional development opportunities in diversified areas such as creative fundraising, personnel management, dealing with delinquent children, community involvement, stress and anger management, and other related topics to continually improve their personal and professional growth (Hawes et al., 2000). It helps that from the outset, district policy supports the best individuals possible to oversee, manage, operate, and teach in the alternative school.

Given these desirable traits and remarkable abilities plus the types of students found in these schools, Paglin and Fager (1997) vehemently argue against mandatory assignments which force teachers to work in alternative schools. All alternative-school teachers should want to be there and apply only on a voluntary basis. Alternative-school teachers should have a vision and desire to work in these environments and be capable of performing tasks well beyond the job descriptions for the traditional public school instructors. It is recommended that alternative-school teachers hold a variety of certifications so that they may teach a variety of subjects, and only those teachers who have a history of receiving exceptional and outstanding performance appraisals should be considered for positions within alternative schools (North Carolina Department of Public Instruction, 2000; Paglin & Fager, 1997). Just as alternative schools should not serve as dumping grounds for "bad" children, they should also not be used as dumping grounds for "bad" teachers. Hawes et al. (2000) recommend that alternative-school teachers work rotating shifts with time spent providing instruction in both the alternative and traditional school environments in order to prevent stress and "burnout." They also suggest providing incentive or bonus pay for alternative-school teachers. Leastwise, there needs to be an effort to develop a competitive package of salary and benefits. The package will bring these teachers to the table; the reward of the work will keep them there.

Encourage and Nurture Committed Staff. The key to establishing and maintaining a successful alternative school may be found in the quality of its leadership, especially its principal. Alternative-school principals must possess genuine concern and caring like the school's teachers, but they must also model these prosocial behaviors on a daily basis. Exceptional administrators keep open doors and are constantly asking their students and staff how they are doing, what is new, what works and does not work, and how we can fix it. Without strong, decisive, caring, and knowledgeable leadership the alternative school is doomed to fail.

Research on and evaluations of alternative schools clearly indicate that the teachers in these schools must show genuine concern, care, and empathy for their students. They must be totally committed and truly believe that the children are our future. Alternative-school teachers must create, and maintain, warm nurturing climates and be capable of patiently providing ample time for individual learning with the students (De La Rosa, 1998). Dugger and Dugger (1998) further note that alternative-school instructors must be able to easily approach at-risk students and establish long-lasting rapport through modeling desirable and appropriate behaviors. Teachers should *demonstrate* the ability to talk with the students and not at them, or worse, talk down to them (Paglin & Fager, 1997). Model alternative-school teachers act as champions, or advocates, for their children and often make home visits and attend sessions in which children are required to attend meetings with juvenile court counselors or other members of the juvenile court, school, and social service systems. Exemplary alternative-school educators make concentrated efforts to know their students' parents and home surroundings. Summarizing what constitutes an effective alternative-school teacher, Hawes et al. (2000) argue, "You can't buy these teachers you must find them" (p. xviii). They also add that alternative-school teachers cannot be created; they are equipped with certain natural, innate abilities that suit them for this work. Alternative schools need teachers with innate abilities who have been well trained to do a difficult job. Teachers who are dedicated, well trained, and well compensated and who share in-school governance will choose to work in an alternative school for a long time. Elimination of any of these features may lead to burnout and consequently a high teacher turnover rate in the school.

Continuously Develop the Alternative School Professional. Dynamic alternative-school staff and teachers eagerly pursue professional development and continuing education opportunities; they should be enthusiastically encouraged. These teachers have an intrinsic desire to learn and improve themselves so that they may better serve their children and their unique interests. The North Carolina Department of Public Instruction (2000) delineates an extensive list of recommended courses for providing staff development for alternative-school educators. Some of the suggested courses are as follows:

- Cooperative learning;
- Using technology for teaching;
- Child development;

- Mastery learning;
- Conflict resolution;
- Character education;
- Gangs and cults;
- Addiction/drug trends and terminology;
- Diversity; and
- Crisis management.

Develop Support Staff as You Develop Teaching Staff. Support staff within alternative schools should ideally possess the same attitudes and beliefs as the alternative-school administrators and teachers. The most successful alternative schools look for the same attributes whether hiring a teacher or a cafeteria worker. Support staff play a vital and integral role in creating, shaping, and maintaining the family or loving atmosphere of the school. Like teacher selection, the selection of support staff should be treated in a similar fashion, with only the most caring staff being selected and employed within the alternative school—being selected because they want to be there for the children. Model alternative schools also employ a school counselor, nurse, social worker, psychologist, physical education instructor, and transition coordinator. If these employees cannot be hired on a full-time, part-time, or contractual basis, the services that they offer should be provided for the students through other means.

Students

As with alternative-school teachers and staff, the students who attend these programs must also want to be there and take advantage of opportunities for getting a second chance at education. Most alternative students really do fit this mold and do realize the importance of their education. Surprisingly, many alternative-school students experience a turnaround during their stay and consequently do not want to return to their home schools—schools in which they experienced problems, were treated less favorably, did not feel like they fit in, and were far more impersonal than the alternative-school setting.

Establish Admissions Policy, Criteria, and Process. Model alternative schools operate with voluntary admissions policies (i.e., students apply to the school upon referral from the traditional public school where the students have been suspended or expelled). Mandating a child's attendance in an alternative school should be avoided as it can create a plethora of problems for the child, other alternative students, and school staff. The most effective enrollment or selection processes use a team review where the student applies for admission and then attends an initial screening interview at the alternative school. This review involves the student, parent(s), and representatives from both the traditional, or referral, school and the alternative school. The child's academic and behavioral records are assessed and if the child is admitted to the alternative school, he or she receives a student contract which outlines an educational plan and is signed and agreed on by all parties. The contract should also specify the length of the child's stay in the alternative school and how the student's transition back to the home school will be accomplished. It is advisable to transition students back at either the end of a school term or the end of a school year, as opposed to arbitrarily sending the child back during the middle or last part of the term or year. The length of a student's stay in an alternative school is directly correlated with academic and behavioral improvements, with longer stays producing more pronounced gains. Brewer et al. (1998) found that students who stayed in an alternative learning program for three or more grading periods demonstrated more academic improvements than did short-term stay students. Our own research indicates that a minimum stay of at least one semester must occur if any improvements are to be realized.

Assess Student Needs. Student assessment should be a continual process that begins when the student enters the alternative-school classroom. It is imperative that academic and behavioral progress be monitored and evaluated on a frequent basis. The best alternative schools reserve one afternoon weekly for teachers and staff to discuss the progress of their students in group or town hall-type meetings. The California Continuation Education Association (2000) provides an excellent five-stage typology for assessing an alternative-school student's progress. This model includes performance measures for assessing the student's impulse control, substance use, self-esteem and confidence levels, attendance, assignment completion, subject mastery, successfully passing courses, and receiving the high school diploma. The model also includes long-term follow-up on such areas as receiving and holding permanent employment. Hawes et al. (2000) identified numerous best practices for assessing alternative-school students, including using a wide and varied number of measures, allowing students to work at their own pace and to work toward subject mastery, using make-up assignments, and, most important, abolishing the traditional grading system in favor of a pass/fail system.

A FEW MORE EFFECTIVE PRACTICES

Involve Parents

The best alternative schools encourage and openly embrace parental involvement in all facets and activities of the school. Parental involvement should occur during the child's entire stay at the alternative school and not end once the child completes the enrollment and selection period. Weekly visitations to school are encouraged, as are parent-teacher conferences. Parents can also assist with school operations such as serving as chaperones on field trips or serving food at picnics. But nearly every one interviewed mentioned how difficult it was to engage the parent of an at-risk child. Parents of these children are invariably struggling with the basics of life and living themselves. That means the effort to engage them has to be redoubled and relentless. Although it is most difficult, those doing it remark that it is worth the effort.

Make Evaluation Part of Daily Business

Outstanding alternative schools not only provide continous assessments of their students, they also evaluate and continually monitor their own operations, processes, and staff. Ongoing data collection and analysis are essential for improving and maintaining the school's performance and its ability to provide effective services to the students. The National Dropout Prevention Center (2001) outlines criteria for evaluating alternative schools with an emphasis on monitoring the school climate, resource allocation, curriculum development, instruction delivery, and leadership. Brewer et al. (1998) suggest involving community members in this evaluation effort as well.

Provide Feedback and Earned Reward

Alternative schools need to recognize and reward their students for academic and behavioral improvements throughout the year and on a frequent basis. Small steps deserve praise, just as do larger accomplishments. Effective alternative schools recognize this fact and implement countless ways of providing positive feedback. Alternative schools that allow students to complete their diploma or GED (General Equivalency Diploma) requirements in their entirety should hold a separate yet equally important graduation ceremony with all students being honored and rewarded.

PROFILES OF MODEL PROGRAMS

Mat-Su Alternative School, Wasilla, Alaska

The nationally recognized Mat-Su school is located in a rural area about forty-five miles from Anchorage and serves at-risk children in the seventh through twelfth grades. The school operates on a year-round basis with all students making a personal decision to attend. The school serves teen parents, homeless children, delinquents, and students who are behind in their coursework.

A variety of services are available to the children, including counseling, onsite day care, and a food and clothes bank. The school works closely with a variety of agencies to provide holistic support for its students. Students are required to keep weekly logs and planners and review them for progress and needed improvement on a routine basis with instructors. Classroom instruction occurs in small classes with individualized and computer-assisted instruction the norm.

All students complete a world-of-work course, which is largely life skills with all alternative high school students being required to work on a part-time basis and all middle school students being required to perform comparable hours of community service. The school is heavily oriented to preparing its students for a vocation by developing skills such as life skills training, basic computer literacy, and keyboarding.

The school faculty members are dedicated to their students and spend all day with them in a warm and personal environment. In addition to ten teachers, a work-study specialist, custodian, and nurse are employed on a full-time basis.

Paglin and Fager (1997) comment on the exceptional track record of the Mat-Su school, noting that 80 percent of the students graduate and 90 percent have steady employment a year after graduation. Setting up a local advisory board, networking with local businesses, and having a strong school-to-work emphasis were identified as keys to program success. To contact this program, call (907) 373-7775.

New Directions Academy, El Paso, Texas

The New Directions Academy serves at-risk teens ages 17 to 21. The school offers a highly flexible schedule with a minimum of two hours of daily classroom attendance being required and supplemented with an additional two to three hours per day of independent study at the school or at home. Operating on a year-round schedule, the school is open from 7 A.M. to 9 P.M. to accommodate the varying needs of its students.

Students are required to complete the standard courses offered in their respective home schools but only work on two courses at a time. Individualized instruction and computer-based training modules are available at all times for the students. It is the responsibility of each student to schedule a weekly performance review with his or her teacher and to request more assignments once others have been completed.

Support services are readily available and include access to a school social worker, job counselor, and pregnancy education program. Teachers offer support and encouragement by modeling responsibility and accountability and encouraging extensive parental involvement. De La Rosa (1998) suggests that the personalized, warm, and caring environment creates a sense of belonging that consequently encourages and empowers children to succeed. To contact this program, call (915) 434-3000.

Discovery II, Jackson County, North Carolina

Discovery II serves at-risk students in the ninth through the twelfth grades and accepts them on a referral basis with those referrals made by home school administrators or parents. Applicants must be assessed by a review team and submit an essay describing why they want to attend the school. Potential students attend the school for two days to observe and be observed with current Discovery II students actively involved in the selection process. Upon acceptance, the student signs an academic and personal improvement contract.

Few formal classes or lectures are held; they are replaced by ample individualized instruction. Students are given copies of their courses' goals and objectives, as outlined in the state's standard course of study, and are expected to check them off once mastery has been demonstrated to the teacher's satisfaction. Experiential learning is encouraged through field trips and other hands-on activities. Days in the classroom begin and end with group meetings to discuss school and student concerns and other germane issues.

Hawes et al. (2000) identified numerous features of this alternative school which they observed as promising practices. The therapeutic environment treats students as responsible and trustworthy adults, which creates a climate that is more conducive to learning. Staff members also act as parents and problem-solving facilitators by listening to their students and helping them help themselves. The small number of students in the school ensures that this practice is continuous and frequent. A good mix of caring teachers contributes greatly to the school's success (the teachers have psychology and social work backgrounds in addition to their teaching credentials). Community involvement is strong; college students serve as volunteer mentors, and the school provides job shadowing programs and student assistance from a local senior citizens' organization. The county school board takes an active interest in the school and its students by being intimately involved and offering strong support and assistance. Finally, the school administrator actively sells the school and its philosophy of "giving students something to do, someone to love and something to hope for" (Hawes et al., 2000, p. 57). To contact this program, call (828) 586-2311.

OFFER VARIOUS ALTERNATIVE-SCHOOL EXPERIENCES

We observed that each community should consider several types of altena tive educational experiences because not all children respond well to regular school. Alterntive programs need to encompass the entire spectrum of children from the child who has only temporary and minor difficulty "fitting in" to the child who has severe adjustment problems. The worst thing to do is to remove the child from the school environment and then have no place for him or her to continue school. It may be expedient to expel, but doing so without an alterntive school setting incurs an inevitable and severe cost. Leaving a child to his own devices, even in an organized and disciplined environment, is a prescription for a bad ending. It may be that a community can afford only one alternative program; so be it. But plan for comprehensive services. There is nothing wrong with combining resources from several municipalities to offer needed services for the range of school experiences needed by children. Begin by reviewing the successes demonstrated by the programs and effective practices mentioned.

References

Black, S. (1997). One last chance. *The American School Board Journal, 184*, 40–42.

Brewer, D., Blackwelder, S., Aragon, A. T., Langmeyer, D., & Cobb, C. (1998). *Alternative learning programs evaluation: 1997–98.* Raleigh, NC: North Carolina Department of Public Instruction.

California Continuation Education Association. (2000). *Stages of development: A way of thinking about alternative schools* [On-line]. Available: *www. cceanet.org/Documents/API/Stages.htm.*

De La Rosa, D. A. (1998). Why alternative education works. *The High School Journal, 81*, 268–272.

Dugger, J. M., & Dugger, C. W. (1998). An evaluation of a successful alternative high school. *The High School Journal, 81*, 218–228.

Duke, D. J., & Griesdorn, J. (1999). Considerations in the design of alternative schools. *EBSCO Clearing House, 73*, 89.

Gregg, S. (1999). Creating effective alternatives for disruptive students. *EBSCO Clearing House, 73*, 107–114.

Hawes, J., Dillard, L., Brewer, D., Cobb, C., & Neenan, P. (2000). *Case studies of best practices: Alternative schools and programs: 1998–99.* Raleigh, NC: North Carolina Department of Public Instruction.

Kellmayer, J. (1998). Building educational alternative for at-risk youth: A primer. *The High School Magazine, 6*, 26–31.

Lange, C. M. (1998). Characteristics of alternative schools and programs serving at-risk students. *The High School Journal, 81*, 183–198.

May, H. E., & Copeland, E. P. (1998). Academic persistence and alternative high schools: Student and site characteristics. *The High School Journal, 81*, 199–208.

National Dropout Prevention Center. (2001). *Alternative schools: An effective strategy to prevent dropouts* [On-line]. Available: *www.dropoutprevention.org/21evelpages/e . . . g/41vlAltSchooling/41vlEffStrAltEdOverview.htm.*

North Carolina Department of Public Instruction. (2000). *Clarification of guidelines for alternative learning programs and schools.* Raleigh, NC: Division of School Improvement.

Paglin, C., & Fager, J. (1997). *Alternative schools: Approaches for students at risk.* Portland, OR: Northwest Regional Educational Laboratory.

Raywid, M. (1999). History and issues of alternative schools. *Education Digest, 64*, 47–51.

Virginia Commonwealth University. (2001). *Effectiveness of alternative schools* [On-line]. Available: *www.vcu.edu/eduweb/merc/briefs/brief%2040%20effectiveness_of_alternative_sch.htm.*

Chapter 14

Planning, Operating, and Expanding an Alternative School

This chapter addresses the three major components of a program, or project's, life cycle. Specifically, preimplementation planning strategies are highlighted, with an emphasis on the necessary components for successfully planning an alternative school program. Once the alternative school is operational, it is imperative to maintain high levels of operational effectiveness and efficiency to ensure continued program success. Key points to consider for maintaining a successful alternative school are discussed. Finally, and perhaps most important, it is advantageous to market, expand, and replicate the successful alternative school strategies and practices in order to provide adequate services to those at-risk target populations and effectively bridge the service-to-needs gap within the municipality.

PHASE ONE: PLANNING AN ALTERNATIVE-SCHOOL PROGRAM

Identify Key Leadership/Establish a Governance Board

Raywid (1999) offers several salient policy and planning questions that must be addressed before an alternative educational program is initiated. These are critical issues; the responses to these questions will ultimately shape the alternative school, its efficiency, and effectiveness. As Raywid (1999) notes, with insight, these programs are malleable; alternative schools will be what one makes them. The following questions must be considered and extensively debated with solid and attainable answers being provided long before the alternative school opens its doors.

- *Target population.* For whom is the alternative school intended? Who are the targeted students? The needs assessment must yield a detailed profile of children in need. These profiles may well define classes of children who need very different alternative schooling responses.
- *Define mission.* Is the school's primary mission to educate or to benefit the feeder schools by removing the most incorrigible and intractable students? From the mission should flow beliefs, objectives, goals, measures, and targets. It also helps to discuss a school's vision.
- *Student selection.* How will the students be selected? Is their attendance

mandated by court or school referrals or will there be a voluntary admissions policy?

- *Academic standards.* Will the alternative school be held to the same academic and other accountability standards as regular public schools?
- *Location.* Where will the school be located? Transportation is a primary determinant of where to put the school. Students must have access that avoids lengthy bus rides.
- *Staffing.* How will teachers be recruited and retained?
- *Purpose.* Is the goal of the alternative school to transition students back into the mainstream public schools or to serve as a separate and distinct educational forum for granting the high school diploma or GED (General Equivalency Diploma)?

There are other crucial planning questions that should not be overlooked. They include and are not limited to the following:

- *Curriculum.* Will the standard public school curriculum be followed or will different curricula be required?
- *Permanent funding.* Where are the funding sources and are they permanent?
- *Transportation.* How will students be transported to, and from, the alternative school?
- *Parental/community involvement.* How will community, and more important parental, involvement be attained and maintained?
- *Performance measurement.* How will student and school performance be monitored?
- *Oversight.* How much flexibility and autonomy will the school administration be allowed to have?

The research on alternative schools clearly documents the need for a governing body, or advisory council, which is composed of the major stakeholders or key players from the community. At a minimum, this governing board should include the following:

- *Educators.* A representative from the school district's central office.
- *The alternative school liaison.* Include your liaison to the appropriate feeder public schools.
- *Public sector.* Consider members of law enforcement, mental health, and social services agencies.

- *Community and business.* You must have community and business members. Don't forget the faith community.

After program implementation the alternative school principal, an alternative-school teacher, an alternative-school student, and the parent of an alternative-school student should be added to this governing body.

Kellmayer (1998) suggests that this group be assembled at least one year prior to school implementation. The formation of this advisory council should not be underestimated. Careful attention to detail must be invested in assigning duties and responsibilities as their deliberations and policy and program decisions will significantly affect the alternative school throughout the entire three phases of the project life cycle. (See Chapter 2, Exhibit 2.1, for a description of the project life cycle.) Certainly, this leadership body is a critical factor that means failure or success. In addition to addressing the aforementioned planning questions, this body should develop the school's vision and mission statements and standard operating policy and procedures, as well as formulate the numerous plans, such as the long-range and implementation plans, which are fully delineated throughout the remaining portions of this chapter.

We strongly recommend that this advisory board attend a professionally facilitated retreat before the group begins its formative and substantive work in outlining the development of a new alternative school. Emphasis should be placed on team development and team-building strategies, as well as enabling the members to learn more about each other and, more important, to experience their group dynamic and ascertain how this body will work best to achieve its goals and objectives. Remember, the people are just as important as the program; thus, the more time that needs to be spent up front on advisory board development the less time waste, resource misuse, and obstacles the board will encounter as it engineers the alternative program.

Conduct a Needs Assessment

As part of its work the advisory board will be responsible for conducting an in-depth needs analysis that will ascertain all relevant, community, human, technological, financial, and curricula characteristics and resources that will be needed to make the alternative school operational. Needs-assessment data should be obtained from a variety of sources and through a variety of means including surveying and holding focus groups with middle and high school principals, school counselors, other existing alternative-school personnel, and representatives from the anticipated feeder schools as well as parents of at-risk children. Existing school and financial data should also be obtained and analyzed as part of this needs assessment. We encourage the use of outside consultants or expert researchers and planners to conduct this assessment and also advocate using local university faculty and students.

Though data needs and availability vary for each different location the following types of data should be analyzed and included in the needs-assessment phase:

- Current and projected student populations;
- Current and projected school suspensions and expulsions;
- Standardized test scores and other locally mandated tests such as competency and end-of-grade tests;
- Data on school absenteeism;
- Current and projected school budgets and potential revenue sources; and
- Demographic data surrounding the target population (i.e., at-risk children).

The collection of target population data is by far the most important piece of information that will be needed to establish and maintain an effective and efficient alternative school. It is imperative to collect data on the attributes of the at-risk children in the entire area that will be served by the alternative school. Data should be collected on those socioeconomic, demographic, educational, and familial factors that are known to be significantly correlated with academic failure, dropping out of school, juvenile delinquency, and other behavioral and emotional disorders. These indicators, or red flags, should at a minimum include the following:

- Single-parent and/or overcrowded homes;
- Substance-abusing family members;
- Lack of parental supervision (i.e., children raising themselves);
- Residing in high-crime areas with a high drug presence;
- Low impulse control;
- Lack of respect for authority figures;
- Low parental educational background; and
- Lack of attention and affection.

As a general rule, the more specific the data, the better. Also, the more historical the data are, the better; and the more predictive the information is (i.e., data projections), the better.

Develop a Mission Statement and Philosophy

Exemplary alternative-school program personnel invest a great deal of time and energy on developing, and constantly promulgating, clear and concise vision and mission statements and guiding philosophies. All these statements reference the desire to provide alternative education, and most include further desires such as producing productive adults, fostering a feeling of love and sense of belonging, and building character in the lives of their targeted youth. As Vasu and Klopovic (2000) note, a program's vision statement should be reviewed periodically in order to make adjustments to program operating policies and procedures. Do not shorten the visioning process; it is worth the agony of doing it well.

Once the vision statement has been formulated, a mission statement should follow. This statement should support and reflect the stated purposes or intentions of the broader vision statement and expound on and clarify the overall purpose of the alternative school. Readers are encouraged to refer to the mission statements of other existing alternative learning schools as one possible jumping off point for their own guiding philosophy. Hawes, Dillard, Brewer, Cobb, and Neenan (2000) enumerate several examples of strong vision and mission statements in their work, and we recognize many of these as outstanding statements. The following mission statement was actually developed by the students of one alternative school:

> Our mission is to make our class be a happy, safe, comfortable, caring place where we have love and belonging, power, freedom and fun. We will be respectful, honest, trustworthy, in control of ourselves and motivated. (Hawes et al., 2000, p. 2)

Other examples include:

> Providing an opportunity for each student to gain the skills needed to function effectively in the world at large. (Hawes et al., 2000, p. 11)

> Providing a student-centered curriculum that meets the needs of students with diverse abilities, problems, backgrounds, and concerns. (Hawes et al., 2000, p. 39)

> Our mission is to empower each student utilizing a systematic approach that maximizes academic potential, promotes life-long learning, and develops skills necessary for re-entry into a traditional setting. (Elton O'Neal, personal communication, March 6, 2001).

Finally, relevant goals and specific, concrete, and measurable objectives should be agreed on and documented. These goals and objectives should possess a logical and structural relationship to the school's broader vision and mission statements and provide explanations as to when, where, why, and how the vision and mission statements will become reality. Again, we encourage communicating with existing alternative school administrators who will more than likely gladly share personal goals and program objectives.

As Welsh and Harris (1999) suggest, goal statements should describe anticipated future changes that have an impact on the problem and allow for execution of the program's ultimate mission. Goal statements should be brief and broad and lack the specificity for measuring actual outcomes, reserving the determination of impact and outcomes for the more precisely defined operational measures outlined in the objective(s) for each program goal.

The program objectives represent the true nuts and bolts of the alternative school and are an essential feature of the school's evaluation plan as discussed in the next section. These are quantifiable and measurable factors that facilitate the assessment of program goals. Hudzik and Cordner (1983) outline numerous attributes of strong program objectives and note that in addition to being measurable and direct extensions of program goals, objectives should be suitable, feasible, acceptable, flexible, and understandable. An example of the relationship between goals and objectives follows:

Goal: Improve the academic performance of the alternative school enrollees.

Objective 1: Maintain an average daily attendance rate of 100 percent.

Objective 2: Maintain a 90 percent completion rate for class assignments.

Objective 3: Raise the average student GPA from 2.7 to 3.0.

Objective 4: Raise passing rates for (end-of-year) EOY tests from 60 percent to 75 percent.

Remember to always check that each objective is linked to each goal and that each goal is linked to the ultimate purpose, which is to develop productive citizens. If the link is unsure, perhaps the objective needs modification or even abandonment. Each objective represents the expenditure of significant resources and especially the rarest resource, time. Make each objective productive.

Conduct a School Evaluation Plan

Why Evaluations Are Critical to School Administration. This is another vital component of the project life cycle (see Chapter 2, Exhibit 2.1). It is imperative that your evaluation plan be prepared before and implemented at the same time the alternative school opens its doors to students. Sooner than later members of the traditional schools, central office administrators, and even members of the community will clamor for "results." It is much easier to evaluate a program from its inception as opposed to performing one retrospectively, after the school has been in existence for some time. The worst situation is to have to scramble and hastily compile an ad hoc evaluation to appease a school board that is questioning program performance during the hectic and final twilight hours of budget deliberations.

What to Measure. Strong school evaluation plans should include measures for assessing impact or outcome of the school and measures for monitoring the internal operations of the school (i.e., process evaluation measures). Duke and Griesdorn (1999) offer an excellent list of suggested impact evaluation measures including:

- *Graduation rates.* Percentage of students who graduated or received a GED;
- *Successful return to home school.* Percentage of students who successfully transitioned back to the feeder school;
- *Aggregate grade point average.* Class grade point average assesses overall school performance;
- *Dropout rates.* Dropout rates for the alternative school versus the entire school district;
- *Assignment completion.* Percentage of students who complete daily assignments;
- *Standardized test performance.* Percentage of students passing or making improvements on standardized tests;
- *Discipline rates/improvements.* School disciplinary infractions are a dramatic indicator especially when compared to previous infraction rates in regular school;
- *Attendance rates.* Daily attendance rates compared to previous rates in regular school; and
- *Self-esteem improvements.* Percentage of students who report feeling better about themselves.

It should be mentioned that, typically, state accountability tests are not powerful enough by themselves to show academic progress in an alternative school. We found that many successful alternative schools administer individualized diagnostic reading, writing, and math tests at least every six months to assess student performance.

Continuous Assessment/Process Evaluation. We strongly advocate process evaluation with an emphasis on continually assessing the alternative school's daily operations within the framework of its stated mission, goals, and objectives. One effective means of achieving this is to create a school improvement team that essentially becomes an oversight committee or the school's best critic. This team should, at a minimum, include teachers, students, and administrative personnel. Expanded school improvement teams would involve support staff, parents, and members of the local business and public service organizations. Regularly scheduled meetings should be conducted in which this group analyzes the school's prescribed process evaluation measures and, most important, makes recommendations for improving the school and removing, or at least minimizing, potential obstacles that would prohibit goal attainment. Many effective alternative schools have elaborate school improvement plans that are developed from, and around, their desired process evaluation measures. These plans guide a successful school evolution and help ensure program success through internal quality control. Suggested process evaluation measures, or questions, should include the following:

- Are school rules, policies, and procedures being followed and enforced consistently, firmly, and fairly?
- Is there adequate and open communication between staff, students, and administrative personnel?
- How involved are parents and community members?
- How strong are the working relationships and communication patterns between the alternative school, the public feeder schools, and the central office?
- What are the school's most effective practices and, conversely, what are its current weaknesses?
- Is the school's student selection process still adequate?
- Are the curricula and teaching methods working?
- Are the staff and students content?
- Are the school's mission statement and its goals and objectives current, and is the school making progress to achieve them?
- Is the school's process of transitioning students back to their respective feeder schools sufficient and efficient?

In addition to using surveys and standardized test score reports, other data collection techniques might involve talking with students, parents, and community members through town hall meetings or focus groups. Transition specialists might conduct longitudinal studies that follow former alternative-school students to assess their reassimilation to the public schools and, just as important, their readjustment to the community. Data collection is quantitative and qualitative. It is an ongoing process that occurs every day by routinely collecting pertinent numbers and observing, listening, and talking about the school and its environment.

There are shelves of textbooks and publications with respect to research design, conducting evaluations, and designing surveys. Sage Publications has an excellent survey resource kit which includes nine volumes that guide readers from designing the survey to presenting the final results (see Fink, 1995; Miller, 1991; Stringer, 1996; Weisburg, Krosnick, & Bowen, 1996; U.S.

General Accounting Office, 1993, for extremely useful and user-friendly information on conducting the types of applied evaluations that alternative-school personnel are urged to perform).

The most difficult part of assessing efficiency (the amount of work done daily) and effectiveness (results) is *to begin*. An evaluation program may not be sophisticated; what matters is that a program has one that works for its situation.

Develop a Resource Plan and Marketing Strategy

Procure Resources. Another obvious issue that the advisory board must address is resource procurement. A plan or strategy for securing initial and permanent funding must be developed. Some alternative schools use the entire advisory board for this purpose; others form a separate subcommittee. Either way, all avenues of funding, including local school district appropriations, state and federal grants, support from nonprofit organizations, and community donations, should be thoroughly investigated. The most successful alternative schools include personnel who eagerly and aggressively rise to the funding challenge. Creative funding is both an art and a science and the advisory board should actively search for, and find, one or more persons who can fulfill this role and find sufficient funds for the school. It is also advisable to obtain copies of existing alternative school budgets as a reference point for determining the magnitude and extent of the necessary resources for starting and maintaining a new alternative-school program.

Market the Concept. As with any new product or service, its success, or conversely its failure, is directly dependent on how well it is marketed and sold to the target populations and the general public. A new alternative school is no different. The most successful alternative schools have a marketing strategy and launch strong public relations campaigns. It is extremely important to identify the key stakeholders, and primary and even secondary groups and organizations that can make or break the school's success. These stakeholders and important organizations must buy into and support the new alternative-school program. Clearly, these people and groups are constantly being approached, even bombarded with new ideas and programs all of which compete for scarce resources and limited public dollars. What can the advisory board do to rise to the top and demonstrate that an alternative school is laudable, needed, and will be advantageous for the community?

The first method is to be prepared and have a plan or marketing strategy in hand before approaching anyone. The needs-assessment study can serve as a major tool for the board to draw on when trying to "sell" the concept of alternative learning. It is recommended that a shotgun approach be taken with an eclectic mix of the community being contacted to receive presentations about creating a new alternative school. The greater the buy-in from a variety of community groups, especially groups with vested interest, the greater the chance of garnering support for the school and bringing the concept to reality.

We found that it is more effective to speak with one or two of the most influential group members first in order to anticipate the types of questions that the larger group will ask. This may seem like extra work but it is worthwhile in that the board will be perceived as totally prepared and knowledgeable about the group receiving the sales pitch. It is also advantageous because different groups will ask different questions germane to their particular interests and functions in the community. Thus the pitch for support appears to be directly aimed at this group and does not come off as a canned presentation being delivered in rote fashion. The following list suggests some of the various types of organizations that can be approached with the alternative- school concept. Each list will vary and should be determined by the need to know plus the ability to contribute to the work of engineering alternative schools:

- Administrators of the public schools that will provide students to the prospective alternative school;
- The district Board of Education;
- The state Board of Education or Department of Instruction;
- County Commission or City Council;
- Chamber of Commerce;
- Local youth boards or councils;
- Leaders and policymakers from the juvenile justice system;
- Professional associations whose members work with children;
- Civic organizations, such as the Rotary or Shriners;
- Mental health professionals;
- Social services professionals;
- Church boards and organizations;
- Private business representatives; and
- Any groups that possess power in the community and have the ability to contribute to the school either financially or through endorsement.

Marketing Tips. Through the course of our research, we have discovered several excellent ways to create a strong and, more important, a winning marketing strategy.

- *Market comprehensive services.* The alternative school should be marketed as a comprehensive service (i.e., it offers full academic instruction, behavior modification, social and vocational skills training, and health and psychological services, and contains a built-in evaluation component).

- *Market school quality.* The quality of the school should be stressed, with an emphasis on documenting the effectiveness and efficacy of existing alternative school programs.
- *Market cost-benefit/effectiveness.* Stress the long-term costs and benefits of providing alternative education as opposed to building more juvenile correctional facilities or placing a greater burden on the already strained hospitals and mental health facilities.
- *Use grassroots networking.* Use a grassroots approach with extensive networking, hand shaking, and forging strong one-to-one working relationships.
- *Market community problem solving.* One of the most profound tips the authors received was to define the issue as a broad community problem and not as a simple and narrow public education problem.
- *Demonstrate usefulness and results.* Demonstrate the utility and impact that an alternative school can have on the entire community with its students eventually becoming productive members of the community who will give back to the community as opposed to preying on it.
- *Market continuously.* Finally, remember that marketing is like evaluation, it needs to be continuous, creative, persistent, and malleable throughout the life cycle of the project.

Developing support, funding, and resources is a strategy for continuous activity on many levels by all stakeholder groups. While the board is the primary mover, the development strategy must include the constant representation of a vital program by community leaders, educators (especially those in the alternative learning program), parents, and students (yes, students). There is nothing that "sells" like the success of an at-risk young citizen.

Formulate a Long-Range or Strategic Plan and an Implementation or Action Plan

As part of its work it is suggested that the advisory board develop a long-range, or strategic, plan which addresses short-term, mid-range, and long-term objectives. Some alternative schools hold an annual planning retreat and involve the board, administrators, faculty, parents, and students to assess where they are on the plan and where they want to go.

Short-term goals are those that need to be achieved within the year, and most commonly revolve around day-to-day operations. Issues to be considered include the following: teacher retention, continuation funding, boosting student academic and behavioral progress, student enrollment criteria, curriculum development, staff-student and student-student relations, parental and community involvement, and school safety concerns.

Mid-range goals are those that need to be achieved within two to five years and typically concern improving the effectiveness and efficiency of the alternative school and planning for growth. Common mid-range goals include expanding student enrollment with an emphasis on determining the types of future students anticipated, building a competent and stable group of administrators and faculty, and addressing key policy issues such as how children transition back to their respective feeder or home schools and beyond. Plan to assess the more long-range impact of alternative school graduates by recording how they do after school. Do they indeed move on to more education or training? Are they gainfully employed? Do they stay away from public dependency and services? Are they productive citizens?

Long-range goals are those that will need to be achieved in the distant future (i.e., five years or more down the road). These goals should be driven by the school's existing needs assessment and results of its internal evaluation. Common long-range goals include expanding the program to include a larger and more varied student body, facilities enhancements, and revisiting the mid-range goals to determine if they have been sufficiently met. This is really the meat and potatoes of planning. Inevitably the initial experiment with an alternative learning program merely illuminates the length, depth, and breadth of the need. Look to expansion to address the true need of a community for alternative schooling options and facilities.

We also recommend that the advisory board develop an implementation or action plan that addresses all the key steps that will be needed for putting the program into action and delineating what will need to be completed before the doors are open and the first students arrive. A detailed Gantt chart, or visual project timeline that outlines major tasks, responsibilities, and due dates, can be helpful for ensuring that all the key steps are occurring, and most important, are occurring as scheduled. The readers are encouraged to review Chapter 5 of Welsh and Harris's (1999) excellent planning book for a thorough treatment of developing an action plan. Welsh and Harris note three important guidelines during this phase of planning:

- Maintain consistency;
- Maintain clear, frequent, and concise lines of communication; and
- Constantly monitor the time line for accuracy and completeness.

Profile Key Staff and Outline Job Duties and Responsibilities

The selection of quality administrators, teachers, and support staff in many ways is the advisory board's greatest challenge and one of the most important tasks the board is charged to complete. Remember, these employees will make the alternative school what it is and will be directly responsible for the school's success or failure. Readers are encouraged to review the attributes of exemplary school personnel, as previously delineated, and actively solicit educators who possess these qualities. First and foremost these school personnel must want to be in the alternative-school environment and demonstrate genuine compassion and concern for their students' successes. Obviously, budgetary constraints will affect the nature of each school's faculty, but it is suggested that the advisory board include the following positions when outlining school personnel allocation and deployment patterns:

- Principal;
- At least one assistant principal;
- Teachers;
- Vocational teachers;
- Transition specialist;
- Crisis intervention/management counselor;
- School psychologist;
- Community/parental liaison;
- Physical education instructor;
- Cafeteria, custodian, and transportation providers;
- Computer specialist/instructor;
- Teachers' assistants;
- School resource officer;
- Secretary/bookkeeper;
- Parental/community volunteers;
- Social worker; and
- Case manager.

Alternative learning work is a tough way to earn a living, made tougher by low pay scales and the students. A nurturing, professional policy for people goes far in attracting and retaining people whose intrinsic motivation must be significant to come to and remain on the job. Much can be done, to a point, which is better than money.

It is highly recommended that all staff receive extensive staff development training and professional and personal development throughout their career in the alternative-school environment. If possible, supplemental, or special duty, pay should be provided. We discovered one innovative technique in which more experienced alternative-school teachers acted as mentors to the newly hired alternative-school teachers during their first year of duty.

It is also highly recommended that all staff be hired and on board at least one month prior to the school's becoming operational. During this month a staff team-building retreat should be conducted with all school personnel interacting with the school's advisory board.

The essential element of planning for staff is the policy set by the board. Personnel policy should establish the process of recruiting, hiring, orienting, developing (professionally), and retaining the best people possible. For example, before the first hiring announcement is made, the duties, responsibilities, and expectations for each position should be written in detail. Likewise, the requisite education, training, and experience should be noted. Hiring policy needs to cover how pools of qualified people will be developed, how interviews will be conducted, and how new hires will be met, oriented, and trained initially. Real effort and time spent on human capital has real return on investment. The time to discuss fine points is during the planning phase, not during the hiring interview.

Site Selection and Defining a Student Admission Policy

Again, readers are encouraged to review and implement those effective practices regarding site selection and the physical aspects of the facility, which were discussed earlier. It is also recommended that a site selection subcommittee of the advisory board members be formed with this as its only purpose. This committee should make extensive site visits to existing alternative schools and determine what best suits their own financial and resource capabilities and limitations. Common questions to address should include the following:

- How old is the facility and how much renovation must occur?
- Should the school have its own separate campus?
- Is there adequate classroom space?
- Is space available for physical and vocational education activities?
- Is ample cafeteria space available?
- Is the site conducive for promoting a safe and orderly learning environment?
- Is there room for future growth?
- Is the site's location easy for students to come to?
- How automated will the school be?
- Is there adequate storage space?

- Is the facility compatible with the Americans With Disabilities Act?

It is equally important to draft a standard policy for student admissions or guidelines for student selection and also exit criteria. Readers are encouraged to review the suggested effective practices in this area. Common issues to consider include the following:

- Will admission be strictly voluntary or will the school take students who have been referred by feeder schools or mandated to attend by the courts?
- What types of students will the school enroll and, conversely, not accept into the program?
- How long will the students remain?
- How will disciplinary problems be addressed?
- How will student progress be measured?
- Will the school transition students back to their home schools or hold a separate graduation track?
- Who will decide if the student should be admitted and how?
- Who will decide when the student is ready to leave the school and under what exit conditions?

There is another important, hidden, aspect to site selection. Having an adequate physical plant is a given. But, remember, the school is also a sales tool. The school will want and have more visitors on a routine basis and more unexpected visitors than is common. Initial impressions are indelible and have important implications. A school that looks like a failure has that much more trouble getting support. Even if the physical plant is an old building, the paint should be fresh and the restrooms should sparkle.

PHASE TWO: OPERATING AN ALTERNATIVE-SCHOOL PROGRAM

The following section offers successful tips and effective strategies from the field for operating an alternative school for at-risk children. This is the natural progression from thorough planning. It is by no means exhaustive and each alternative school's operations will vary based on the physical location of the school, its students and staff, and local and state educational requirements. It is not our intent to instruct alternative-school educators on how to run their respective schools; however, we have found these generic or global suggestions to be particularly effective and meritorious. They form the framework of the site-specific style that evolves from tough analysis and that greatest teacher, *experience*.

Develop an Operational Plan and Administrative Structure

Immediately prior to the school's opening its doors to students an operational plan, or set of established alternative school policies and procedures, should be prepared and thoroughly reviewed with the entire school staff. It is recommended that the policies and procedures manual be concise, thorough, and, most important, user-friendly. The manual should completely address the following major questions or issues related to the school's primary objective of providing quality education for those at-risk students who do not perform adequately within the traditional public school environment. These questions or issues relevant to students are as follows:

- Who is eligible to attend and how do they get there?
- What will happen to the students from their first day until their last day?
- What will staff do to achieve the school's stated mission, goals, and objectives?
- How will staff instruct the students?
- How will behavioral problems be managed?
- Who is eligible to exit the school and what criteria determine their departure?

At a minimum the alternative school's policies and procedures manual should address all relevant administrative procedures, student admissions and departures, behavior management, daily operations, and issues related to curriculum design and revision. Remember that the policies and procedures manual will be one of the most used, and widely perused, documents in the school. It should be viewed as a living and malleable instrument; consequently, we recommend that it contain an index which will facilitate its use and allow staff to locate information in an expedient manner. Obviously, a good point of departure is the operations manual developed from site surveys done during the planning phase.

Teacher and Staff Retention. An important issue that the alternative school's administrative staff should immediately address is teacher/staff retention. One of the most common discussions in which we participated during the course of visiting alternative schools dealt with the importance of hiring and maintaining a devoted, competent, and professional staff. The most effective alternative schools make human capital development a priority, with each staff member pursuing an individualized professional growth or career development plan. It is not enough to simply possess such a plan; exceptional alternative school administrators include staff training and development in their annual budgets and actively encourage, and often reward, their staff for doggedly pursuing self-improvement and professional growth (readers are encouraged to consult the North Carolina Department of Public Instruction, 2000, clarification of guidelines document for an excellent example of the various types of activities and courses which can be delineated in a career development plan for alternative-school educators). The best follow the natural progression of prescribed and suggested initial, intermediate, and advanced training, education, and professional development. Note that support of professional development is a significant motivator and goes a long way to answer a short package of wages and benefits.

We favor, whenever possible, offering incentive pay or extra financial compensation to alternative-school staff who take the greater challenge when compared to the regular public school environment. Exceptional alternative-school administrators provide continual support and offer considerable praise to their staff in order to keep them motivated and to prevent "burnout." Like possessing the ability to exercise creative funding, good alternative-school administrators have a built-in knack for finding diverse and numerous nonfinancial ways to develop, motivate, and retain their staff. Staff development and motivation is certainly an art and a science.

Information/Records Management. As in any public-service organization, recordkeeping and management play a crucial role in organizational operations, and it is no different for the operation of an alternative school. Efficient records management techniques are arguably perhaps an even greater issue for the alternative school given the sensitive nature of student psychological, medical, and behavioral information and their nexus with strict security and confidentiality demands. Consequently, alternative-school administrators must delicately balance what information will be maintained on each student and who will have access to that information.

We suggest that a holistic case-based system of records management be used, with each alternative-school student being assigned a unique numeric case identifier upon enrollment into the school. This identifying number will permit electronic tracking of the students' records. It can also be helpful for maintaining student confidentiality in the event that student data are ever subject to court subpoena or needed for research purposes (i.e., information can be extracted from a database with all of the student's relevant information remaining together as one single case record which does not include the student's name).

This case-based system of managing student information should be systematic and contain extensive documentation on the student's entire stay within the alternative school. Individual alternative-school administrators will need to decide what types of student information to compile based on local and state educational mandates, school district policies and legal obligations, and school-specific needs, goals, and objectives. We recommend that at least the following types of student information be collected and maintained:

- *Referral file.* The complete and entire student file as maintained by the referring school;
- *Admission form and signatures.* Admission form to the alternative school with parental and student signatures;
- *Contract and plan of instruction.* Student contract, academic and behavioral goals, and a plan of instruction for attaining them;
- *Academic progress.* Academic progress data, including attendance, work assignments, grades, and standardized test scores;
- *Behavioral progress.* Behavioral data including disciplinary infractions as well as positive behavioral improvements; and
- *Miscellaneous notes and comments.* Notes/comments from the school psychologist, social workers, and teachers on any relevant issues that staff have to address to effectively educate and manage the child.

Perhaps the most important document is the student contract or personalized education plan (PEP). Each student must have one. Its value is that when the contract is violated or the PEP is not followed, it offers a chance to renegotiate with the student and at the same time teaches the child to learn socially acceptable behaviors and processes.

Alternative-school administrators are urged to seek out professionally developed school information records management software packages that are flexible, user-friendly, and capable of manipulating data in a simple, straightforward manner so that complex ad hoc reports can be quickly produced. This capability is a lifesaver, especially during the budgetary season. Open system platforms and universal operating systems should be considered in the event that the school might desire to upgrade or expand the software or engage in data-sharing projects with other schools or public service agencies in the future.

Automation. Data sharing through integrated computer systems is especially relevant in light of the fact that many at-risk students are transient and may attend numerous schools within many different school districts during their educational career. Thus educators will not have to delay enrollment until the student's records arrive, admit students blindly, or, worse, create a new record from scratch. Integrated systems are also encouraged so that the alternative school can freely exchange data with its numerous feeder schools. If an existing districtwide or statewide student information management system is already operational, the alternative school should ensure that its system is directly linked into these existing systems.

Administrators may wish to explore the feasibility of using a transmission control protocol/Internet protocol (TCP/IP) platform that permits staff to access student records through an Intranet or Internet application. Fortunately, data security protocols and standards have seen significant advances and thus permit secure access to records through encrypted log-ins and protected passwords. Administrators should at least consider a school Intranet or local area network, irrespective of the issue of accessing student records, which can be useful for sharing information among staff and/or between staff and students. School calendars, announcements, newsletters, awards, handbooks, manuals, and plans would then be easily accessible to all relevant parties. A school Internet web site could also be developed and used by students to keep parents and community members abreast of school activities. Once automation is in place, creativity and utility take over, making it well worth the sweat and expense.

Daily Operations Management. We asked numerous alternative-school administrators and other staff members to elaborate and share strategies on how to troubleshoot, problem-solve, and narrow the scope of their operations in order to make their work manageable. Numerous comments were offered with an overriding theme of "one day at a time" emerging. Staff should focus on daily operations and offer lavish praise to the students, as well as each other, on a frequent and even excessive basis. Staff commented on how a simple "thank you," "good job," or pat on the back goes a long way and quickly rectifies problems or deescalates a crisis. Proactive problem solving works best. We were told that keeping tabs on the rumor mill and simply being good at looking, listening, and observing will enable alternative school staff to create a safe environment conducive to learning.

As in any workplace, tension and problems often occur between staff members. Exceptional alternative-school administrators do not remain invisible to, or ignore, staff dissension and act quickly to resolve the tension before it escalates. These administrators know that it does not take long for student radar to pick up signals regarding disagreements between staff. Students often use this knowledge to their advantage and usually to the disadvantage of the school environment. Other ideas for problem solving include developing a school improvement team consisting of administrators, teachers, students, and support staff as well as making counseling services available for staff.

Justify Resources and Foster Key Service Provision

Market Resources. Despite the rigors, demands, and challenges of operating an alternative school "one day at a time", insightful comments and helpful suggestions were obtained regarding a vital activity that the alternative-school administrator might neglect to perform adequately and frequently. We were reminded about the importance of justifying the school and its resources and the relevancy of emphasizing and obtaining continuous and eventually permanent funding. Numerous successful strategies exist for continually selling and marketing the alternative school in order to guarantee its continued existence and acceptance as an important community and educational institution. We suggest there be a continuous information feedback loop between the alternative school and its key stakeholders, including the feeder schools, the central school district, the community, parents, and members of the business sector. The school board requires special attention. Do not fear asking what and how the board members like their information. Timing is everything; remember to get it to them when they need it.

It is important to maintain open and frequent lines of communication with the feeder schools and the central school district office regarding both individual student performance and school performance as a whole. The reporting of the process and impact evaluation data, as compiled in the school's evaluation plan, should occur on a frequent basis with student enrollment, attendance, grade point averages, and transition results being openly shared as a barometer of the school's progress.

The result of the school improvement team's work is another way to maintain visibility with the alternative school's key stakeholders. Remember, the school improvement plan is as important to the alternative school's success as the PEP is for the students' success. Continually documenting school and student success stories offers promise for demonstrating the staff's commitment to students and the school's mission, goals, and objectives. Alternative-school staff should not be afraid to report—or worse, try to cover up—failures or issues that have not been adequately resolved. Being forthright with the stakeholders should not be underestimated. Nothing or no one is perfect; openly discussing problems and accepting constructive criticism actually increases credibility in the eyes of those who are judging the program. Adopting a defensive posture only exacerbates tensions between alternative-school staff and its stakeholders.

Do not be deluded into thinking that the longer the alternative school has been operational and the more at-risk students it has served, the easier it may be to justify its continued existence. This may be true for some alternative schools but certainly not all. Alternative-school administrators are encouraged to revisit their needs-assessment studies and especially their marketing plans continuously and not file them away on a bookshelf to collect dust. The more successful principals see these documents and tasks as "living, breathing" things.

One effective practice we found especially productive was to revisit the section of the marketing plan that discusses the negative results of what happens if the alternative school is not established. Contrasting the number of students who remained in the educational environment because of the alternative school with those who would have been left on the streets profoundly documents school efficacy. If possible, cost savings estimates should be calculated and used to justify school resources. Documenting cost savings—that is, showing the total dollar amount that the school has saved taxpayers since its inception versus spending funds on juvenile corrections—is highly encouraged. The strategy is to prove and continuously restate not how much the program costs but how much it saves.

Successful alternative-school administrators realize that the act of justifying resources goes far beyond crunching numbers and making boring fiscal presentations. These administrators astutely realize that this can be an exciting endeavor and actually make selling the school fun! Inviting key stakeholders, including parents, members of local businesses, and the advisory board, to school functions can become the most effective way to demonstrate the school's utility and consequently remind stakeholders of the vital role that the school performs for the community. Inviting stakeholders to school field trips, student presentations, and graduation ceremonies is essential and is far more productive than only having the stakeholders, especially parents, show up at the school when problems arise. One innovative alternative-school administrator hosts an annual cookout at which students prepare and serve food to the school's key stakeholders. The phrase "if you build it they will come" does not apply to alternative schools. Thus, if the school is to survive, staff and students must actively encourage visitation and involvement from the community and its members.

Deliver Key Services. Service delivery is critical. The school's primary and most salient service is providing education to those at-risk students who do not perform adequately in the traditional classroom setting or public school environment. Three dimensions of service delivery that alternative-school educators should address include the following: stability, accessibility, and quality. Tips for maintaining a stable alternative school learning environment include minimizing student "downtime" and maintaining a structured environment in which the students have little free time that can invite misbehavior. Stability can also be attained, and maintained, by addressing problem behaviors immediately and/or before the teaching process begins and by enforcing school policy firmly, fairly, and uniformly. One alternative-school administrator insightfully noted the importance of maintaining clean and working school facilities and amenities. If a window is broken or unsightly trash is visible, it is promptly repaired or removed, thus minimizing the potential for more of the same that could quickly lead to instability and even chaos.

Maintaining an accessible or visible school presence can be attained through many of the previously discussed strategies for justifying the school and its resources. Alternative schools should have an open-door policy and work closely with the media to showcase their school and its service delivery. The media is surprisingly cooperative and favorable in its coverage if approached well ahead of a controversial piece of news. Implementing the previously suggested strategies regarding site selection and student admissions can also ensure a greater degree of visibility, and consequently, accessibility to the alternative school.

Maintaining quality may be the most difficult, but also the most important, aspect of service delivery. Alternative-school administrators may vary in terms of how they work to achieve quality education for their students, with some preferring total quality management (TQM), which utilizes a team approach to constantly monitor program processes to maintain them within acceptable standards of efficiency. This focus on process efficiency augments overall program effectiveness. Other administrators may favor management by objectives (MBO) which focuses time, money, and other resources on mutually agreed upon goals and objectives that are designed to enhance program efficiency and achieve real results. It is certainly not our intent to recommend how alternative-school administrators should manage their respective schools; however, several excellent suggestions were noted during our research and site visits to alternative schools. Revisiting the school's evaluation plan and employing school improvement teams appear to be effective strategies for maintaining an ongoing level of quality service delivery. Alternative-school administrators are encouraged to stay abreast of the most effective school management techniques and be willing to modify their behaviors and beliefs (i.e., be flexible and open to change). It is argued that the quality of the school is directly correlated with the quality of the staff. Thus, staff recruitment, retention, and professional development should be continually emphasized.

Communication Within the Alternative School

Effective and, perhaps more important, timely communication should be encouraged and constantly maintained within the alternative-school environment. This is vital and extremely important given the types of children who are attending the school. One effective practice that we discovered was simply scheduling weekly group discussion sessions or a school town hall meeting in which staff and students address any problems or concerns they may have. It is also effective for staff to meet separately and at least weekly to discuss student progress and to inform each other about what is going on with the students, especially regarding any problems students may be having academically, personally, or behaviorally. It was also suggested that staff-parent communications be frequent, timely, and mandatory and go beyond the ordinary parent-teacher conference. Given that many of the school's students come from dysfunctional households, staff-parent communication is most important yet may be difficult to achieve when facing complacent or reticent parents. Home visits appear to be effective for breaking down parental resistance and maintaining parental interest and involvement in the child's life and education.

What makes communications work within an agency and what factors are associated with effective and efficient communications? Watson Wyatt Worldwide (1999) surveyed various personnel from 913 organizations that were involved in a variety of different service industries.

The study identified ten highly effective communication attributes that exist in exemplary organizations. Among the most salient findings the researchers found were that successful communications are highly dependent on the extent to which senior management recognizes the importance of effective communications, consistently sells this to all employees, and relates communication initiatives to the organization's mission, goals, and business strategies. Successful alternative-school administrators are constantly interpreting and relating their vision for the school. A written and well-defined communications strategy or plan is imperative and at a minimum should include information on how the agency is performing and feedback mechanisms and take a proactive approach to resolving communication problems.

Finally, successful communications should be rewarded with continual emphasis placed on motivating and encouraging all employees to follow the communications plan that will ultimately improve job performance. Watson Wyatt Worldwide (1999) concludes that the single most important factor for successful organizational communications is the integration of communications into the agency's particular business strategy or mission by and with senior management. Remember, effective alternative-school administrators spend a large portion of their day in the halls and classrooms talking with other staff and students. They sell the school and promote positive communications by example and not by dictate or mandate.

Other Salient Operational Issues

Standard Operating Plans. In addition to the various plans discussed previously, it is advisable to have a safe school plan that outlines daily security measures and provides contingency scenarios for potential school crises such as a shooting or natural disaster. It is inevitable that there will be a crisis; be ready for it. If not included in the school's policy and procedures manual, it is recommended that a personnel selection and retention plan be developed. A school improvement plan is also recommended that will guide the work of the school improvement team. Technology plans and a student/parent handbook are also used by successful alternative schools.

Operational Factors. When asked, "What operational factors produce a successful and effective alternative school?" the following items or components were mentioned:

- Having a full complement of motivated and competent teachers who care;
- Having a strong group and individual counseling component;

- Emphasizing instruction through technology;
- Hiring and keeping a school resource officer who truly likes children, especially at-risk young men and women;
- Hiring the best principal available;
- Have an outside adult mentor for each student;
- Having active parental and community involvement;
- Maintaining low staff-to-student ratios;
- Making sure all students have a voice in school affairs; and
- Establishing stable and permanent funding.

There are many measures of success at this stage: a full and qualified staff, a well informed and involved board and community, well-oiled daily operations, and services that change young lives. The tendency is to focus on these worthy purposes at the expense of stability (i.e., the funding stream). We are not saying neglect services; we do say conduct business and even define business in light of the campaign for justification. It is easy to put the genuinely Herculean task of getting through the day first; that is a mistake. The quest for support must be part of the fiber of getting through the day. It is too late and tragic to the program to have to backtrack to demonstrate, in facts and figures, when the questions are asked. At that time it matters not how good the day goes and how many young lives are improves because the school may cease to exist.

There is also another important purpose to being stable and delivering a good service to a defined population of need. These are the foundations for what all public services should be in a position to do: Grow to meet real need. This is when a communitywide, demonstrable difference is made.

EXPANDING THE ALTERNATIVE SCHOOL: CLOSE THE SERVICE-TO-NEEDS GAP

The final section of this chapter addresses the issue of expanding alternative learning programs to close, or at least bridge, the gap between service provision and the need for more alternative educational programs for at-risk youth who are not currently being served in these programs. All previous work prepares a municipality for expansion. In fact, it should be a stated purpose from the outset.

Conduct a Readiness Assessment

Decide to Expand. When discussing the expansion of the number of alternative schools, the types of services provided, and/or the types of students who receive these services it is important to first ask the following: "Do we need to expand?" If the answer is in the affirmative, then logically the next question to ask is the following: "Are we ready to expand?" This question can be answered by conducting a readiness assessment that should involve reanalyzing much of the data previously collected in the needs assessment and ongoing process evaluation. Key stakeholders should be involved in this readiness assessment, including existing alternative-school staff, the school's advisory board, members of the central school district, affected feeder public schools, and community representatives. Zingheim and Schuster (1995) cogently note that a readiness assessment gauges where a program is now and where it needs to go in the future. The readiness assessment provides a justification and foundation for positive growth and future change. During the expansion phase it is not necessary, or productive, to reinvent the proverbial wheel. Much of the work for expanding service delivery can piggy back on the work that was conducted during the planning phase and use many of the same processes, data collection strategies, and program plans on record.

The Retreat. If feasible, an expansion planning retreat should be held and should involve the major stakeholders and members of the alternative school and its advisory board. The emphasis should be on reviewing the work of the school improvement team and its plan as well as assessing relevant information from the school's process and impact evaluation. If the expansion goal is to open another separate facility, much of the work done for the initial alternative school can be replicated. If the expansion goal is to provide a new service and/or educate a different type of student than those the school is currently serving, more work will be involved. Experts from the educational, mental health, and criminal justice systems should be consulted and included in this type of expansion. It is also most worthwhile to have the retreat professionally facilitated, preferably by the strategist who helped initially; choose carefully.

Update Existing Documents

One often overlooked practice that occurs after an alternative school has been in existence, and expansion is anticipated, is updating the school's current documentation, vital plans, and related mission and vision statements as well as goals and objectives. All these items should be reviewed periodically, whether or not expansion is planned for, but certainly must be updated to reflect any new expansion initiatives. It is significant that several leading alternative-school principals speak of their vision, mission, beliefs, and goals as "living" things. They really work on being the vision. New facilities, different students, and new course offerings necessitate new or additional policies and procedures, operating practices, admission requirements, and a more focused mission statement. Remember, expanding service delivery also requires expanding the role of the alternative school and consequently its guiding documents.

Determine the Service-to-Needs Gap

During the expansion planning stage the original needs-assessment study should be updated and revisited. Attention should be directed toward trends and data projections. A notable effective practice here involves using feeder school review boards that periodically assess their students for potential academic failure and/or behavioral problems that may be manifested later. Feeder school administrators and teachers know their children with difficulties and should be encouraged to report information to the alternative school on both the number of at-risk children and the varying types of problem behaviors. Providing alternative school administrators with this information will enable them to have an accurate account of how many students might be heading in their direction within the next month or year. Combine these numbers with a cost-effectiveness computation for a strong statement of need for growth. A "canned" electronic presentation should always be ready. A simple update to answer the question of the moment and you are ready for just about any audience.

Other relevant data and their projected numbers should be examined and at least include information on the following:

- Projected student enrollments;
- Suspension and expulsion data;
- Feeder school disciplinary records;
- Dropout rates;
- School crime data;
- Juvenile delinquency petition orders filed in the juvenile courts; and
- End-of-year and end-of-grade test results.

Analyzing these data and projected trends will enable alternative-school personnel to visually see the service-to-needs gap and expand accordingly. It is also recommended that at least one focus group be held for the purpose of assessing this gap and for determining the appropriate expansion response. All stakeholders and the wider community should be included. One disregarded but loud voice can be particularly nettlesome.

Keys for Successful Expansion

Numerous critical issues must be addressed and certain situations must be present to ensure a greater degree of future success and to guarantee that expanding the alternative school and/or its services will not fail. The most obvious, and yet sometimes ignored, key to expansion is that there must be a need to expand. Expanding without studying the service-to-needs gap can be deleterious and also counterproductive to the current school's existence. Expansion should not be considered until the alternative school is operating efficiently and effectively and has an acceptable and firm record of success. Again, success is real improvement in the lives of the youngsters in the classrooms. Other keys to successfully expanding the concept of alternative education as suggested by current alternative school administrators and teachers should consider the following:

- Strong and current data on which to base decisions;
- Support from the central school district and feeder schools;
- Buy-in and support from all alternative school staff;
- Securing permanent funding for the existing program;
- Knowing exactly where you are and exactly where you want to be; and
- Expanding judiciously, incrementally, and only as each additional program or site is firmly successful.

ALTERNATIVE SCHOOL IS ONLY PART OF THE SOLUTION

Planning for and establishing an alternative school is formidable. It is a task that offers as many challenges as rewards for educators, students, parents, and community members. Paglin and Fagler (1997) delineate some of these challenges which include the inappropriate placement of students into the alternative school with the alternative school being erroneously perceived as an all purpose solution for dealing with all troubled children irrespective of the types of problems they have. The lack of stable funding is perhaps the greatest challenge for the continued existence of an alternative school. Insufficient funds and resources force administrators to prioritize, and in many cases eliminate, some school materials, supplies, and other needed services thus compromising quality service delivery. The loss of a charismatic leader or talented staff member as well as political and economic changes or crises can also affect the alternative school and its successful existence (Paglin and Fager, 1997). Offsetting these challenges and obstacles to success is the school's ability to effectively "save" at least some of the community's children that the authors argue is most rewarding to everyone.

Zero tolerance legislation that permits feeder schools to suspend or terminally expel children who engage in drug activity or possess weapons will force school administrators and central district officials to face the harsh reality of what to do with these children. As your programs expand and grow their nature and content will also need to become more flexible and adaptive with more specific and focused programs being developed and implemented which address unique adolescent problem behaviors. Problem specific alternative schools, such as those which serve only children with behavioral disorders or only children with criminal histories, will bridge the service to needs gap and further the much needed goal of offering a full continuum of care for at-risk children.

The education, supervision, and management of troubled teens pose both challenges and extra demands beyond those associated with the traditional public school environment and its standardized methods of classroom instruction. The preceding chapters on planning, operating, and expanding an alternative learning program can be viewed as a guide for both educational administrators and teachers who have chosen to devote their careers to working with at-risk youth within the public educational system. Successful programs are there to guide any attempt at beginning alternative programming. We have attempted to compile effective practices in a generalized manner, which, when combined with local expertise, dedication, and determination, can be replicated to implement new programs or incorporated into exising ones. Readers are encouraged and challenged to think outside of the proverbial "box" and adopt those strategies and practices which are best suited for their respective programs and students, with the ultimate goal of removing the "troubled" and "at-risk" labels and replacing them with more prosocial descriptors such as "graduates," "college-bound," and "promising young leaders of tomorrow."

References

Duke, D. J., & Griesdorn, J. (1999). Considerations in the design of alternative schools. *EBSCO Clearing House, 73,* 89.

Fink, A. (1995). *The survey kit.* Thousand Oaks: CA. Sage.

Hawes, J., Dillard, L., Brewer, D., Cobb, C., & Neenan, P. (2000). *Case studies of best practices: Alternative schools and programs: 1998–99.* Raleigh, NC: North Carolina Department of Public Instruction.

Hudzik, J. K., & Cordner, G. W. (1983). *Planning in criminal justice organizations and systems.* New York: Macmillan.

Kellmayer, J. (1998). Building educational alternative for at-risk youth: A primer. *The High School Magazine, 6,* 26–31.

Miller, D. C. (1991). *Handbook of research design and social measurement* (5th ed.). Newbury Park, CA: Sage.

North Carolina Department of Public Instruction. (2001). *Clarification of guidelines for alternative learning programs and schools.* Raleigh, NC: Division of School Improvement.

Raywid, M. (1999). History and issues of alternative schools. *Education Digest, 64,* 47–51.

Stringer, E. T. (1996). *Action research: A handbook for practitioners.* Thousand Oaks: CA. Sage.

U.S. General Accounting Office. (1993). *Developing and using questionnaires.* Washington, DC: Program Evaluation and Methodology Division.

Vasu, M. L., & Klopovic, J. (2000). *Promising and effective practices in juvenile day treatment.* Raleigh, NC: Governor's Crime Commission.

Watson Wyatt Worldwide. (1999). *1999 communications study: Linking communications with strategy to achieve business goals.* Washington, DC: International Association of Business Communicators.

Weisburg, H. F., Krosnick, J. A., & Bowen, B. D. (1996). *An introduction to survey research, polling and data aAnalysis* (3rd ed.). Thousand Oaks, CA: Sage.

Welsh, W. N., & Harris, P. W. (1999). *Criminal justice policy and planning.* Cincinnati, OH: Anderson.

Zingheim, P. K., & Schuster, J. R. (1995). Exploring three pay transition tools: Readiness Assessment, benchmarking, and piloting. *Compensation and Benefits Review*, *27*, 40–45.

Part V

Promising and Effective Practices in Juvenile Day Treatment

by James R. Brunet, Ph.D., Michael L. Vasu, Ph.D., Meredith B. Weinstein, Ph.D., and James Klopovic, M.A., M.P.A.

Part V is organized to give maximum benefit to policymakers and administrators who are exploring alternative programming for at-risk youth. The chapters are presented in a sequence that follows a program from the earliest planning and design stages through implementation and performance monitoring (see Albert, Faro, & Lawson, 1998; McGarry & Carter, 1993). It is not our intention to provide detailed instructions on the day-to-day operations of a juvenile day treatment program (see, e.g., the accreditation standards in American Correctional Association, 1993). Instead, we highlight key questions that should be considered at various stages in a program's development and the responses that other programs have taken to address these issues.

At each point in the program's progression, we offer a series of promising and effective practices. For ease of use, we briefly describe each effective practice and provide support from the research literature. We offer specific examples from three North Carolina pilot sites and exemplary programs in other states and then further explain the effective practice. This format provides the reader with support for the effective practice based both on the research literature and the actual experiences of others.

Juvenile day treatment is distinguished from a juvenile day reporting program for a reason. Day treatment is one of the main factors that distinguishes a day program for older youth from those programs that are commonly referred to as alternative learning programs. Treatment is the key. Treatment is part of a larger offering of services for youth as they are prepared for independence as young adults. There is a clear-cut reason for the focus on treatment as there are distinct populations of young people who need specific help beyond what is offered via traditional classroom curricula and extracurricular activities. Chapter 15 discusses these distinctions and makes the case for having an array of treatments available for children who need them. Juvenile day treatment, then, is one of the services that need to be offered in a comprehensive spectrum of services for children who may have difficulty in the regular classroom.

Juvenile day treatment is offered in the context of the juvenile day reporting program.

Chapter 16 begins the process of thinking about how to offer juvenile day treatment. In keeping with the concept of the "life cycle" it considers key activities necessary to plan thoroughly. Naturally, the focus is on building the vital business foundation under the contemplated services. It will be some necessary time before the community is in a position to have even the first student in a day treatment program. Under planning, then, Chapter 16 considers such topics as appropriate leadership, consensus building, data analysis, and identifying service gaps. As the effort progresses, development considers vision and mission, targeting service populations, building public support, and the all important topic of money. Even before a single treatment service is offered there must be designs for administration, management, the facility, staffing, and logistics. The point is that the success of this or any service offering is determined by the thought put into it. But appropriate thought must lead to determined action.

Planning has to end in operational action or there is no progress. As with planning, implementing and expanding juvenile day treatment involves specific activities. Chapter 17 discusses how day treatment integrates into the existing environment via collaboration with other service entities. When there are students actually in the program, treatment should be rooted in proven methods and be delivered after comprehensive assessment; there should be continuous case management, and specific needs of community youth should be met. Furthermore, Chapter 17 makes the point that program monitoring and evaluation be part of the fabric of every day operation.

In essence, Part V completes the discussion of programs that exemplify a continuum of developmentally appropriate services for our youth from prenatal to young adulthood. We make the point again that the choice of programs is locally determined. But those programs must be built on a solid business foundation, be performance oriented, answer a specific, assessed need for a specific population of children, and be built with the view to expanding to an assessed need in the local community. Another point that needs reiteration is that it is futile to begin any one of these programs without proper preparation, preparation that aims to make a permanent presence of the service. It is slow and meticulous and worthwhile work, the results of which are easy to see in the smiles of successful children, children who otherwise may not succeed. No one program is *the* answer, but in concert many programs begin to make a difference. Over time their collective effect is incalculable.

References

Albert, L. H., Faro, F. C., & Lawson, R. H. (1998). *Critical elements in the planning, development, and implementation of successful correctional options.* Washington, DC: U.S. Department of Justice.

American Correctional Association. (1993). *Standards for juvenile day treatment programs.* Lanham, MD: Author.

McGarry, P., & Carter, M. M. (Eds.). (1993). *The intermediate sanctions handbook: Experiences and tools for policymakers.* Washington, DC: U.S. Department of Justice.

Chapter 15

Considerations for Developing Juvenile Day Treatment Programs

WHAT IS JUVENILE DAY TREATMENT?

Defining the Concept

Juvenile day treatment has emerged as a popular community-based alternative for court-involved youth. Since the early 1970s, the universe of day treatment programs has expanded from a handful of initiatives in Colorado, Florida, and Kentucky to dozens of centers located throughout the country.[1] For purposes of this chapter, day treatment is defined *as a community-based program that includes intensive supervision, sanctions, and treatment of a juvenile offender in a nonresidential setting.* Juveniles assigned to day treatment (often as a condition of probation) report to a specific location on a daily basis, remain at the center for the duration of the day, and return home at night. While at the center, juveniles receive a variety of treatment and educational services, as well as intensive supervision and sanctions for inappropriate behavior.

Usual services include individual and group counseling, drug assessment and treatment, life skills training, academic coursework, and supervised recreation. Typically, a juvenile participates in a juvenile day treatment program for six months; however, some programs vary this period from forty-five days to nine months. The intervention begins with an assessment of needs and risks and development of an individualized treatment plan. Services are delivered on-site by center staff or contracted providers. Case managers continuously monitor the juvenile's progress toward meeting the objectives set out in the treatment plan.

Program Goals

What do these programs seek to accomplish? The primary goal of day treatment is to reintegrate rehabilitated juveniles into their schools and communities. Some jurisdictions also see a fiscal benefit from the use of juvenile day treatment programs. For example, in Alabama, the Community Intensive Treatment for Youth (CITY) program is viewed as a cost-effective alternative to secure custody that reduces crime and the demand on institutional bed space (Earnest, 1996). Similarly, Kentucky's extensive system of juvenile day treatment facilities has been credited with allowing the state to maintain one of the nation's lowest per capita number of secure juvenile residential beds (Wolford, Jordan, & Murphy, 1997).

Key Characteristics

Perhaps the most distinguishing feature of juvenile day treatment is the variety of approaches taken to implement the concept. Some programs emphasize the vocational needs of older juveniles; others focus on the educational needs of preteens. Some programs are functionally part of a county or city government; others are run by private (non- and for-profit) organizations. Underlying this diversity, however, are four crosscutting characteristics shared by all day treatment programs.

Juvenile day treatment programs function as *intermediate sanctions*. They are less severe than incarceration but more restrictive than regular probation (Morris & Tonry, 1990). Day treatment is commonly used as a "front-end" diversion from detention. Judges order juveniles to attend day treatment as an alternative to incarceration. In other communities, day treatment serves as a "back-end" or aftercare program for juveniles who are leaving secured facilities (see Tonry, 1997, pp. 2–3). The overarching goal in both cases (diversion and aftercare) is to keep individuals in the community in order to conserve institutional resources for higher-risk juveniles.

Juvenile day treatment programs blend intensive treatment services with close surveillance of the juvenile over an extended period. The key here is the *balance* between rehabilitative programming and supervision. The balance is achieved through the use of rigorous reporting requirements (up to six days a week over six months) and low staff-to-student ratios that reinforce positive behavioral changes in a closely monitored setting.

Most programs target *high-risk juvenile offenders* for service provision.

The term "offender" signifies that most juveniles have been involved with the court system in some manner. Some day treatment programs do take client referrals directly from the local school district (e.g., children in long-term suspension). However, court-adjudicated youth comprise the greatest number of program participants.

Day treatment is a strategy for keeping the juvenile in the community, or, more specifically, in the home. Juveniles go to the center during the day but return home in the evening. The most comprehensive programs offer family counseling as a part of the overall treatment approach. Day treatment programs are *nonresidential*.

In summary, juvenile day treatment is distinguished by its status as an intermediate sanction, balance between treatment and control, focus on court-adjudicated youth, and extension of services into the juvenile's home environment.

Day Treatment Process

Another way to describe juvenile day treatment is to follow a client from the time the juvenile enters the program through program exit. Figure 15.1 offers a graphical representation of this process.[2] The process begins with the juvenile appearing before a family court judge as a result of delinquent behavior. The judge orders the juvenile to probation with a juvenile court counselor. A requirement of the juvenile's probation is participation in juvenile day treatment. The juvenile court counselor meets with the day treatment center staff to ascertain the juvenile's status and success in meeting set goals. The court counselor is available to the day treatment staff for any necessary sanctions.

As a participant at the juvenile day treatment program, the juvenile takes part in an array of services and programs. Center staff monitor participant progress and broker services with outside providers (the case management function). A juvenile may exit the program in one of three ways: successful completion, negative termination, or neutral termination. A successful completion is one in which the juvenile has met the program requirements and his or her individual goals and is deemed to be ready to return to home school and community. The juvenile remains under the supervision of the juvenile court counselor until the term of probation expires. A negative termination is one whereby the juvenile is unable to meet the set goals or has committed continuous and serious violations of program rules. When a juvenile is negatively terminated, a return to court for a more restrictive sanction such as placement in juvenile detention or wilderness camp occurs. The third potential outcome is a neutral program exit. There are numerous reasons outside the juvenile's positive or negative behavior at the center that can lead to the juvenile's premature exit from the program. The juvenile's family may relocate to another jurisdiction or the juvenile may be ordered to a residential program as other prior charges are adjudicated. Figure 15.1 demonstrates the placement of juvenile day treatment in the larger juvenile justice system.

Figure 15.1
Juvenile Day Treatment Model

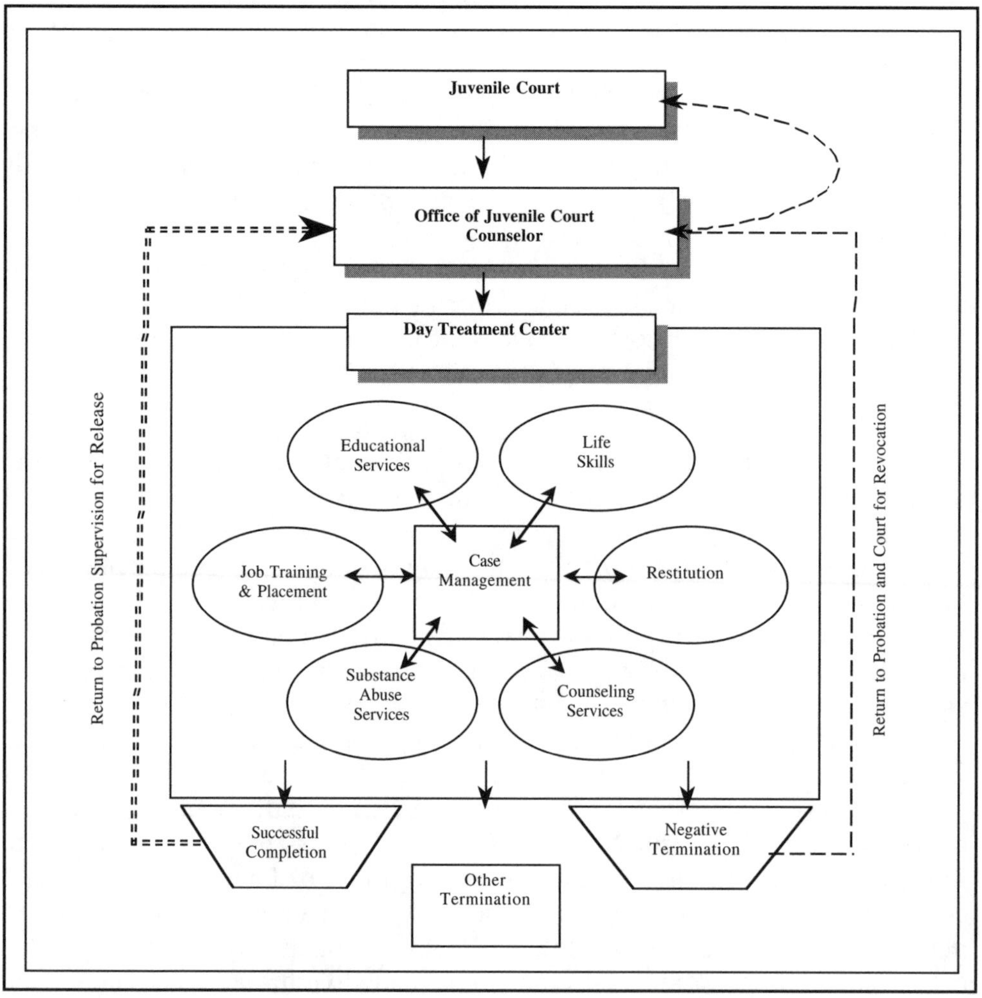

WHAT DOES THE RESEARCH LITERATURE SAY ABOUT JUVENILE DAY TREATMENT?

After almost three decades of experience with juvenile day treatment centers in the United States, there is a surprising lack of published research on this subject. Much of the available information pertains to the operation, replication, and evaluation of the Project New Pride program in Denver, Colorado. Although Project New Pride was not called "day treatment" when it was first created in the early 1970s, its original programmatic approach is strikingly similar to today's day treatment programs. Contemporary programs retain key elements of the New Pride model, including the population targeted for service (inner-city teens with criminal histories) and complement of services (education, counseling, employment, and cultural awareness). Interest in juvenile day treatment reached an apex in the late-1970s with the expansion of Project New Pride to ten test cities. By the mid-1980s, enthusiasm for the concept waned in response to two factors: (1) the end of federal funding for such programs and (2) evaluations that painted conflicting pictures of the intervention's effectiveness (see Blew, McGillis, & Bryant, 1977; Gruenewald, Laurence, & West, 1985). While Project New Pride (now called Fresh Start) still exists today, it appears that many of the replicated sites have since closed their doors.

The more contemporary research literature does contain several references to day treatment. The National Council on Crime and Delinquency's (NCCD) database of promising juvenile treatment and prevention programs is one of the few sources of descriptive information about day treatment programs. Using the NCCD data, Howell (1998) identified several day treatment programs that appear to reduce the likelihood of recidivism among program participants. While informative, no organized effort is made to compare and contrast day treatment programs on key philosophical and operational variables. What is missing from the analysis is an examination of common practices that distinguish truly effective programs from the rest of the field. In addition, the "snapshot" program description used in the NCCD database trades historical context (and the important lessons that may be learned from its study) for brevity. As such, little is known about the recent development and implementation of juvenile day treatment programs.

In addition, not much is known about the effectiveness of day treatment. The most rigorous impact study was conducted on the ten sites replicating the New Pride program. The study concluded that the "preponderance of the evidence indicated no differences between comparison and treatment group recidivism rates overall" (Gruenewald et al., 1985, p. 8-1). In contrast to expectations, participation in the New Pride program did not result in a significant decrease in rates of adjudication and commitment to correctional institutions. A recent compilation of effective criminal justice programs recognized the "potential promise" for juvenile day reporting programs but noted the lack of studies that show the effectiveness of these programs (Sherman et al., 1997). Several studies using less robust research designs (i.e., nonexperimental designs with no control groups) cast day treatment in a more positive light. A preliminary study of a day treatment program in Bethesda, Pennsylvania revealed a recidivism rate of only 5 percent in the first year after discharge. Although this is an impressive finding, the study author warns that the result "must be viewed with extreme caution because the sample size was very small ($n = 20$), and the study did not incorporate a control group" (Howell, 1998, p. 145). Likewise, the recidivism rate for persons leaving day treatment services in Kentucky was 25 percent (Bowling & Hobbs, 1990).

In short, the scholarly literature offers little in the way of process or outcome information about juvenile day treatment. This is due to several possible reasons including too few programs with established performance records, problems in defining what a day treatment center is, and difficulties in creating equivalent control groups for comparison.

WHY STUDY THE IMPLEMENTATION OF DAY TREATMENT PROGRAMS?

The primary goal of this investigation is to identify "promising and effective practices" that will guide the future development of juvenile day treatment facilities. Part V of this book summarizes important "lessons learned" from both new and more established programs. It is meant to provide practical guidance to those who are actively considering the creation of juvenile day treatment programs in their communities. Some communities will find, after moving through the earliest stages of program planning, that day treatment matches identified public safety and programming needs. Others will uncover gaps in their existing service delivery system that are more appropriately addressed by interventions other than juvenile day treatment. This document seeks to assist community leaders as they make these important resource allocation decisions.

This research was undertaken with three goals in mind:

- To outline an emerging sequence of promising and effective practices in juvenile day treatment;
- To assess the implementation of pilot sites in North Carolina; and
- To identify baseline measures of program effectiveness that will become the foundation for the future study of program impact.

The intended audience for this chapter includes judges, law enforcement officials, court personnel, criminal justice planners, city and county administrators, and citizens responsible for developing, implementing, and operating juvenile day treatment programs. This chapter is designed to assist decision makers in the preplanning stage by outlining the issues involved in establishing a juvenile day treatment program in a community.

HOW INFORMATION WAS COLLECTED FOR THIS STUDY

Our research design encompasses several different strategies including implementation evaluation, developmental evaluation, and effective practice identification. We define each of these approaches subsequently.

Implementation evaluation is a common technique for studying new programs. It compares planned program components against those that are actually implemented. Implementation studies often focus on the characteristics and quality of services delivered. We also include elements of what Patton (1997) has termed "developmental evaluation." The evaluation process in developmental studies involves the active participation of those who are being evaluated. For example, program staff and evaluators may jointly formulate operational definitions and collect data. What is unique about developmental evaluation is its purpose: to facilitate ongoing improvements in the program under study.

As a final component in our research design, we identify program components that are associated with certain desired outcomes. This tactic, often called "effective" or "best" practices, is a derivative concept of benchmarking. Like benchmarks, effective practices provide a useful performance metric for interagency or intersector comparison. Peters and Waterman (1982) conducted detailed case studies of "high performing" companies, and identified characteristics that distinguished them from less successful ventures. In similar fashion, the effective practices in this study were developed by observing the operations of exemplary programs throughout the United States and by reviewing studies that describe successful juvenile treatment programs.

The research team used multiple methods to collect information for this study. The five data collection strategies are described in detail next.

- *Literature review.* A detailed review of the existing research was undertaken. The literature review focused on three subject areas—community-based juvenile delinquency programs, juvenile crime and delinquency, and program implementation. The review played a prominent role in our identification of exemplary programs.
- *Direct observation.* The research team visited five juvenile day treatment centers outside North Carolina. We toured the facilities, witnessed the delivery of educational and other treatment interventions, and attended staff meetings. In addition, the research team visited the three North Carolina pilot sites on numerous occasions to view the operation and management during the first year of program startup.
- *Documentation review.* Researchers reviewed a variety of program documents including funding requests, policy and procedures manuals, performance data, job descriptions, annual reports, student handbooks, educational and treatment materials, risk and needs assessment instruments, and court records.
- *Structured and semistructured interviews.* Researchers conducted structured and semistructured interviews with program directors, staff members, and stakeholders. Most interviews were conducted on site at the day treatment centers. In several cases, telephone interviews were used to accommodate the schedules of key policymakers and to make contacts

with established programs in other parts of the country. Instruments used open-ended questions to capture the complexities of program design and implementation. Seventeen interviews were conducted with day treatment managers and staff in four states (Alabama, Colorado, Kentucky, and Pennsylvania). Research staff also interviewed day treatment staff members and key stakeholders at the North Carolina pilot sites (more than twenty individuals).

- *Focus groups.* Two separate focus groups were conducted at each North Carolina site. The first focus group included persons who make decisions affecting the local juvenile justice system. These "stakeholder" groups typically included judges, chief juvenile court counselors, law enforcement officials, representatives from the business community, county administrators, and school district officials. The second focus group consisted of program staff and service providers. These focus groups were designed to gain a general understanding of the planning and implementation processes as well as to identify individuals for subsequent interviews. The focus groups were important in providing the researchers with specific examples of promising practices and consistent problems involved in establishing a juvenile day treatment center. A number of important findings emerged from the collective knowledge of the participants in the focus groups.

PROGRAMS THAT CONTRIBUTED TO THE STUDY

This study reports on the early experiences of three pilot day treatment programs in North Carolina. One program is located in Wilmington (New Hanover County), a midsize city along the state's southeast coast. The other two programs are located in the Research Triangle region of central North Carolina in the cities of Raleigh (Wake County) and Durham (Durham County). Though these programs are alike in many ways, they display unique qualities that distinguish them from their sister sites. We identify important similarities and differences in the programs as a way to briefly introduce these initial efforts. More detailed descriptions are provided throughout Part V.

Early Stage North Carolina Programs

The North Carolina day treatment centers share several common characteristics. First, all three programs received startup funding from the same granting agent—the Governor's Crime Commission. The Crime Commission typically provides "seed money" to help new programs get started. This funding stream is time-limited (one to two years) after which program administrators must secure alternative sources of operating funds. Second, each center is located in an urban setting. Larger cities are more likely to have a critical mass of juveniles who will benefit from day treatment, as well as the existing infrastructure (i.e., transportation and treatment services) necessary to carry out the program. Third, all three programs began accepting clients at approximately the same time. Wilmington was the first to open its doors in December 1997, followed closely by Raleigh (March 1998) and Durham (July 1998). Fourth, each county had prior experience in developing and implementing community-based correctional programs for adults. Advisory boards consisting of key members of the local criminal justice system carried out much of the work that led to the establishment of these adult programs. These boards were already in place in the counties that wished to start juvenile day treatment programs. As such, there was a level of cooperation in these counties and familiarity with intermediate sanctions that cannot be presupposed in other locales.

The North Carolina programs vary in several important respects. First, a different type of organization runs each juvenile day treatment program. A local nonprofit agency with experience operating intermediate adult programs oversees the program in Raleigh. A national nonprofit organization that specializes in youth recreation and mentoring services houses the day treatment program in Wilmington. The Durham program is run by the county agency that is also responsible for the adult day reporting center. Second, each county took a different approach to finding a physical location for the program. Some invested heavily in refurbishing facilities while others used existing structures with little modification. Third, the mix of services available varies from program to program. In Wilmington, education is the primary on-site activity while Durham stresses a balance of behavioral and educational programming. Fourth, the programs target different juvenile groups for service provision (age range) and receive clients from different sources (court referred, school referred).

Establishing Programs

The research team also learned about juvenile day treatment through site visits and consultations with exemplary programs in other parts of the United States. Researchers visited five day treatment centers operated by three providers (CITY Program in Birmingham and Tuscaloosa, Alabama; Bethesda Program in East Milton and Williamsport, Pennsylvania; and, Cornell Abraxas in Harrisburg, Pennsylvania). These programs were selected because of their national reputations for delivering quality services and their different approaches to day treatment.

Alabama's CITY program is a sanction that is available to juveniles in eight urban and rural counties. In a unique arrangement between the CITY program and local school districts, certified schoolteachers provide instructional services to clients at each program site. Bethesda day treatment centers provide school day and after-school programs for court-involved youth in several states. What distinguishes Bethesda from the other approaches is its use of intensive individual and family counseling to reduce delinquent behavior.

Before its recent merger with the for-profit Cornell Corrections, Abraxas had a long history of running various types of residential and nonresidential programs for juveniles. The day treatment center in Harrisburg is a relatively new venture for the company (began operations in 1995).

In addition, program directors and senior staff members at three other facilities in Lexington (Kentucky), Denver (Colorado), and western Pennsylvania (Adelphoi Village) were consulted. Most of these programs have been in existence for well over ten years.

Readers are encouraged to consult Exhibit 15.1 for a detailed comparison of day treatment centers on several different program variables (e.g., hours of operation, target population, staffing, facilities).

JUVENILE TREATMENT IS A SPECIFIC SERVICE IN A RANGE OF SERVICES

The "treatment" in juvenile day treatment programs, at the local level of government, is what distinguishes this service from other institutional choices for the juvenile. It is an alternative to court action and it is a choice when perhaps alternative schooling is inappropriate. The community is better equipped to handle the diverse, sometimes extreme needs of its youth when actual treatment is offered. Treatment in this case is an accepted psychological therapy. It is not mere counseling. It is therapy that addresses a certain diagnosed psychological need. Otherwise, the program or service has the trappings of addressing needs when it is not actually doing so. Most programs offer orientation, education, and counseling; the pitfall is to mistake these services for therapeutic treatment. Thus, juvenile day treatment is offered in the day reporting setting, for example, as part of a package of services. Furthermore, the juvenile day reporting program is not complete without a treatment component.

This is a necessary distinction to make from the very beginning of program planning. To do otherwise is to miss the opportunity to serve a population of youth. Again, it is with negative consequences to the community. Yes, the obvious consequence is the progressive failure of the child in the home, in the community, in the school, and then, possibly the most dramatic failure, emergence as a criminal. The less dramatic, but more dire, result is the greater number of youngsters who become failures as adults and then meander through life on the fringes of society. We don't "see" them because they don't offend with a crime or commit some other affront to society. They could have done better but they didn't. They have marginal lives, whether it is as inadequate parents of their own families, or in a subsistence-level job, or by being off and on the public services network for a lifetime. Treatment at the appropriate time may not be entirely effective for all who need it, but it is effective enough to make a difference in many lives that otherwise would be less than they could have been. The right touch at the right moment is life changing.

Footnotes

[1] There is no comprehensive listing of juvenile day treatment centers in the United States. An extensive search conducted by the National Council on Crime and Delinquency located juvenile day treatment programs in Pennsylvania, Alabama, Louisiana, Florida, New Jersey, Missouri, and Texas (see Howell, 1998). Within the last several years, other states have added juvenile day treatment programs including North Carolina, Oklahoma, Michigan, and Maryland.

[2] A model, by its very nature, is a simplification of reality. It is included here to provide a general description of a typical flow of juveniles into and through day treatment (see Brunet, 2002, for a similar description of adult day reporting centers). Distinctive features of individual programs are not captured in the generic model shown. Figure 15.1 also has the added benefit of showing the critical linkages between juvenile day treatment and other key actors in the larger juvenile justice system.

References

Blew, C. H., McGillis, D., & Bryant, G. (1977). *An exemplary project: Project New Pride.* Washington, DC: U.S. Department of Justice.

Bowling, L., & Hobbs, L. (1990). Day treatment services. In B. Wolford, C. J. Miller, & P. Lawrenz (Eds.), *Transitional services for troubled youth* (pp. 45–50). Richmond, KY: Department of Correctional Services, Eastern Kentucky University.

Brunet, J. R. (2002). Day reporting centers in North Carolina: Implementation lessons for policymakers. *Justice System Journal, 23*, 135–156.

Earnest, E. (1996, August). Youth day treatment program works for Alabama. *Corrections Today*, pp. 70–73, 140–141.

Gruenewald, P. J., Laurence, S. E., & West, B. R. (1985). *National evaluation of the New Pride replication program, Final report, Volume II: Client impact evaluation.* Walnut Creek, CA: Pacific Institute for Research and Evaluation.

Howell, J. C. (Ed.). (1998). *Guide for implementing the comprehensive strategy for serious, violent, and chronic juvenile offenders* (2nd printing). Washington, DC: U.S. Department of Justice.

Morris, N., & Tonry, M. (1990). *Between prison and probation: Intermediate punishments in a rational sentencing system.* New York: Oxford University Press.

Patton, M. Q. (1997). *Utilization-focused evaluation* (3rd ed.). Thousand Oaks, CA: Sage.

Peters, T. J., & Waterman, Jr., R. H. (1982). *In search of excellence: Lessons from America's best-run companies.* New York: Warner Books.

Sherman, L. W., Gottfredson, D., MacKenzie, D., Eck, J., Reuter, P., & Bushway, S. (1997). *Preventing crime: What works, what doesn't, what's promising*. Washington, DC: U.S. Department of Justice.

Tonry, M. (1997). *Intermediate sanctions in sentencing guidelines.* Washington, DC: U.S. Department of Justice.

Wolford, B. I., Jordan, F., & Murphy, K. (1997). Day treatment: Community-based partnerships for delinquent and at-risk youth. *Juvenile and Family Court Judges*, *48*, 35–42.

Exhibit 15.1
Comparison of Juvenile Day Treatment Programs

Program Characteristics	CITY Program (AL)	Bethesda (PA)	Cornell Abraxas (PA)	Wake County JDRC (NC)	New Hanover County (NC)	Durham Day Program (NC)
Operations						
1. Capacity	30	25–40	30	20–25	60	25
2. Hours of operation	M–F 8–4:30	M–F 8–8 Sat. 9–1:30	M–F 8–8 Sat. 8–8	M–F 8:30–4	M–F 9–3 Wed. 3–6	M–F 8:30–5
3. Services	• Individual counseling • Group counseling • Substance abuse referral to outside provider • Home visits (infrequent) • Education (3 subjects, self-paced) • Recreation • Food (1 meal)	• Individual counseling • Group counseling • Family counseling (home visits) • Victim restitution • Community service • Intensive outpatient drug and alcohol abuse counseling • Education (all subjects, self-paced) • Anger management • Recreation • Career and vocational counseling • Crisis intervention (24-hour beeper) • Food (1–3 meals) • Student transportation	• Individual counseling • Group counseling • Community service substance abuse referrals to outside vendor • Education (all subjects, traditional classroom) • Recreation • Food (2–3 meals) • Student transportation	• Individual and group counseling • Family counseling • Education (non-certified) • Recreation • Life skills training • Food (1 lunch) • Student transportation (bus fare, van pickup) • Mental health referrals	• Individual and group counseling • Family counseling • Education (New Hanover County schools) • Community college provides self-esteem, communication skills, and life skills training • Recreation • Food (1 lunch from adjoining school) • Transportation (2 vans)	• Group counseling • Substance abuse education and counseling • Education (GED provided by community college) • Rational behavior classes • Recreation • Job skills classes • Employment skills • Food (1 meal) • Transportation (bus fare) • Mental health referrals
4. Treatment philosophy	• Cognitive • Behavioral	• Cognitive • Behavioral • Affective/emotional	• Cognitive • Behavioral	• Cognitive • Behavioral aspects	• No clear treatment approach—aspects of cognitive-behavioral	• Cognitive • Behavioral aspects
5. Program start	1981	1983	1995	1998 (March)	1997 (December)	1998 (July)

Program Characteristics	CITY Program (AL)	Bethesda (PA)	Cornell Abraxas (PA)	Wake County JDRC (NC)	New Hanover County (NC)	Durham Day Program (NC)
Target Population						
1. Gender/age	M&F 14–18 yo	M&F 10–18 yo Preadolescents at 3 sites	M&F 12–18 yo	M&F 12–15 yo	M&F 11–15 yo	M&F 16–18 yo
2. Admissions policy	Open. Notes limited success with low-IQ children (under 70)	Open. Will take persons with violent crimes and histories. Also serves those with mental illness, mental retardation, and sex offenses	Open. Will serve sex offenders and persons with violent crimes and histories. Denied admission to one child with serious mental issues.	Court-referred.	Persons on juvenile probation or long-term suspension from school.	Court-referred.
3. Client source	• Direct sentence	• Direct sentence (detention diversion) • Probation violations (detention diversion) • Aftercare to detention	• Direct sentence • Aftercare to detention	• Direct sentence • Probation violations	• Direct sentence • School district	• Direct sentence • Probation violations
4. Average length of stay	6.3 months	6 months	6–9 months	6 months	6 months	6 months
Administration						
1. Personnel	• Program coordinator (1) • Educational coordinator (1) • Teachers (2) • Teacher aide (1) • Counselors (3) • Recreation coordinator (1) • Office manager (1) • 3:1 ratio (child:staff)	• Program director (1) • Day treatment supervisor (1) • Prep school supervisor (1) • Counselors (3) • Psychologist (1, part time) • Substance abuse counselor (1) • Teachers (2) • Van drivers (3, part time) • Secretary (1) • 5:1 ratio (child:staff)	• Program director (1) • Assistant director (1) • Teacher supervisor (1) • Teachers (3) • Counselors (3) • Life skills workers (5) • Probation officers (2) • 2:1 ratio (child:staff)	• Program director • Teacher • Social worker • Human services technician • Administrative assistant • Haven House contractor	• Boys & Girls Club director (25%) • Assistant school principal • Teachers (4) • Teacher's aide (4) • Contracted case manager • Administrative assistant (25%) • School resource officer • Van drivers (2)	• Program director • Assistant director • Case managers (2) • Certified substance abuse counselor • GED instructor • ESC offender specialist • Administrative assistant • Contractors: rational behavior teacher, anger management teacher, and drama therapist

Program Characteristics	CITY Program (AL)	Bethesda (PA)	Cornell Abraxas (PA)	Wake County JDRC (NC)	New Hanover County (NC)	Durham Day Program (NC)
2. Educational/professional background	• Teachers: state certified • Counselors: MA + 1 yr. or BA + 1 yr.	• Teachers: state certified • Counselors: BA + 2 yrs. of experience	• Teachers: state certified • Counselors: BA + 1 yr. of experience	• Teachers: not certified • Social worker: MA in counseling + experience	• Teachers all certified • Counselor certified in counseling and substance abuse	• Teacher uses GED curriculum • Counselors certified
3. Cost	$43/day $424,617 (start-up and 1 yr. operations)	$46/day (80% state and 20% county)	Reimbursed $80/day from probation and $30/day from school	$320,520 annual	$571,757 1st yr. $284,000 1st yr. school district in-kind contribution $422,000 2nd yr.	$125,000 annual $95,000 Crime Commission $30,000 county match
4. Evaluation	Retention: unknown Impact: 32% new adjudications 1 yr. after completion	Retention: unknown Impact: 28% recidivism (1996)	Retention: 50% (many terminated for curfew violations) Impact: unknown	Implementation study in progress	Implementation study in progress	Implementation study in progress
Program Operations						
1. Phases	No. Progress measured by compliance with individual goals	Normative system Family system	3–4 phases	No	No	3 phases
2. Discipline	Three rules for termination: drugs, weapons, or fighting. Big group: staff and clients make the rules Behavior is evaluated 6 times a day (incentive store-privilege system)	Graduated sanctions 8 levels of confrontation (friendly nonverbal–passive physical restraint)	Privilege system Passive restraint	Written rules	Written rules Reasons for dismissal 1. Constant disruption 2. Possession of guns, drugs 3. Any threat of violence	Written rules
3. Local advisory board	Yes, limited role	No	No	Yes	Yes	Yes
Facilities						
1. Location	Urban and rural areas 9 sites in Alabama	Urban and rural 9 sites in Pennsylvania	10 sites in Oklahoma Others in Texas, Miami, Baltimore, and Detroit	Urban 1 site (Harrisburg, PA)	Urban	Urban
2. Building	School district surplus properties	Leased space	Rent from state for $1, former mental hospital	Leased space	Facility owned by Boys & Girls Club	Leased space

Chapter 16

The Formative Stages of a Day Treatment Program

For a juvenile day treatment program to be successful, many components must be considered prior to actually serving clients. These key issues should be addressed as the program is being conceptualized by policymakers. The formative stages of program planning, development, and design are critical to the creation of a successful day treatment program.

EFFECTIVE PRACTICES IN PROGRAM PLANNING

Identify Local Leadership

• ***Effective Practice.*** A community group composed of criminal justice practitioners (judges, juvenile court counselors, attorneys), mental health professionals, educators, and concerned citizens should come together and discuss the problems of at-risk youth in the local community.

• ***Support in Literature.*** A community must identify the "critical mass" of local leadership who can strategically plan for the needs of juveniles. Because the problem of addressing the needs of juveniles is system- and community wide, the organizational response needs to be broadly inclusive of all major interests. It is an effective practice for the development of a juvenile day treatment program to be coordinated through a communitywide executive board. Communities using this approach should locate their juvenile day treatment program under a policy board that guides the director and staff. The executive board needs to be selected based on members' knowledge of and involvement with the problems of juveniles in the community. The members ideally are stakeholders who provide a "service integration" approach, in which different service agencies coordinate efforts to address the issue under consideration (Burt, Resnick, & Matheson, 1992).

The first order of business is to identify the program's "customers" or "stakeholders." These are the individuals and institutions that have some measure of influence over the program. The influence can be direct (e.g, a county commission's approval of an agency's budget) or indirect (e.g., citizen concern about juvenile crime leading judges to order more clients to intermediate sanctions). The primary actors in the juvenile justice system include sentencing judges, prosecutors, defense attorneys, law enforcement officials, service providers, juvenile probation officers, and elected officials, among others. For programs that depend on the court for client referrals, the most important customer tends to be the sentencing judge (Petersilia, 1990).

The composition of the board must be organized such that members are able to identify and assess the needs of the juveniles in the community. Likewise, the executive board members should have the background to assess whether a juvenile day treatment program is appropriate for the needs of the community. Because the juvenile day treatment program must interact with other community agencies and actors, the most important of whom are court counselors and representatives of the school district, it is vital for representatives from the school district and juvenile probation to be a part of the executive board.

• ***Support in Practice.*** In our research, we have seen the composition of this board vary. In New Hanover County, North Carolina, for example, the community group that started the juvenile day treatment program included representatives from the public schools, the courts (chief court counselor, district attorney), the assistant county manager, a member of the press, law enforcement, and a private citizen, among others. In our site visits to more mature programs that have been in existence for over a decade (e.g., CITY and Bethesda programs; see Exhibit 15.1), we observed close connections and frequent interactions specifically with judges, court counselors, and the business community. As programs develop, the role of the board will tend to decrease; however, program management should maintain close contact with relevant stakeholders.

Make Explicit the Motivations Underlying the Planning Process

• ***Effective Practice.*** From the outset, the motivation to adopt a new program must be sincere and locally initiated.

• ***Support in Literature.*** In their seminal study of criminal justice program implementation, Ellickson and Petersilia (1983) identified sincere motivation at the time of program adoption as a correlate of implementation success. They found that locally initiated programs, as opposed to those programs that were externally imposed (e.g., through mandates), had the highest levels of implementation success. The motivation to create a new program is considered sincere if the innovation addresses a "pressing local problem" (Petersilia 1990). Stated another way, program survival is less likely if the initiative is either "imposed from above" or adopted primarily as a mechanism for attracting extra revenue. In sum, the ability of a program to succeed is in part determined by the motivation underlying its creation.

• ***Support in Practice.*** The practical experiences of our exemplary programs support the literature on the importance of motivation. Two of the earliest day treatment programs in the country, CITY and Bethesda, began at the grassroots level. The CITY program grew out of an initiative sponsored by the University of Alabama (Tuscaloosa). Relying heavily on faculty and student volunteers, the center operated out of a modest building on campus. The Bethesda program was initiated by a former chief probation officer in reaction to the lack of community-based interventions for juveniles in central Pennsylvania. These programs are linked by a common motivation—to turn troubled youth away from delinquency through intensive treatment and supervision in the community. The underlying motivation for creating these programs was altruistic, not financial.

All three programs in North Carolina were locally initiated. The idea to create day treatment programs emerged from existing criminal justice work groups (advisory boards) in each county. These work groups, comprised of representatives from the local criminal justice system, were responsible for the development of adult day reporting centers a few years earlier. For the most part, juvenile and adult day reporting centers are similar in structure and programming. The boards viewed the adult and juvenile centers in the same way; that is, as a way to fill a gap in the continuum of available services/sanctions. As such, the board's prior experience with the adult programs facilitated the adoption of the juvenile version in the three pilot counties. For example, in New Hanover County, a community board, the New Hanover County Citizens Crime Commission, was formed to address the needs of the juveniles in the community. This board determined that there was a need for a day program to keep juveniles who were suspended from school long term and on probation off the streets. This board sought out funding and developed the Pathways program. The development of this program was based on members of the community assessing their needs and identifying a problem.

Achieve Consensus on the Problem and Its Significance

• ***Effective Practice.*** Persons involved in the program planning process must agree on the nature of the problem as well as the means the community wishes to use to address the problem.

• ***Support in Literature.*** Those who are involved in program development and design must work as a team to create an intervention that not only meets the needs of the community but also meets the needs of all involved agencies. Because this type of program draws from resources of numerous agencies, from mental health to the school district to juvenile probation, all persons involved must be satisfied with the overall design of the program as well as the individual program elements. By creating consensus in the planning process, the full range of persons involved in the operation of the program will be more apt to work as a team to fulfill the entire range of services program participants need.

One problem facing many communities is the changing composition of American families. Females who are at or just above the poverty line head many families. Moreover, in those families in which both a mother and father are present, the dual-income family is becoming a modal category, producing a generation of latchkey children. Finally, our nation's children are exposed to a media culture that is enamored with explicit violence.

One clear consequence of the foregoing trends is a "diminished capacity" of many families to deal, in general, with the problems of adolescent development. In fact, some of the factors previously mentioned—poverty, single-parent homes, and lack of adequate parental supervision—are themselves correlates of delinquency (Greenwood, 1995). In other words, inadequate childrearing practices are strong predictors of delinquent behavior. Children must learn from their families the ability to exercise self-control, that is, the ability to defer gratification in favor of long-term projects or prospects (Hirschi, 1995). The diminished capacity of the family to instill these values in some children produces enormous pressures on society. Clearly, some of these pressures are felt in terms of students unmotivated to learn and difficult to discipline and are ultimately expressed in school violence. Significantly, according to a national study of American teachers, "students' lack of interest" and "discipline" are two of the most serious problems facing American public education today (Harris & Associates, 1984). Public schools systems are acting quickly and quite correctly in removing these students from regular public schools. However, there is a real danger to society if these at-risk juveniles are expelled to the street.

Communities need to provide a safety net to deal with at-risk youth. To do this, the community clearly needs to determine the nature and scope of its juvenile problem and ascertain where a day treatment program fits into the programmatic mix. Without a clear understanding of the nature and scope of its juvenile problem, the community cannot design adequate interventions.

For example:

- Is the problem with adjudicated juveniles between the ages of 11 to 15 who are suspended long term and need to be reintegrated into the school system?
- What proportion of these juveniles are court adjudicated?
- What is their family situation?
- Is the problem in the community with juveniles in the in-between years of 16 to 18 who need to be reintegrated into society rather than reintegrated into the schools?
- Is the problem with short-term suspensions of both adjudicated and non-adjudicated youths?

• ***Support in Practice.*** Each of the in-state and out-of-state programs we looked at had a clear sense of the nature and scope of its juvenile problem. In addition, this information was central to planning the scope of sources provided in all but one of the juvenile day treatment programs we investigated. In the Bethesda program, the issue of the "diminished capacity" of the family to socialize adolescent youth was built into the program's treatment paradigm. A family service component specially provided support to the parents of the at-risk juveniles in the program. It was clearly recognized that stabilizing and enhancing the home environment was imperative if any long-term program effects were to be realized. We strongly suggest that some form of family services be a part of any juvenile day treatment program.

In Wake County, North Carolina, consensus was not achieved between the juvenile court system and the school administration. The school district did not see a need for a juvenile day treatment program in the county because the school provided alternative schools for students suspended long-term. However, the court felt there was a need. As such, the number of long-term students participating in the program was unexpectedly low, resulting in the shift of emphasis to a non-treatment-oriented program for youth suspended short term.

Analyze Relevant Data for Decision Making

• ***Effective Practice.*** Decisions in the planning process should be based on quantitative and qualitative information about the target population and existing service capacity in the community. At a minimum, stakeholders should consider how many juveniles are on probation, what the risk and needs levels are of targeted youth, how many children are suspended from school, and what programs are currently available in the community to address the needs of these individuals.

• ***Support in Literature.*** To implement any effective juvenile intervention program, a community must understand the dimensions of the problem it faces. To do this, decision makers must develop "a common frame of reference" (McGarry, 1993a) that is based on a shared understanding of the problem. McGarry identified four categories of baseline information for policy groups to consider: (1) a flow chart of the disposition process; (2) the number of cases at each decision point and the length of time between steps in the process; (3) an inventory of available sanctions; and, (4) profiles of juveniles at each stage of the sanctioning process.

• ***Support in Practice.*** The first step in this process is to gather relevant data. Durham's juvenile day treatment center, for example, reported in its application for funding that its Department of Probation had 118 offenders younger than 18 years of age under its supervision, and Juvenile Court had an additional 78 individuals ages 16–18 under supervision. Almost 500 students dropped out of school in the 1994–1995 school year. These data were employed in their program design and helped to determine the goals they sought to achieve with their program. A data-driven approach will be the cornerstone of any successful program implementation because so much is derivative of the data it will provide. For example, some communities we visited had a system of alternative schools in place that could accommodate specific types of students (e.g., those suspended from the regular school system). For such communities, a day treatment program was an additional resource (referred to locally as "alternative school plus") designed to deal with adjudicated juveniles in a day treatment environment. In another community, no such system of alternative schools was provided by the local school system, and the day treatment program, in effect, served the dual purpose of an alternative school program and a treatment resource. Knowing this information at the program planning stage was essential to the design of these communities' juvenile day treatment programs.

Identify Gaps in the Continuum of Services and Select a Programmatic Response to Meet the Need

• ***Effective Practice.*** Decision makers should identify gaps in the existing continuum of interventions for at-risk youth in their community and then agree on appropriate responses to bridge the gaps.

• ***Support in Literature.*** Although our research shows that a juvenile day treatment program is an important program element in a comprehensive strategy designed to deal with the problems of at-risk youth, it is just that, one element in such a strategy. Our research found that communities are best advised to conceptualize the problem of at-risk juveniles as a combination of related strategies expressed in the programs or resources available to the community to deal with juvenile problems. Collectively, these programs constitute what we call a pyramid of services for at-risk youth (see Chapter 1). What the community needs to do is to determine how many layers of the pyramid they currently have available to it and what if any gaps exist.

Looking at the pyramid of services for at-risk youth, the bottom of the pyramid is anchored by Head Start and Smart Start. Both represent "upstream" interventions that can have a dramatic impact on juvenile behavior by providing academic and behavioral interventions early enough to make a lasting difference. The next layer of the pyramid is school and community programs designed to provide resources to the community and to juveniles. These programs include, but are not limited to, peer mediation, conflict resolution, and so on, which are increasingly offered through the public schools or community health organizations in many communities. All these programs attempt to deal with issues of adolescent development.

The next level in the pyramid is after-school programming. According to a recent study sponsored by the North Carolina Governor's Crime Commission (Whitaker, Gray, & Roole, 1998), a number of different sponsors for such programs currently exist, including public school systems, nonprofit organizations (Boys and Girls Clubs of America), county governments, and local government housing authorities. Moreover, at the state level, the North Carolina Department of Public Instruction provides funding for such programs. At the federal level, the Juvenile Justice and Delinquency Prevention Act of 1974 provides funds for after-school programs. Most after-school programs have goals designed to develop character, provide structured supervision, prevent delinquency, and improve academic skills. Clearly, all such programs provide a potential resource for at-risk youth.

The next level of the pyramid is alternative schools. However, as we have noted previously, not all school systems have this resource at the time of this writing. At least one site we evaluated used the day treatment center to serve both adjudicated and non-adjudicated juveniles who had been suspended from the schools. In fact, the day treatment center was called "alternative school plus." The final level of the pyramid is the Juvenile Day Treatment Center, which we have defined as an intermediate sanction that emphasizes both treatment and supervision of the juvenile offender in a nonresidential setting.

Finally, our research has found that communities are best advised to conceptualize the problem of at-risk juveniles in terms of a combination of related strategies expressed in the programs or resources available to the community to deal with juvenile problems. Once this is done, gaps in services can be identified and a strategic plan designed to eliminate those gaps established. We believe that for many communities (but not all) a juvenile day treatment center will fill a gap in the community's continuum of services.

• ***Support in Practice.*** In all the sites we visited, the position of the juvenile day treatment program in the continuum of services was clearly understood by staff. Moreover, they used this knowledge in promoting their own day treatment programs as preventing juvenile delinquency, providing social control, and providing a cost-effective alternative to the more expensive and invasive alternative of institutional incarceration. However, this is not to imply that all sites had the full range of services expressed in the pyramid.

EFFECTIVE PRACTICES IN PROGRAM DEVELOPMENT

Agree on a Vision, Mission, and Goals for the Program

• ***Effective Practice.*** Stakeholders should formulate a shared vision, mission, and goals for the planned intervention.

• ***Support in Literature.*** Some commentators (Peters & Waterman, 1982) note that it has become a common practice for business organizations to define a shared vision. It is imperative that juvenile day treatment programs first define a vision that guides their activities. This vision should exist in a written format and should incorporate the strategic aims of the organization and dictate how people and other resources are used in the pursuit of that vision. This vision should then be revisited periodically and used as a criterion for establishing program and policies. Much research from the private sector underscores the importance of an organization having a strategic vision that guides operational decisions.

After identifying a vision, the planning board should formulate a mission statement that clarifies the purpose of the planned program without spelling out the method for achieving it (Boone & Fulton, 1996). The mission statement is a reflection of the values and intentions that emerged during the vision definition process. The mission is a succinct statement of purpose that inspires the organization.

The next step is to agree on realistic and measurable goals for the program. At this critical stage, the mission statement is divided into more specific areas of planned program impact. The research literature notes the importance of goal formulation. Petersilia (1990) found that effective program implementation is facilitated by "clearly articulated goals that reflect the needs and desires of the customer" (p. 130). Others note that the lack of specificity about goals often leads to confusion, conflict, and inappropriate decision making (Harris & Smith, 1996).

The goal-setting process, especially for intermediate sanctions such as day treatment, is not easy for several reasons. First, community-based offender programs often pursue multiple (and sometimes contradictory) goals at the same time. For example, day treatment centers seek to punish (through intensive control) and rehabilitate offenders. Second, stakeholders may hold different expectations about the program (see Petersilia 1990). In the case of day treatment, prosecutors would likely emphasize the surveillance component of the program while members of the defense bar would champion the program's more therapeutic aspects. Third, new programs lack historical referents for developing measurable goals. Ellickson and Petersilia (1983) note that many programs begin with vague goals but develop more specific ones as the level of program information (e.g., inputs, outputs, productivity, and quality of services) builds over time. Fourth, goals may not be plausible. Programs that speak of ending delinquency or achieving perfect success are simply unrealistic. Even if the goals are plausible, it may not be possible to track goal attainment. New programs often do not have the information systems or staffing resources necessary to develop and maintain performance monitoring systems.

We reproduce five clearly-stated operational goals that were first developed for an intensive aftercare program for high-risk juveniles (Altschuler & Armstrong, 1994, p. 11). They are instructive for emerging day treatment programs:

- Prepare youth for progressively increased responsibility and freedom in the community.
- Facilitate youth-community interaction and involvement.
- Work with both the offender and targeted community support systems (families, schools) on qualities needed for constructive interaction and the youth's successful community adjustment.
- Develop new resources and supports where needed.
- Monitor and test the youth and the community on their ability to deal with each other productively.

• ***Support in Practice.*** The community is best served by conceptualizing its approach to juvenile problems the way that many American corporations see their business, by first defining a vision. An example is to divert as many at-risk youths as possible from delinquent behavior and to make them productive citizens. This vision leads logically to a mission; for example, develop a continuum of community alternatives targeted and sequenced to the developmental stage and individual need(s) of at-risk juveniles. From this mission, goals should be established; for example, establish programs that will return juveniles to school, integrate them into society, reduce recidivism, and so on. Finally, a plan can be forthcoming that is performance based with specific criteria and a positive cost-benefit return to the community, permanently funded, and long range in focus. The program must be institutionalized and be able to grow and adapt to close the service-to-needs gap. Finally, the program must be targeted to those who need and can benefit from the program(s). An example of the mission of the juvenile day treatment program in New Hanover County is "to provide a positive, structured environment to enhance educational, social, and emotional development for students (ages 11–14) with high risk behaviors."

The external sites offer two different models for specifying program goals. In the first case, the CITY program presents a set of three goals on which to evaluate its success: (1) 70 percent of current program enrollees and recent graduates will have no new offenses charged within one year after discharge; (2) 80 percent of current enrollees and recent graduates will avoid commitment to detention facilities; and (3) the CITY program will cost 50 percent less than comparable programs. The program seeks to make an impact in three measurable areas: recidivism, diversion, and cost- effectiveness. The CITY program has taken a different approach to goal setting by incorporating quantifiable performance standards into their goals. There is some indication that these goals are based on historical data which no doubt provide a base figure from which to work.

A second approach to goal setting is used by the Bethesda program. Program success is determined by the juvenile's achievement of four "meta-goals." These goals (retribution, restitution, reconciliation, and restoration) focus on individual accountability and relational healing. Once these goals are achieved, the likelihood of recidivism is reduced.

The goals for the three North Carolina centers are still evolving at this point in their programmatic development. As noted earlier, this is not an unusual finding. New programs have no experience on which to develop goals. New Hanover has broadly stated goals that may be hard to measure in the future (e.g., to increase parent involvement with high-risk youth and to bring about behavioral changes in students that will ensure continuation in their educational program). Some of the goals relate to organizational initiatives rather than juvenile goals (e.g., to implement new educational strategies for high-risk students). In contrast, Durham has established a succinct goal statement:

"reduce recidivism and probation revocations among youthful offenders in Durham County and thus reduce crime committed by 16 to 18 year olds in Durham County." This is a good example of a long-term goal (to reduce recidivism and crime). It is recommended that the long-term focus be supported by goals that can be achieved in the short term (to secure appropriate treatment that addresses criminogenic factors). As the programs mature, we expect the goals to be directed toward well-specified short- and long-term objectives.

Specify the Group Targeted for Service Provision

• ***Effective Practice.*** Based on the goals established earlier, a target population with well-defined characteristics should be identified. The characteristics of juveniles in the target group should be clearly described in the program's admissions policy.

• ***Support in Literature.*** This stage in the program's development is a natural outgrowth of the goal setting and data analysis that occurred earlier in the planning process. Several examples best illustrate the important link between programmatic goals and the identification of a group for service provision. If the goal is to reduce incarceration costs, the day treatment program must be designed to divert juveniles from detention or to reduce the length of their stay while in detention (see Albert, Faro, & Lawson, 1998). As such, the target group should include juveniles who would typically receive a disposition requiring some form of incarceration. Cost-effective goals cannot be achieved if the program admits large numbers of low-risk juveniles who are not eligible for institutional placements. If another goal is to reduce the level of drug and alcohol addiction and abuse in a certain class of juvenile delinquents, the target group should include individuals who have certain drug charges or histories of substance abuse. Also, if the program seeks to reintegrate youth back into their home schools, a younger class of program participants (e.g., middle school age) should be sought out rather than older teens who may be directed toward vocational opportunities and the General Equivalency Diploma (GED). The profile of eligible candidates for day treatment ultimately forms the basis for the program's admissions policy.

• ***Support in Practice.*** The policy group should consider several issues when developing a target profile. First, the specific sociodemographic and criminal backgrounds of potential program participants need to be identified. It is not our purpose to provide an exhaustive list, but characteristics such as age, gender, mental capacity, family cohesiveness, history of abuse, current offense, risk level, and prior criminal record are typically incorporated into a target profile. Second, the source of client referrals needs to be determined. Will the judge order the juvenile to day treatment directly? Is day treatment an option for juveniles who are in danger of having their probation revoked? That is, can the juvenile probation department initiate the referral? Can day treatment serve as a structured aftercare program for juveniles exiting detention facilities? Can a school district refer students to day treatment even if they are not court involved? In the programs studied, we found instances of referrals from all four sources (judges, juvenile probation department, detention, and school district). The referral source varies by program. The Bethesda program takes clients from three sources. In New Hanover County, the day treatment program receives approximately half of its clients from the court and half from the school district.

Once these items have been decided, the policy group can move on to the third issue: establishing the program's capacity. Many factors influence this decision, including financial resources, space considerations, and numbers of juveniles who match the other targeted characteristics. Programs typically serve twenty to thirty clients at any one time. However, some programs work with more clients (e.g., the day treatment center in Lexington, Kentucky oversees fifty-five juveniles while the New Hanover program has a rated capacity of sixty).

After describing the target population, the program's admission criteria can be formally stated. The programs outside North Carolina maintained fairly open policies. Some even accept sex offenders. In general, day treatment centers admit boys and girls between the ages of 10 and 18. They do not typically deny entry to persons based on current charge or prior criminal history. A notable exception is Wake County, which does not admit juveniles who have committed violent crimes. The CITY program has found that its intervention does not work well with individuals with an IQ below an established threshold.

Build Public Support for the Program

• ***Effective Practice.*** Community-based programs such as day treatment, by definition, require the support of the community. The day treatment program needs to create a message about its vision and mission. It must make sure that the community receives the message.

• ***Support in Literature.*** Stakeholders are those actors in community decision making who are in a position to influence or be influenced by a decision (Vasu, Stewart, & Garson, 1999). As a new program, day treatment needs stakeholder support to develop and become institutionalized. Because these programs are new, their place in the combination of strategies designed to deal with at-risk juveniles can become "blurred." They can become just another public program with a new acronym. The message that needs to be conveyed is that day treatment is a sanction that emphasizes both treatment and supervision of the juvenile offender in a nonresidential setting. What also must be conveyed is the fact that for many communities, the day treatment program is a vital element in a comprehensive wraparound approach to juvenile delinquency that fills a gap in the community response to at-risk youth. Albert et al.

(1998) suggest that programs may be promoted through the media by describing such successes as cost savings, goal achievements, and public safety, as well as individual success stories.

• ***Support in Practice.*** All three efforts in North Carolina were locally initiated. As we have noted, they emerged from existing criminal justice work groups and drew their initial stakeholder support from this nucleus of people. In New Hanover, the deputy county manager took a strong leadership role in promoting the need for juvenile day treatment and was successful in securing county funding. In addition, the district attorney, a representative of the school district, the chief court counselor, a member of the mental health community, a concerned citizen, and a member of the press (among others) were active in the policy board that developed the center. The presence of a member of the media provided a firsthand mechanism for keeping the public educated about the program's development and projected benefits.

As previously stated, numerous stakeholders should be included in the planning of the program; one of these stakeholders should be a member of the media. This will help provide "good press" for the program. New Hanover County indicated the importance of selling the program to the local community, especially those residents living near the location of the center. The name given to the program is important. Programs should avoid referencing the fact that they are dealing with adjudicated youth. Thus, New Hanover County decided to call its program "Pathways."

There are other approaches to building public support for the program. Some invite members of the local community to an open house and tour of the facility. Programs in Kentucky and elsewhere use volunteers at the center in an effort to establish good rapport with the immediate neighborhood. In addition, juveniles clean local schools and engage in other work projects that benefit the community. These kinds of endeavors, which can be sold as "payback"-type programs, have a tremendous amount of public relations value. They place the juveniles in a good light and help build support in the community for juvenile day treatment.

Provide Adequate and Stable Financial Resources

• ***Effective Practice.*** A reliable, long-term funding stream should be identified to ensure the complete implementation (and institutionalization) of the day treatment program.

• ***Support in Literature.*** We found few references in the academic literature to support this effective practice. One article identified "plentiful resources" as a correlate of successful program implementation (Petersilia, 1990). The more important literature for our purposes is found in the historical description of the Project New Pride expansion in the mid-1980s (Laurence & West, 1985).

The Project New Pride day treatment program in Denver received national recognition as an exemplary program in the late 1970s. After much fanfare (and some question about its effectiveness), the New Pride model was replicated in ten sites throughout the country. The new programs received three to four years of operational funding from the federal government. After the federal financial commitment ended, seven of the ten programs ceased operations. The three remaining programs were able to continue on in a severely diminished capacity by tapping other revenue sources (e.g., education funding). The program in Pensacola, Florida, turned into an intervention for educationally and emotionally handicapped students (Laurence & West, 1985). The Pensacola program had to change its entire focus in order to keep its doors open. The relatively high cost of juvenile day treatment ($350,000 a year in 1983 dollars), when combined with a general decline in interest in delinquency programs, made it exceedingly difficult for these programs to continue functioning. Most of these programs did not achieve a level of institutionalization within their parent agency or within the larger juvenile justice system that would have improved their competitive standing for scarce funds.

• ***Support in Practice.*** How are existing day treatment centers funded? The most successful programs diversify their sources of revenue, thereby adding a level of stability that is absent in programs that rely solely on a single funding stream.

- Two programs in Pennsylvania, Cornell Abraxas and Bethesda, receive funds from two primary sources—probation and the school districts. These day treatment centers collect the per diem allocations that are usually given to probation departments and schools for providing similar services. The juvenile day treatment programs in Pennsylvania also bill Medicaid for case management and mental health services.
- Kentucky day treatment funding is divided into two general sources—educational and treatment. Educational funding is primarily provided by the state department of education and is based on average daily attendance (Wolford, Jordan, & Murphy, 1997). The state juvenile justice department funds the treatment portion of day treatment.
- The North Carolina pilots rely heavily on state funds with some matching funds provided by the county (Durham) and in-kind contributions provided by the local school district (New Hanover). The source of future funding after the initial planning/operating grants expire is uncertain at this time.

We offer one final word about the financial commitment necessary to operate a juvenile day treatment program. These programs are resource intensive. For the programs considered in this study, annual operating costs averaged between $350,000 to $500,000. First-year start-up expenses are even higher due to one-time equipment and refurbishment costs. Durham's expenses ($125,000) are significantly lower due to the economies produced through a sharing of resources (personnel, rent, service providers) with an adult day reporting center. Cornell Abraxas came in at the high end (over $600,000). Policymakers need to be aware of the costs involved in running a comprehensive day treatment program.

EFFECTIVE PRACTICES IN PROGRAM DESIGN

Choose an Administrative Structure to Oversee the Program

• ***Effective Practice.*** An agency should be selected to administer the program after an exhaustive survey of current community resources.

• ***Support in Literature.*** Policymakers have to choose an agency to operate the day treatment program. The first step is to identify the agencies in the community that may have an interest in operating a program. The public administration literature is helpful in its identification of the strengths and weaknesses of the different sectors in delivering similar services. Osborne (1992) explained that the public sector is better at regulating industry and ensuring equity while the private sector is more adept at innovating and adapting to rapid change. Tasks that demand compassion and commitment, require extensive trust on behalf of clients, or involve the enforcement of individual responsibility and behavior are best handled by nonprofit organizations. Bendick (1984) concluded that the available research shows that business is better at providing services that are "straightforward, simple, and technological," but it has less success with programs that are "complex, long-run, and sociological" (p. 154). Examples do exist of private companies providing services traditionally delivered by government including prisons, housing, and other social services (see Savas, 1987).

• ***Support in Practice.*** Once again, there is a lot of variety in the administrative structures used to oversee day treatment programs. There does not appear to be a standard administrative structure used within or between states. We learned of day treatment programs that were administered by public, private for-profit, and private nonprofit organizations.

In fact, the three external sites that were visited by the research team employ different administrative structures. Bethesda is a nonprofit organization, CITY is a governmental entity, and Cornell Abraxas is a for-profit company. The diversity may be due to variances in existing organizational capacity to run a program.

Kentucky exhibits a full range of administrative approaches to day treatment. The eighteen day treatment centers in Kentucky follow one of three administrative models (Wolford et al., 1997):

- *State operated.* Day treatment staff are employees of the state Department for Juvenile Justice. Educators work for the local school district.
- *School operated.* Under a contract with the state, the local school district assumes administrative responsibility for the entire program. Both treatment and educational personnel are employees of the school district. Half of the programs are administered by school districts.
- *Nonprofit operated.* Treatment staff are employees of a nonprofit agency that has a contract with the state to provide services. Teachers work for and are supervised by the local school district.

It is important to note that since 1983, all new juvenile day treatment centers in Kentucky have opted for the school-operated approach. School-operated programs typically use one director to oversee both treatment and educational program components. This reduces administrative costs.

North Carolina is much like her sister states in the diversity of administrative approaches taken to manage day treatment. The Durham day treatment program is administered by the same county agency that oversees the adult day reporting center. A local nonprofit operates Wake County's program while New Hanover's center is run by the local chapter of a national nonprofit organization (Community Boys' & Girls' Club of America).

At this point, it is too early to determine which approach appears to be the most effective. It is recommended that decision makers consider all alternatives that are currently available in the community.

Select a "Leader" Rather Than Simply a "Manager" to Direct the Program

• ***Effective Practice.*** The juvenile day treatment program needs a leader/leadership team to champion the idea and develop practical strategies for implementing it.

• ***Support in literature.*** Leadership is one of the most popular and important topics in organizational behavior. A great deal of the popular business literature throughout the world deals with the topic. For over fifty years, in both the public and private sector, research has been conducted about the relationship of leadership to organizational effectiveness. Leadership is thinking outside the box. It is inherently a proactive activity that is results oriented. Leading and managing are not synonymous. Managing is a series of functions—scanning the environment, planning (organizing and staffing), implementing, and evaluating. Leading is only one part of the management process. Not all managers are leaders. Leadership goes beyond simple management. The idea that people need both task skills and people skills to be effective is now firmly accepted. Leadership and management require working with and through people to achieve organizational goals. As we have indicated previously, the nature of those goals or outcomes affects managerial style. In addition, the maturity level of the employees does as well. An ultimate objective of all leaders and managers must be to empower their subordinates to do the job. However, managers must realize that in order to get their employees to a given level of maturity (i.e., increase their willingness and abilities), they need to employ different behaviors in different situations. Moreover, managers need to set a vision. They need to think in terms of "we," and they need to "walk their talk." Finally, leaders need to know the importance of the symbolic aspects of the organization and to encourage the heart. Leadership is both art and science (Vasu et al., 1999).

The literature is replete with studies that stress the need for dynamic leadership to oversee organizational or systematic change. Scheirer (1996) notes that effective organizations have a single person who has overall authority for managing the organization, as well as the charisma to articulate the mission both internally and externally. Likewise, intensive supervision programs that tend to survive have "a leader who is vitally committed to the objectives, values, and implications of the project and who can devise practical strategies to motivate and effect change" (Petersilia, 1990, p. 136). What we recommend is a leader who is both politically savvy and technically competent.

Ellickson and Petersilia (1983) found that programs with active leaders were the most successful. Active leaders "spearheaded project initiation and then continued to make key policy or staffing decisions or fought for funding whenever its availability became problematic" (p. 26). After the project has been adopted, it is not uncommon for active leaders to become supportive leaders. Supportive leaders are less involved in the day-to-day operations of a program, but they still provide general support for the decisions and funding requests of the program director. Ellickson and Petersilia postulate that the transition from active to supportive leadership is a sign of the program's "routinization"—its ability to operate smoothly without high-level intervention (p. 27). Thus, the continuous support of leaders throughout the program's early development and implementation is a prerequisite of success.

Leaders are identified as either single individuals or groups of policymakers. Petersilia (1990) seems to side with the single-leader approach. She acknowledges the need for a team of top managers to oversee the proper implementation of the leader's policies; however, the team does not have a role in setting those policies. Others see an important role for a group of leaders. For McGarry (1993b), a group of high-level policymakers from the local criminal justice system is an essential component of the intermediate sanction process. "The goals, values, and judgments of this decision-making body will guide the entire process" (p. 21). Except for differences in the composition of the leadership function, all authors seem to agree that it is important for program management and leaders to remain in harmony, with clearly differentiated roles (Scheirer, 1996).

• ***Support in Practice.*** At our exemplary sites a number of people were responsible for the development of these centers; however, two individuals assumed significant leadership roles—Ed Earnest (CITY) and Dominic Herbst (Bethesda). These two leaders share similar characteristics including: a charismatic personality; a sincere dedication to improving the lives of troubled youth; and an aptitude for handling political and technical matters. They serve as the principal spokespersons for their respective programs. As to their dedication, both men have worked with juveniles for most of their professional lives. Their political acumen is evidenced, in part, by their ability to expand their programs during a period of modest growth in state expenditures. Bethesda now operates in seven states while CITY runs nine programs throughout Alabama. Beyond the political aspects of the job, these two leaders are responsible for various managerial (e.g., personnel, budgeting, and contracting for services) and programmatic (e.g., counseling and mentoring) tasks.

By our earlier definition, Earnest and Herbst are best classified as active leaders. As their programs have grown (become "routinized"), these leaders have delegated certain operational decisions to an increasingly large program staff. Thus, there is some support for Ellickson and Petersilia's contention that leadership support tends to move from active to supportive as programs mature. Interestingly, advisory boards play a minor role in the exemplary programs studied. They do exist, but their role is limited. The local advisory board for the CITY program in Birmingham meets infrequently and does not have formal procedures or duties. Individual board members are tapped for support on an "as needed" basis. Instead, most of the success is driven by the charismatic leader who is able to marshal the support of local leaders (judges, city council members) without the routine intervention of formal organizations such as advisory boards.

No single leader or group of individuals is instantly identified with the juvenile day treatment concept in North Carolina. This may be due, in part, to the preexistence of criminal justice advisory boards. Unlike the exemplary programs, the process is not driven by a dynamic leader seeking to institute changes in the local criminal justice system. Instead, the initiative has developed through a more formalized process involving staff work, advisory board deliberations, submission of grant applications to the Governor's Crime Commission for start-up funding, and the hiring of a project director to oversee implementation. In contrast to the active leadership style prominent in other states, the advisory board members are best characterized as supportive leaders. While the board members are not generally involved in the daily operations of the program, they support the program through other means (e.g., referring clients to the program and approving the program director's annual spending priorities). This is not to say that certain individuals have not played important roles in fostering these programs. By way of example, the deputy county manager in New Hanover County actively promoted the concept early in the process. In addition, in Durham, the credibility of the program director resulted in the juvenile day treatment program being asked by the county manager to develop a similar program for younger youths. It is unclear whether the lack of active leadership (individual or group) during the developmental stages of the project will have a long-term impact on program success and survival.

Identify an Appropriate Facility to House the Program

• ***Effective Practice.*** Policymakers should consider a number of options for siting the program, including the use of existing facilities and rental agreements.

• ***Support in Literature.*** Specific technical standards are spelled out by the American Correctional Association (1993). The second part of the manual discusses physical plant requirements in subsections titled building and safety codes, sanitation and hygiene, and safety and emergency procedures.

• ***Support in Practice.*** When finding a physical facility, a number of considerations must be taken into account. First, as a result of the stipulations of many schools' "zero tolerance" policies, the target population may not be allowed on school grounds. As such, a new program must find a facility off school property or develop an arrangement with the school district to locate the program. Second, the cost of the facility being used must be considered. Every dollar spent on rent for facilities is one less dollar spent on direct service provision. Thus, program developers should attempt to locate state or county property that can be used for minimal cost. For example, the Cornell Abraxas program rents space in an old mental health facility from the state of Pennsylvania for $1 a year. The third consideration is whether to co-locate the program with other existing programs. This is important because of the unique characteristics of the population being served. It is important to isolate the juveniles from adult offenders if the programs are to be co-located with other programs for adult offenders. In addition, one must also consider the implications of locating the program where the participants may have contact with nonoffenders. Each of these two situations has been seen in the North Carolina pilot sites. For instance, in Durham the juvenile day treatment program is located at the site of the adult day reporting center. As a result, program staff must be sure the distinct populations do not come into contact with one another; moreover, scheduling must be such that physical space can be split between the two populations. In contrast, New Hanover County co-located its program at the Community Boys' and Girls' Club. The difficulty with this arrangement is isolating the juvenile day treatment participants from other children attending the Boys' and Girls' Club.

Hire Staff With Proper Qualifications, Experience, and Disposition to Work With Target Population

• ***Effective Practice.*** Staff with the expertise and desire to work in both aspects of juvenile day treatment—the social control and treatment dimensions—should be retained.

• ***Support in Literature.*** The staff in day treatment programs can be categorized into three professions: educators, treatment providers (substance abuse counselors, behavior therapists), and case managers. Each profession, to a varying degree, has its own set of internal standards as to the necessary educational and experiential requirements for practitioners. These standards are fairly well established for educators (minimum of a bachelor's degree, state licensure) and therapists (state licensure and certification, continuing education requirements). For therapists, these standards ensure an appropriate level of "therapeutic integrity" (Gendreau, 1996). However, case managers do not share the same level of professionalization as the others. There are no state standards, certifications, or training requirements that dictate entry into the profession. This may explain the diversity in how various programs define the roles and responsibilities of case managers.

• ***Support in Practice.*** Because the qualifications for educators and therapists are well defined, we focused our field research on the backgrounds of case managers. We found some commonalities and differences. Most had a bachelor's degree, typically in the behavioral and social sciences (criminal justice, social work, or political science). The previous occupations held by case managers ranged widely from military officers to schoolteachers. Some employed recently graduated college students (Wake). No site mandated that case managers maintain certain professional credentials. The case managers were generally viewed as the disciplinarians on staff.

What we found to be the most important quality among all staff classifications was the dedication to working with this difficult population. Interviewers repeatedly asked staff members at various sites why they worked at the center under some unfavorable conditions at times. A common response heard was that they truly enjoyed their work, especially when they have an impact on a juvenile (e.g., a marked change in attitude). Staff members who do not bring this missionary zeal to work do not stay long in their position.

Consider Other Important (and Often Overlooked) Logistical Issues

• ***Effective Practice.*** When designing a program, it is necessary to thoroughly consider issues related to the transportation of clients, liability insurance, and licensure of the facility to provide substance and alcohol abuse services.

• ***Support in the Literature.*** Because most of these operational issues go beyond the scope of this chapter, we refer our readers to *Standards for Juvenile Day Treatment Programs* (American Correctional Association, 1993) for a discussion of many day-to-day operational issues. However, our research has isolated certain logistical issues that emerged in one form or another in all the sites we visited. We found that these issues are much better addressed early in the planning stage for a program because they have an impact on the ability to deliver the service on the first day of operation. How these issues are resolved will vary from site to site. For example, if a day treatment center is located in an urban area that draws its clientele from a ten-block adjacent area, the "transportation issue" may involve no more than providing an activities van. However, if the center is located in the county seat of a rural community, transportation may be the driving force in the ability to provide the service. Finally, if the school district is an active participant in day treatment, its transportation resources may be used. At any rate, a basic issue that should be addressed early in the planning is how the clientele will get to the day treatment center.

Also, given the fact that the clientele of day treatment are at-risk youth, a variety of liability issues (in addition to those involved in transporting juveniles to and from the site) may also present themselves. Clearly, legal advice should be sought early in the planning process about liability issues. Finally, licensure of the facility to provide substance and alcohol services must also be addressed. However, how it is addressed will vary depending on whether the program chooses to be a direct provider of these services or to "contract" out for these services with a local mental health agency or nonprofit organization.

• ***Support in Practice.*** Most sites tried to resolve the previously mentioned business and logistical issues in the planning stage. For example, Durham draws its clientele from an area adjacent to its program and consequently transportation to the site was not a major issue. Conversely, in New Hanover, transportation was required and provided using vans of the Boys' and Girls' Club to get the clientele to the center. Moreover, in New Hanover, treatment services were contracted out with a local mental health facility. In Wake County, specific treatment services were also contracted out (e.g., family services). The Durham program used the treatment services already available on contract through its adult day reporting center, including some unique services such as drama therapy. Resolving transportation, liability insurance, and licensure issues early in the planning process will facilitate its smooth implementation.

THE RECURRING NATURE OF THE BUSINESS OF MAKING YOUR IDEA WORK

Viewing a project in terms of its life cycle allows project staff to anticipate and plan for the maturation of action items. This is important because project staff have a tendency to neglect the underlying business of service delivery and focus on the service itself, in this case, treatment. Every key activity matures with the project, especially activities such as leadership, staffing, funds development, and building collaborative relationships. Project staff have a tendency to assume, for example, that leadership does not need tending as a project changes from start-up to an expansion enterprise. In the beginning, funding will probably be from a one-time grant. It is a real evil to try to begin an idea that is meant to answer a problem that has taken years if not decades to fester in the community and have only one year of dollars to do something "lasting and positive." But most often the choice is to start with terminal grant money or not start at all. The goal is to obtain and use one-time funding but not depend on it.

Planning, for example, focuses on courting grantors. But when up and running, the project must find more stable funding sources. Thus the operational project, perhaps a juvenile day treatment program again, needs to develop grants and possibly a line item in the local budget or perhaps fee for service. In fact, the grant should be viewed as a lucky and undependable funding source. The mature, established project in the expansion phase of the life cycle would perhaps look to developing a giving program in addition to the search for permanent budgetary status from a municipality. The point is, the viable project does not approach resources development, or any other critical function, only in the planning stage. The activity changes as the organizational focus changes; it is not ignored and expected to be "okay" just because it had a one-time active status. The business of service delivery is more important than the service itself. It does not matter if your program offers one of the most successful treatment modalities ever recorded if it is canceled for lack of funding, leadership support, or collaborative agreement. So leadership must make sure they understand the business of offering juvenile day treatment before they offer it at all.

References

Albert, L. H., Faro, F. C., & Lawson, R. H. (1998). *Critical elements in the planning, development, and implementation of successful correctional options.* Washington, DC: U.S. Department of Justice.

Altschuler, D. M., & Armstrong, T. L. (1984). Intervening with serious juvenile offenders. In R. Mathias, P. DeMuro, & R. Allinson (Eds.), *Violent juvenile offenders* (pp. 187–206). San Francisco: National Council on Crime and Delinquency.

Altschuler, D. M., & Armstrong, T. L. (1994). *Intensive aftercare for high-risk juveniles: A community care model.* Washington, DC: U.S. Department of Justice.

American Correctional Association. (1993). *Standards for juvenile day treatment programs.* Lanham, MD: Author.

Bendick, M. (1984). Privatization of public services: Recent experience. In H. Brooks, L. Liebman, & C. S. Snelling (Eds.), *Public-private partnership: New opportunities for meeting social needs* (pp. 153–171). Cambridge, MA: Ballinger.

Boone, H. N., & Fulton, B. A. (1996). *Implementing performance-based measures in community corrections* [National Institute of Justice Research in Brief]. Washington, DC: U.S. Department of Justice.

Burt, M. R., Resnick, G., & Matheson, N. (1992). *Comprehensive service integration programs for at-risk youth: Final report.* Washington, DC: Urban Institute.

Ellickson, P., & Petersilia, J. (1983). *Implementing new ideas in criminal justice.* Santa Monica, CA: Rand.

Gendreau, P. (1996). Principles of effective intervention with offenders. In A. J. Harland (Ed.), *Choosing correctional options that work: Defining the demand and evaluating the supply* (pp. 117–130). Thousand Oaks, CA: Sage.

Greenwood, P. W. (1995). Juvenile crime and juvenile justice. In J. Q. Wilson & J. Petersilia (Eds), *Crime: Twenty-eight leading experts look at the most pressing problem of our time* (pp. 91–117). San Francisco, CA: ICS Press.

Harris, L., & Associates. (1984). *The Metropolitan Life survey of the American teacher.* New York: Metropolitan Life Insurance Company.

Harris, P., & Smith, S. (1996). Developing community corrections: An implementation perspective. In A. J. Harland (Ed.), *Choosing correctional options that work: Defining the demand and evaluating the supply* (pp. 183–222). Thousand Oaks, CA: Sage.

Hirschi, T. (1995). The family. In J. Q. Wilson & J. Petersilia (Eds.), *Crime: Twenty-eight leading experts look at the most pressing problem of our time* (pp. 121–140). San Francisco, CA: ICS Press.

Laurence, S. E., & West, B. R. (1985). *National evaluation of the New Pride replication program, Final report, Volume I: Organization, implementation, and results of the replication process.* Walnut Creek, CA: Pacific Institute for Research and Evaluation.

McGarry, P. (1993a). Developing a common frame of reference. In P. McGarry & M. M. Carter, (Eds.), *The intermediate sanctions handbook: Experiences and tools for policymakers* (pp. 71–77). Washington, DC: U.S. Department of Justice.

McGarry, P. (1993b). Essential ingredients for success. In P. McGarry & M. M. Carter, (Eds.), *The intermediate sanctions handbook: Experiences and tools for policymakers* (pp. 21–26). Washington, DC: U.S. Department of Justice.

Osborne, D. (1992, April). Privatization: One answer, not the answer. *Governing*, 83.

Petersilia, J. (1990). Conditions that permit intensive supervision programs to survive. *Crime and Delinquency*, *36*, 126–145.

Peters, T. J., & Waterman, Jr., R. H. (1982). *In search of excellence: Lessons from America's best-run companies*. New York: Warner Books.

Savas, E. S. (1987). *Privatization: The key to better government.* Chatham, NJ: Chatham House.

Scheirer, M. (1996). A template for assessing the organizational base for program implementation. In M. Scheirer (Ed.), *A user's guide to program templates: A new tool for evaluating program content* (pp. 61–79). San Francisco, CA: Jossey-Bass.

Vasu, M. L., Stewart, D., & Garson, G.D. (1999). *Organizational behavior for public managers.* New York: Marcel Dekker.

Whitaker, G., Gray, K., & Roole, B. (1998). *Developmental analysis of after-school programs.* Chapel Hill, NC: Center for Urban and Regional Studies.

Wolford, B. I., Jordan, F., & Murphy, K. (1997). Day treatment: Community-based partnerships for delinquent and at-risk youth. *Juvenile and Family Court Judges*, *48*, 35–42.

Chapter 17

Program Implementation and Operation

After agreeing on a conceptual approach to day treatment, the next step is to bring the vision to reality. The focus here is on the more practical concerns of running a day treatment center. This chapter begins by highlighting issues that should be considered as the program moves from design to implementation. This is followed by strategies for delivering effective services. The chapter concludes with the identification of effective practices related to the management of a program after it has been implemented.

EFFECTIVE IMPLEMENTATION STRATEGIES

Continue Commitment to Day Treatment as the Program Moves From Concept to Reality

• ***Effective Practice.*** Stakeholders and program staff should have a long-term commitment to the mission and goals of juvenile day treatment.

• ***Support in Literature.*** There is a tendency for the initial enthusiasm generated for a new idea to wane in the face of other competing priorities and difficulties experienced during implementation. The key is to make sure that a long-term commitment is made to the program at all levels including stakeholders, program managers, and staff (see Harris & Smith, 1996). External stakeholder commitment is especially important in order to keep (and in some cases expand) program funding. Program director commitment is critical for day treatment programs. The researchers in the New Pride evaluation described in Chapter 15 wrote about the deleterious effects of turnover in the director's position (Laurence & West, 1985). Such turnover typically spelled the demise of the program. Others note the importance of "secure administrators" and "low staff turnover" for successful program implementation (Petersilia, 1990). Finally, the level of support that the program enjoys among program management and staff is an important correlate of successful implementation. The degree to which program staff supports the initiative is referred to as "street-level commitment" (Harris & Smith, 1996, p. 210). Not surprisingly, Ellickson and Petersilia (1983) found that overall program success is related to the degree of project director and staff commitment to the program. In sum, successfully implemented programs have high levels of stakeholder and street-level commitment.

• ***Support in Practice.*** All the successful day treatment programs we studied are characterized by a long-term commitment to the mission and vision of juvenile day treatment. There has been considerable stability in the top leadership at Bethesda and CITY. The two leaders have been with their respective programs since the early 1980s. The Cornell Abraxas day treatment center experienced a change in leadership recently. In fact, the entire Abraxas program has undergone a significant transformation, from a nonprofit to for-profit corporation. One of the most repeated recommendations that existing programs had for new programs was to have a unified staff. All staff members must work together to achieve a common goal (see Chapter 15, Exhibit 15.1, in this volume for a description of these programs).

The North Carolina sites have not enjoyed the same measure of leadership stability as their out-of-state counterparts. The Hanover County, North Carolina, program recently replaced the person responsible for overseeing the day treatment center. The Wake County, North Carolina, program had three directors in its first year of operation.

Integrate Program Into Existing Environment

• ***Effective Practice.*** Juvenile day treatment centers should be fully integrated into the existing educational and juvenile justice systems.

• ***Support in Literature.*** Harris and Smith (1996) view implementation as a "process of mutual adaptation between the vision and goals of those who initiate development or adoption of an innovation and the organizational or system environments in which the innovation is applied" (p. 183). This definition recognizes the importance of two environments for new programs—internal (organizational) and external (system). Incomplete integration into either of these two environments may undermine the program.

Internal integration is a challenge when a new program is administratively located within another organization. For example, intensive supervision probation units have often failed to receive the support from other probation and parole staff (Petersilia, 1990). External integration is a concern for all new interventions. Frequent information exchanges with other criminal justice system players help build political support and promote greater coordination of resources (see Lawrence's, 1997, discussion on the relationships between probation and schools). The most successful programs have the strong support of the local judiciary. In short, judges need to be involved (Petersilia, 1990). The same case can be made for school districts. If the goal of day treatment is to reintegrate juveniles back into their home communities and schools, it is highly desirable to have a good relationship with the school district. Schools have much discretion in determining who will attend classes at a particular site.

An overreliance on the support of external actors may also be problematic to a program. Implementation may fail if a project depends on others who lack a sense of urgency in the project (Pressman & Wildavsky, 1984). Individuals or organizations may be called on because of their expertise or jurisdictional authority, yet they may lack a real commitment to the program.

Agencies work together more cooperatively when the personnel of the organizations respect each other in terms of competence and job performance; when they share regular, positive communication; and when they share compatible objectives and philosophies (Hall, Clark, Giordano, Johnson, & Van Roekel, 1981). This human resource development has to be a part of the operation.

The need for close collaboration among various system players is especially important for integrating the juvenile back into his or her home community and school (Armstrong & Altschuler, 1997; Cook, 1990). Procedures for handling the transfer of school records and communication about the juvenile's academic and behavioral progress should be in place early.

• ***Support in Practice.*** There are numerous examples of successful program integration into the local criminal justice and educational systems. An effective device is to appoint key officials to the local day treatment advisory board. The Chief Juvenile Probation Officer sits on the CITY advisory board in Tuscaloosa. This relationship opens the lines of communication between the two programs. By and large, the exemplary programs have good working relationships with the court. Judges and probation officers are well aware of the program and are willing to refer juveniles to it. The CITY program is also well integrated into the local education system. School districts provide surplus school property for CITY day treatment facilities and transport students via school buses. Also, teachers at CITY work for the school district, not the day treatment program.

In New Hanover, the school district is an active partner with the center. Teachers work for the school district and are supervised by an on-site assistant principal. Lunches are brought over from an adjacent school. Wake County offers some educational services, but the instructors are not state certified. Durham refined its target population in response to the reluctance of some school officials who oppose the reintegration of high-risk juveniles back into their home schools. Durham serves older adolescents who qualify for General Equivalency Diploma (GED) classes offered through the local community college. There are signs that the North Carolina pilot programs are not well integrated into the local criminal justice system. The New Hanover and Wake sites have had difficulty enrolling students into their programs. Judges have been reluctant to refer juveniles either for lack of knowledge about the program or because of dissatisfaction with the program. Also, attendance is sometimes spotty, perhaps indicating that juvenile court counselors are not backing lapses in juvenile reporting with proportional and timely sanctions.

Establish Collaborative Service Arrangements

• ***Effective Practice.*** Service arrangements with other agencies should be secured in order to expand programmatic options while holding the line on costs.

• ***Support in Literature.*** Few programs can realistically hope to provide a full range of services themselves. Thus, there is a strong need for securing services that already exist in the community. This may involve contracting for services or using community volunteers.

• ***Support in Practice.*** We note several examples of collaborative service arrangements. Durham has an agreement with the local YMCA that allows the program participants to use the YMCA's recreational facilities. Durham also uses independent contractors to provide drama therapy and behavior modification classes. Other programs have established ties with the local department of health to provide educational programming. The CITY program in Birmingham uses volunteers in innovative ways to teach sportsmanship and discipline. A member of the local advisory board teaches the juveniles how to play golf. Bethesda has established a unique arrangement with the federal Bureau of Prisons to help day treatment participants and adult male prisoners work through parenting issues together.

EFFECTIVE SERVICE DELIVERY

Ensure That Treatment Is Rooted in Proven Methods

Effective Practice. The rehabilitation component of day treatment should be based on empirically validated strategies for changing juvenile values and behaviors.

Support in Literature. Over the last fifteen years, the "what works" literature has produced a series of studies that identify characteristics of effective juvenile delinquency programs. Following is a list of the components most relevant to juvenile day treatment:

- *Structure.* Effective rehabilitation programs "[a]re structured and focused, use multiple treatment components, focus on developing skills (social relations, academic, and employment skills), and use behavioral and cognitive-behavioral methods with reinforcements for clearly identified, overt behaviors" (Sherman et al., 1997, 9–49).
- *Treatment modalities.* Lipsey (1992) found that employment, multimodal, behavioral, and skill-oriented treatment modalities had the largest impact on juvenile recidivism. Also, effective programs provide large amounts of meaningful contact and are longer in duration.
- *Key program elements.* For Altschuler and Armstrong (1984), successful programs for delinquent youth possess the following key elements: continuous case management, emphasis on reintegration services, opportunities for youth achievement, and involvement in program decision making; clear and consistent consequences for misconduct; enriched educational and vocational programming; and a variety of counseling matched to youth's needs.
- *Key treatment components.* Greenwood and Zimring (1985) list the following components in successful youth programs: opportunities for success and development of positive self-image; youth bonding to prosocial adults and institutions; frequent, timely, and accurate feedback for both positive and negative behavior; reduced influence of negative role models; recognition and understanding of thought processes that rationalize negative behavior; opportunities for juveniles to discuss childhood problems; and program components adapted to the needs of individual youth.

There are several noteworthy similarities within these studies. The intervention strategies most favored by the reviewers are behavioral or cognitive-behavioral approaches. At the core of the behavioral approach is the concept of reinforcement, "which refers to the strengthening or increasing of a behavior so that it will continue to be performed in the future" (Gendreau, 1996, pp. 120–121).

These approaches appear especially effective when delivered within the community because they are more amenable to certain interventions (e.g., family counseling) that are generally not available in institutional settings (see Clements, 1988). Several researchers also note the importance of programming that improves the academic and vocational skills of juveniles. Finally, researchers agree that the use of multiple interventions appears to reduce the likelihood of future delinquency.

• ***Support in Practice.*** Many of these recommended intervention strategies are used in the exemplary programs. Three examples illustrate the practical application of these strategies. First, the Bethesda and CITY programs make excellent use of token economies to change behaviors. Juveniles earn points for positive attitudes and prosocial activities and lose points for negative behaviors (e.g., flashing a gang sign and unexcused absence). Staff assesses student behaviors at multiple points during the day. Points can be cashed in at the "incentive store" for food and games. Accumulated points may also be used in some places to buy the right to go on a field trip or take a Friday afternoon off. Both programs use a 4:1 positive to negative reinforcement approach.

Second, children at the CITY and Bethesda programs take part in establishing and enforcing center rules. At infrequent intervals, all CITY staff members and students come together in a "big group" to reaffirm the boundaries of appropriate behavior at the center. Through a free and open exchange of ideas, the big group is responsible for establishing center rules and sanctions for violators. The group does not disband until all members agree on a new set of rules. At Bethesda, juveniles help to enforce positive group norms through modeling of appropriate behaviors and pressure from fellow participants to conform.

Third, the multimodal approach to treatment is a hallmark of the Bethesda day treatment program. An array of services is available based on the individual needs of the juvenile. The Bethesda menu of interventions includes counseling (individual, group, and family), victim restitution, community service, intensive outpatient drug and alcohol treatment, education, anger management, career and vocational counseling, and recreation.

Taken together, the North Carolina pilot sites are perhaps weakest in their usage of theoretically supported interventions. A behavioral approach is evident in both Wake and Durham (emphasis on positive and negative reinforcement, attitude/behavior classes). However, the use of token economies, modeling, and other behavioral approaches is not as pervasive in these organizations as is the case in the exemplary programs. During its first year of operation, there was no discernible treatment philosophy in New Hanover. The center engaged in minimal behavioral programming. The sole intervention is educational. Finally, a multimodal strategy has been implemented with mixed results in the North Carolina programs. The Durham program uses the widest selection of interventions, including individual and group counseling, life skills training, GED classes, recreation, and a variety of other skill and behavioral classes.

Conduct Immediate and Comprehensive Assessments

• ***Effective Practice.*** Within the first two weeks after entering the program, the juvenile's needs and risk level should be assessed and translated into an individualized treatment plan.

• ***Support in Literature.*** Other sources provide a good overview of risk and needs assessment (see Altschuler & Armstrong, 1994; Howell, 1998). For day treatment programs, the needs assessment is especially important because it looks for the "correct match between the offender's underlying problems and the appropriate intervention strategy" (Altschuler & Armstrong, 1994, p. 6). It provides the basis for the programming decisions directed toward the juvenile's rehabilitation.

The results of these assessments are incorporated into an individualized treatment plan. What is a treatment plan? "The treatment plan is a personalized program for each juvenile and family. It is the agenda for change. A comprehensive treatment plan is completed within the first two weeks of admission. Treatment plans discuss problematic behaviors to be resolved through measurable goals and objectives. Each task is assigned to a specific individual with a time schedule for achievement or progress review. All members of the team contribute to the formulation and revision of treatment plans" (Bowling & Hobbs, 1990, p. 48).

Many commentators recommend that the juvenile and family must be involved in setting goals in the treatment plan. The juvenile signs a contract stating a willingness to comply with the treatment regimen and all program rules.

• ***Support in Practice.*** North Carolina programs did not use risk and needs assessment instruments. They used other screening mechanisms, such as interviews with a substance abuse counselor to determine programmatic needs. In other states, the juvenile probation officers complete risk assessment.

As a result of assessment, it was found that 80–90 percent of Durham clients were substance abusers/addicts. Thus, Durham directed its attention toward substance abuse programming. Bethesda has found that the root of juvenile problems lie, in part, with poor relations with the father. As a result, it has developed a program in which juveniles receive intensive family counseling.

Provide Continuous Case Management

• ***Effective Practice.*** Case managers should coordinate services and intensively monitor the juvenile's progress toward achieving treatment and behavioral goals.

• ***Support in Literature.*** Case management involves a series of activities, rather than a single function. The five sequential activities in traditional case management are as follows:

- Assessing the client's needs;
- Developing a service plan;
- Linking the client to appropriate services;
- Monitoring client progress; and
- Advocating for the client as needed (Healey, 1999, p. 2).

The traditional approach to case management viewed case managers as "service brokers," not service providers. More modern conceptualizations of case management allow case managers to provide informal counseling to clients. This improves the relationship between case manager and client. Today, the line between service broker and treatment provider is usually blurred (Healey, 1999).

Finally, in comparison to caseloads historically experienced in other parts of the criminal justice system, the recommended caseloads for intensive juvenile programs are significantly lower. Howell (1998) suggests that case managers maintain caseloads of no more than fifteen to twenty serious offenders.

• ***Support in Practice.*** The exemplary programs have well-established case management systems in place. Case managers are alternatively referred to as "case managers" and "counselors" (sometimes both descriptors are used within the same program). In most programs, case managers serve as service brokers and therapists. For example, the case managers in the CITY program coordinate services and conduct individual and group discussion sessions with juveniles under their supervision. Discussion topics range from sexual education to conflict resolution.

The case management process followed by most day treatment programs closely mirrors the prescribed method in the research literature. We describe a generalized case management process found in many programs. To begin, prospective program participants are screened by day treatment personnel (in many places by the program director) to determine the appropriateness of the client for the intervention. If the juvenile meets the eligibility criteria, the juvenile and his or her family are provided with an orientation to the program. At this time, the program rules and client expectations are spelled out. General information about the juvenile (e.g., address, family information, and history of prior delinquent behavior) may also be gathered at this time. Following multiple assessments and development of a written treatment plan (see previous "Effective Practice" section for greater detail), the case manager refers the juvenile to specific programs. Most treatment programming is provided on site, but the case manager handles referrals to services off site as well. The case manager also coordinates client transportation to off-site programs.

The case manager monitors the juvenile's progress in each treatment area. He or she receives reports from other service providers (substance abuse, education) and meets regularly with the juvenile to discuss achievements and areas for improvement. The case manager plays a critical role in reinforcing positive behaviors and sanctioning misconduct. The case manager's evaluation of the juvenile's progress while at the center is a key factor in determining whether the juvenile will be successfully promoted out of the program.

In the end, the official case manager job description does not accurately describe all the responsibilities that actually define the position. Case managers serve as the center's liaison with parents and probation officers, appear in court on the juvenile's behalf, supervise field trips, help juveniles find jobs, serve as mentors, transport clients to and from the center, and supervise recreational activities among other duties.

Case management is typically the primary responsibility of a single case manager. However, the entire staff, including educators, treatment professionals, and program administrators, contribute to the case management function. This is evidenced in a common technique that is used in the field—the case debriefing. At the end of the day, all staff members consult on the progress of individual clients. As a group, they decide how to work with the juvenile so that positive behaviors are supported in a consistent manner.

The ratio of case managers to program participants varies from program to program. For the most part, they all comply with the recommended levels in the literature. Bethesda and CITY maintained low case manager-to-client ratios, typically one case manager for every seven to ten clients. The case manager caseload in Durham was slightly higher (approximately one to twelve), while the recommended caseload for Kentucky day treatment counselors is approximately one to fifteen.

Provide Services That Address the Needs of Juveniles and the Community

• ***Effective Practice.*** The juvenile should receive services that are specified in the individualized treatment plan. The juvenile may receive services on site or by delivery of off-site contractors.

• ***Support in Literature.*** "Criminogenic needs are the intermediary links to recidivism . . . If criminogenic needs are not targeted, then reductions in recidivism are unlikely" (Bonta, 1996, p. 29). The services provided at the center must be directed to the underlying causes of delinquency or else the program will have little long-term impact.

• ***Support in Practice.*** Day treatment centers provide a variety of services both on and off site. Most programs offer education, supervision, substance and alcohol abuse counseling, behavior therapy, recreation, community service, and mental health services.

- *Educational services.* Programs use many different educational approaches. Some municipalities establish alternative schools (Bethesda). Others use teachers from the local school district (most popular method used in Kentucky, Alabama, and New Hanover County). Some instruction is delivered in a traditional classroom setting (Cornell Abraxas), while other programs use a self-paced method of individualized study (Bethesda and CITY). Almost 40 percent of day treatment participants in Kentucky are enrolled in special education programs (Wolford, Jordan, & Murphy, 1997). The school district must be an active participant in the educational program of the day treatment program because integration back into the schools is the prime objective of day treatment.
- *Supervision.* Day treatment staff closely monitor all client activities. Some programs serve as de facto probation departments; that is, they locate juveniles who do not come to the center.
- *Substance and alcohol abuse education and treatment.* A large range of programs are offered including intensive outpatient treatment, referrals to inpatient (residential) programs, and Alcoholic Anonymous/Narcotics Anonymous meetings. Drug testing must also be performed at the center. Many at-risk juveniles have a variety of problems whose basic expression is found in substance abuse.
- *Counseling.* Counseling can include individual, group, and family. As we noted previously, the role of the family is central to having real, long-term impact on the juvenile. In some cases, the juvenile's major problem may be his or her family environment.
- *Recreation and leisure.* Recreation and leisure activities can occur on and off site. Boys' and Girls' Clubs have a gymnasium and recreation room. Other programming includes field trips, guest speakers, and golf lessons (Birmingham, Alabama).
- *Restitution.* Restitution is not a primary service area supported by juvenile day treatment centers in North Carolina. It is a critical element in day treatment programming elsewhere, however (Freshstart). Bethesda uses a restorative justice approach where the juvenile offender publicly apolo-

gizes to his or her victim. The "restoration" includes financial payments for damages incurred. Saturday morning is often reserved for community service activities such as cleaning school buildings or maintaining the grounds around the day treatment center.

Before incorporating restitution requirements into day treatment programming, administrators should consider the following operational issues (see Rubin, 1988):

1. Do we have the proper insurance coverage for community service?
2. What tax deductions may be required from restitution earnings?
3. Are proper procedures in place for obtaining restitution monies from juveniles' earnings?
4. What percentage of earnings will be used for restitution?
5. How will noncompliance with restitution requirements be handled?

- *Job training and placement.* CITY emphasizes workforce readiness. This programmatic intervention is evident in Durham, where an employment specialist assists clients to secure employment.
- *Mental health services.* Typically, mental health referrals are made to services that are delivered off site. Mental health services broadly defined are imperative to the prevention goal of juvenile day treatment.
- *Other types of programs.* An array of other programs are offered, including drama therapy in Durham. Other programming found in day treatment programs includes anger management, health, consumer credit counseling, parenting, mentoring, and cultural awareness (New Pride).

EFFECTIVE PROGRAM MANAGEMENT

Develop Information Systems to Allow for Program Monitoring and Evaluation

• ***Effective Practice.*** One of the first tasks for the day treatment director should be to develop an information system that facilitates case management, provides for program monitoring, and facilitates program evaluation.

• ***Support in Literature.*** Study of the implementation of computer information systems is inherently multidisciplinary in nature. In a widely circulated essay, Caudle (1987) urged public managers to focus on several basic questions. What is information for? Does it support the organization's mission? Who uses information and for what decisions? What types of reports are wanted? Who are the external users? Where does information come from? How is reliability assured? How is confidentially assured? What provisions are made for data archiving, for data elimination, and to maintain data integrity? How are data linked for retrieval?

While the objectives of organizations vary, all organizations share a primary need to acquire the control necessary to discharge their functions. In fact, the drive for control over environmental factors is at the core of the manager's responsibility for strategic planning (Vasu, Stewart, & Garson, 1999). Strategic planning tools associated with communication have become progressively more important and today they are the most significant category from the point of view of control.

• ***Support in Practice.*** A quick look at our comparison of juvenile day treatment centers points to the fact that the most developed and mature of these programs, Bethesda and CITY, report some positive impacts. Without a well-developed information system, program operations, monitoring, and evaluation are jeopardized. Moreover, our research in North Carolina underscores one important fact. It is far easier to develop an information system prior to serving the first client than it is to implement an information system once the program is under way. As a part of the process of targeting whom the clients for the day treatment center are, the advisory board should consider the design of its information system.

How do you use the information that is collected? Program staff needs to have regular (weekly) progress meetings to discuss each individual participant. These meetings should include the case manager, service providers, teachers, and juvenile court counselors. As a team, this group should determine when a juvenile is adequately prepared to successfully complete the program.

Measure Performance

• ***Effective Practice.*** For a juvenile day treatment center to adapt to the needs of the community and program participants, continuous performance measurement must be conducted.

• ***Support in Literature.*** For successful program continuation there is an ever-present need for continuous measurement of program performance. Measurement and self-evaluation of the program must be a consistent process whereby the information gained from self-evaluations is used to ensure that the juvenile day treatment center is meeting its program goals and mission as well as providing support for continued funding. Although service delivery is the fundamental purpose of a juvenile day treatment center, recordkeeping is an important managerial component of a program. There are numerous aspects of performance measurement that should be included in the continuous program and participant evaluation process. A good introduction to implementing performance measures in community-based programs is provided in Boone and Fulton (1996).

Maintain Accurate Records. The juvenile day treatment center should maintain records for each participant in the program. Necessary data elements include demographic information such as participant's name, date of birth, gender, and race; date entered and terminated, as well as the reason for program termination; name of court counselor; educational information such as school last attended, grade level, and academic testing scores; drug history information; arrest information; and behavioral information. The participant's file should also contain emergency contact information, any necessary parental release information, as well as any disciplinary actions taken while the juvenile is a participant in the program. Further, the record should contain a comprehensive listing of the services the participant received while in the program as well as any referrals to other agencies that were made. This information will facilitate the center by simply knowing the characteristics of program participants as well as facilitating strategic planning of what services may be needed for the population in question. Finally, by compiling a listing of participants and services, the program is in a better position to justify the need for continued funding as well as potential program expansion.

Measure Academic Performance. Academic performance should be measured based on the individual characteristics of the population being served. Academic performance should be measured upon program entry as well as throughout the juvenile's stay in the program and finally on program completion. Academic performance can be measured using any of a number of standardized tests that could determine the juvenile's grade level, reading ability, and math ability. Academic performance for programs which are oriented to an older population, one in which the participants are working toward their GED rather than to be returned to the public school system, should use GED practice tests to track the juvenile's improvement throughout the program as well as to determine if the juvenile is adequately prepared to take the GED exam. Continued measurement would facilitate the program in determining how the participant is progressing and the extent of academic learning while in the program.

Measure Social Behavior. Social behavior should be measured initially by means of risk and needs assessments. This assessment process will assist in the determination of what services each participant needs. Another manner of measuring changes in social behavior is to have the participant assist in the development of goals in the overall treatment plan. The participant's success or lack of success in meeting his or her goals can be used as an indicator of changes in social behavior. By allowing the participant to participate in the goal-setting process, the participant has "bought into" the stated goal(s) and should have some level of willingness to successfully complete the stated goals. An example of the measurement of social behavior is the point card used by the New Hanover County Pathways Program. Each day participants set a goal and are evaluated on a 1–3-point system in each activity during the day in relation to attendance, participation, listening, cooperation, and respect. If the participant has worked toward his or her goal and receives a minimum number of points, he or she is rewarded at the end of the day with recreational activities. In addition, one goal of a juvenile day treatment center is to help the participants improve their social skills through counseling, group cohesiveness activities, and life skills training. By measuring social behavior the program is better prepared to determine when a juvenile is adequately prepared to become a more productive member of society as well as being able to readjust to a public school setting. As indicated earlier in this chapter, a juvenile should successfully complete the program when program services have resulted in the juvenile's being better prepared to be in a traditional setting. By tracking social behavior, the juvenile day treatment staff and administration are better prepared to determine when a participant has successfully completed the program.

Measure Delinquency. Delinquency can be measured on two fronts: criminal behavior and program disciplinary actions. Disciplinary recordkeeping allows the program staff to assess the level of conformity to rules for each juvenile. Success can be measured by examining the level and extent of delinquent behavior. Moreover, by having access to records regarding delinquent behavior, the program, is able to develop services to match the population being served. In addition, by maintaining disciplinary records the staff is in the position to determine if a participant needs to be negatively terminated as a result of repeated disciplinary problems. Delinquent acts can be measured by looking at new arrests while in the program as well as after successful completion of the program (one year later). Further measures of delinquency could include program suspensions, drug relapses, and other disciplinary actions. It is important to track program graduates as the program's goal is not to simply prevent delinquent acts while the juvenile is a participant but to provide juveniles with skills necessary to refrain from delinquent behavior once they have been returned to the community.

Measure Treatment Success. Each person having any treatment relationship with the individual should maintain treatment success information. Each counselor, whether it be for drug treatment, life skills training, or individual/group counseling, should keep a record of contacts with participants. This information can be used to determine how the juvenile has changed behaviorally and emotionally throughout the program. Examples of information that should be maintained include the number of days sober, the results of drug screens, and other treatment assessment tools used in assessing the participant.

Measure Job Placement Success. For programs serving an older population, job placement and job preparedness skills are extremely important. If a juvenile will not be returning to school, he or she should be adequately prepared to enter the job market. Records should be maintained regarding the participant's skills training and interview skills, as well as jobs applied for and obtained. If the program is assisting juveniles in securing employment, contact should be made with the employer to ascertain whether the participant is able to maintain the position over time.

Conduct Program Assessment Surveys. As with any program, there must be some level of self-assessment. Those who oversee the program should continuously conduct evaluations regarding whether the program is meeting its purpose and goals. Without this reflection, problems will not be discovered until it is too late to fix them in a simple and straightforward manner. By finding program weaknesses early in the process, the program can mend the problems and continue without considerable program reconfiguration. Moreover, the program should survey program participants (past and current), staff, and other stakeholders within the community to determine their satisfaction with the program.

Analyze Financial Data. For continued success of any program, meeting desired goals could be overshadowed by financial needs. Program management must consciously consider the financial costs of operating the program. Detailed records should be kept detailing all program costs. Financial limitations must be considered when making day-to-day operational decisions. Provision of service should be the most important goal; therefore, program management may need to find creative solutions to funding needs. For instance, Cornell Abraxas leases its physical facility from the state for $1. This reduces operating costs, which in turn allows more resources for service provision. Becausee juvenile day treatment programs are one alternative for juveniles, the costs of operating the program should be compared to those of other institutional and community-based programs. In addition to providing quality services, it is important for a program to deliver those services in a manner that is financially competitive to other program alternatives.

From the experience of exemplary programs, we have compiled a suggested list of performance measures for various juvenile day treatment activities (see Exhibit 17.1).

PROJECT EXPANSION: YOUR ULTIMATE ACCOMPLISHMENT

The point cannot be made too many times: You must expand to make a noticeable impact on the community. Yet few, very few, projects in the public sector ever get past the initial number of clients served. Your idea must move from startup, to stabilization to addressing the needs of your entire target clientele if it is to begin making the kind of difference the community expects and needs. In other words, expansion is when your project begins making the kind of impact people in the community can see and feel.

The "how" of expansion is simple; just apply your plan, which has now been updated by the experience of daily operation. Key activities are ever present and reflect the maturity of the idea in action. Key stakeholders have moved from the confusion of beginning to relative routine. For example, leadership has moved from the idea-creation mode to that of keepers of the vision. Partners, collaborators, and staff understand their evolving roles and are ready for additional clientele and project sites. Money—that is, its acquisition—is part of daily operations; everyone works on resource procurement as part of their job. And funds development is not speculative, it is put in terms of return on investment; the idea now "makes money" it does not cost. And as important, the project, that is, everyone in it, understands who is being served. All know where the client is, how he can be reached, and how many of them there are. In other words, the project is ready to reach out.

One last point concerning reaching out; it is not a haphazard thing. Expanding is done, not necessarily at the best time, nor even when all the resources are in place, but rather when there is the collective will to do so. The important thing is to move forward to increasing levels of service in increments that preserve beliefs, vision, mission, and goals as they have evolved. Expand with the view to form a services delivery system that can serve as a model for other local public services. Expand with success in mind, and expand yet again until there is enough permanent infrastructure to address the true needs of those you serve.

References

Altschuler, D. M., & Armstrong, T. L. (1984). Intervening with serious juvenile offenders. In R. Mathias, P. DeMuro, & R. Allinson, (Eds.), *Violent juvenile offenders* (pp. 187–206). San Francisco: National Council on Crime and Delinquency.

Altschuler, D. M., & Armstrong, T. L. (1994). *Intensive aftercare for high-risk juveniles: A community care model.* Washington, DC: U.S. Department of Justice.

Armstrong, T. L., & Altschuler, D. M. (1997). Reintegrating juvenile offenders into schools. *School Safety*, *3*, 25–29.

Bonta, J. (1996). Risk-needs assessment and treatment. In A. J. Harland (Ed.), *Choosing correctional options that work: Defining the demand and evaluating the supply* (pp. 18–32). Thousand Oaks, CA: Sage.

Boone, H. N., & Fulton, B. A. (1996). *Implementing performance-based measures in community corrections* [National Institute of Justice Research in Brief]. Washington, DC: U.S. Department of Justice.

Bowling, L., & Hobbs, L. (1990). Day treatment services. In B. Wolford, C. J. Miller, & P. Lawrenz (Eds.), *Transitional services for troubled youth* (pp. 45–50). Richmond, KY: Department of Correctional Services, Eastern Kentucky University.

Caudle, S. L. (1987, Spring). High tech to better effect. *The Bureaucrat*, pp. 47–51.

Clements, C. B. (1988). Delinquency prevention and treatment: A community-centered perspective. *Criminal Justice and Behavior*, *15*, 286–305.

Cook, L. A. (1990). Collaboration and cooperation: Key elements in bridging transition gaps for adjudicated youth. In B. Wolford, C. J. Miller, & P. Lawrenz (Eds.), *Transitional services for troubled youth* (pp. 15–21). Richmond, KY: Department of Correctional Services, Eastern Kentucky University.

Ellickson, P., & Petersilia, J. (1983). *Implementing new ideas in criminal justice.* Santa Monica, CA: Rand.

Gendreau, P. (1996). Principles of effective intervention with offenders. In A. J. Harland (Ed.), *Choosing correctional options that work: Defining the demand and evaluating the supply* (pp. 117–130). Thousand Oaks, CA: Sage.

Greenwood, P., & Zimring, F. (1985). *One more chance: The pursuit of promising intervention strategies for chronic juvenile offenders.* Santa Monica, CA: Rand.

Hall, R. H., Clark, J. P., Giordano, P. C., Johnson, P. V., & Van Roekel, M. (1981). Patterns of interorganizational relationships. In O. Grusky & G. A. Miller (Eds.), *The sociology of organizations: Basic studies* (pp. 477–494). New York: Free Press.

Harris, P., & Smith, S. (1996). Developing community corrections: An implementation perspective. In A. J. Harland (Ed.), *Choosing correctional options that work: Defining the demand and evaluating the supply* (pp. 183–222). Thousand Oaks, CA: Sage.

Healy, K. M. (1999). *Case management in the criminal justice system* [National Institute of Justice Research in Action]. Washington, DC: U.S. Department of Justice.

Howell, J. C. (Ed.). (1998). *Guide for implementing the comprehensive strategy for serious, violent, and chronic juvenile offenders* (2nd printing). Washington, DC: U.S. Department of Justice.

Laurence, S. E., & West, B. R. (1985). *National evaluation of the New Pride replication program, Final report, Volume I: Organization, implementation, and results of the replication process.* Walnut Creek, CA: Pacific Institute for Research and Evaluation.

Lawrence, R. (1997). Shared goals, resources unite probation, schools. *School Safety, 3*, 25–26.

Lipsey, M. W. (1992). Juvenile delinquency treatment: A meta-analytic inquiry into the variability of effects. In T. Cook et al. (Eds.), *Meta-analysis for explanation: A casebook* (pp. 83–127). New York: Russell Sage Foundation.

Petersilia, J. (1990). Conditions that permit intensive supervision programs to survive. *Crime and Delinquency, 36*, 126–145.

Pressman, J. L., & Wildavsky, A. (1984). *Implementation* (3rd ed.). Berkeley: University of California Press.

Rubin, H. T. (1988). Fulfilling juvenile restitution requirements in community correctional programs. *Federal Probation, 52*, 32–42.

Sherman, L. W., Gottfredson, D., MacKenzie, D., Eck, J., Reuter, P., & Bushway, S. (1997). *Preventing crime: What works, what doesn't, what's promising.* Washington, DC: U.S. Department of Justice.

Vasu, M. L., Stewart, D., & Garson, G. D. (1999). *Organizational behavior for public managers.* New York: Marcel Dekker.

Wolford, B. I., Jordan, F., & Murphy, K. (1997). Day treatment: Community-based partnerships for delinquent and at-risk youth. *Juvenile and Family Court Judges, 48*, 35–42.

Exhibit 17.1
Program Goals, Activities, and Performance Measures

Goals	Activities	Performance Measures
1. Receive appropriate program referrals	1-1. Market program to court personnel 1-2. Conduct assessments	1-1-a. Achieve 100% appropriate referrals 1-1-b. Receive # juveniles into program during year 1-1-c. Operate at program capacity (25 juveniles) 1-2-a. Percent of assessments completed within two weeks
2. Protect the community	2-1. Conduct personal contacts with juvenile 2-2. Conduct telephone contacts 2-3. Monitor arrest records	2-1-a. Number of personal contacts 2-1-b. Percent successful/missed 2-2-a. Number of phone contacts with juvenile 2-2-b. Number of phone contacts with employer and school 2-3-a. Number and type of arrests
3. Assist juveniles to change	3-1. Provide drug/alcohol treatment 3-2. Provide educational/vocational activities 3-3. Provide counseling (mental health, anger) 3-4. Refer to job services 3-5. Encourage socially acceptable behavior	3-1-a. Hours/days of treatment received 3-1-b. Number of days free during and after supervision 3-1-c. Number of positive/negative drug tests 3-1-d. Successful terminations by treatment type 3-2-a. Number of classes offered 3-2-b. Number of student hours received 3-2-c. Percent of successful completions (GED, grade advance) 3-2-d. Hours of vocational training received 3-3-a. Hours of counseling received by type 3-4-a. Hours of job counseling provided 3-4-b. Number of successful placements 3-4-c. Percent of successful placements 3-4-d. Average length of employment 3-4-e. Wages earned 3-5-a. Number and rate of major/minor technical violations 3-5-b. Number and rate of probation revocations 3-5-c. Rearrest rates during and after program completion 3-5-d. Sanctions for negative behavior
4. Restore crime victims	4-1. Monitor restitution payments 4-2. Monitor community service work projects	4-1-a. Number of restitution payments made 4-1-b. Percent of total funds restored 4-2-a. Hours of work completed 4-2-b. Value of work completed

Index

[References are to pages.]

[References are to pages.]

[References are to pages.]

[References are to pages.]

[References are to pages.]

[References are to pages.]

[References are to pages.]

[References are to pages.]

[References are to pages.]

[References are to pages.]

[References are to pages.]